Unfitting Stories

UNFITTING STORIES
Narrative Approaches to Disease, Disability, and Trauma

VALERIE RAOUL
CONNIE CANAM
ANGELA HENDERSON
CARLA PATERSON
editors

Wilfrid Laurier University Press

We acknowledge the financial support of the Government of Canada through the Book Publishing Industry Development Program for our publishing activities.

Library and Archives Canada Cataloguing in Publication

Unfitting stories : narrative approaches to disease, disability, and trauma / edited by Valerie Raoul ... [et al.].

Includes contributions made to the research project funded by the Peter Wall Institute of Advanced Studies, 1999–2004, and presentations at a conference held in May 2002.
Includes bibliographical references and index.
ISBN-13: 978-0-88920-509-3
ISBN-10: 0-88920-509-4

1. Sick—Biography—History and criticism. 2. People with disabilities—Biography—History and criticism. 3. Victims—Biography—History and criticism. 4. Narrative inquiry (Research method). 5. Narrative medicine. 6. Sick—Psychology. 7. People with disabilities—Psychology. 8. Victims—Psychology. I. Raoul, Valerie, 1941–

R702.U54 2007   362.19   C2007-900701-5

Cover design by P.J. Woodland. Text design by Catharine Bonas-Taylor.

© 2007 Wilfrid Laurier University Press
Waterloo, Ontario, Canada
www.wlupress.wlu.ca

∞
This book is printed on Ancient Forest Friendly paper (100% post-consumer recycled).
Printed in Canada

Every reasonable effort has been made to acquire permission for copyright material used in this text, and to acknowledge all such indebtedness accurately. Any errors and omissions called to the publisher's attention will be corrected in future printings.

No part of this publication may be reproduced, stored in a retrieval system or transmitted, in any form or by any means, without the prior written consent of the publisher or a licence from The Canadian Copyright Licensing Agency (Access Copyright). For an Access Copyright licence, visit www.accesscopyright.ca or call toll free to 1-800-893-5777.

In memory of Gabriele Helms (1966–2004)

A specialist in autobiography, Gabi was an invaluable member of the UBC Wall project on Narratives of Disease, Disability, and Trauma, both as a postdoctoral fellow and as co-organizer of the conference at which many of the essays in this volume were first presented. She became our colleague in the English department at UBC, and served on the advisory board of SAGA (the Centre for Studies in Autobiography, Gender, and Age). Her energy, intellect, and commitment to the project inspired us all. When she began to work on women's illness narratives, Gabi had no idea that she soon would have her own story of pain and courage. Co-founder of a support group in Vancouver called The Young and the Breastless, she died of cancer on December 31, 2004, after giving premature birth to a daughter, Hana. Hana is flourishing.

Contents

Acknowledgements xi
The Editors xiii

Introduction: Narrative Frames

Making Sense of Disease, Disability, and Trauma: Normative and Disruptive Stories • *The Editors* 3

Interdisciplinarity and Postdisciplinarity in Health Research in Canada
Judy Z. Segal 11

Part I: Public Framing of Personal Narratives

Introduction: Aesthetics, Authenticity, and Audience • *The Editors* 25

Authorizing the Memoir Form: Lauren Slater's Three Memoirs of Mental Illness • *Helen M. Buss* 33

Telling Trauma: Two Narratives of Psychiatric Hospitalization
Hilary Clark 45

Between Two Deaths: AIDS, Trauma, and Temporality in the Work of Paul Monette • *Lisa Diedrich* 53

Paper Thin: Agency and Anorexia in Geneviève Brisac's *Petite*
Barbara Havercroft 61

The Incomprehensible Density of Being: Aestheticizing Cancer
Ulrich Teucher 71

Challenging Subjects: Ruth Sienkiewicz-Mercer, Christopher Nolan, and Autobiography • *Heidi Janz and Julie Rak* 79

The Tectonics of Trauma: Father–Daughter Incest in Film • *Gail Finney* 89

The Silvering Screen: Age and Trauma in Akira Kurosawa's *Rhapsody in August*
Sally Chivers 97

PART II: REPRESENTING THE SUBJECT

Introduction: Narrative in Qualitative Research and Therapeutics
The Editors 107

Writing about Illness: Therapy? Or Testimony? • *Anne Hunsaker Hawkins* 113

Constructing a "Schizophrenic" Identity • *Barbara Schneider* 129

Space, Temporality, and Subjectivity in a Narrative of Psychotic Experience
Lourdes Rodriguez del Barrio 139

Re-sounding Images: Outsiders in Persimmon Blackbridge's *Sunnybrook*
Joy James 149

(Story-)Telling It like It Is: How Narratives Teach at L'Arche
Pamela Cushing 159

Disrupting the Academic Self: Living with Lupus • *Janet MacArthur* 171

Women Surviving Hemorrhagic Stroke: Narratives of Meaning
Sharon Dale Stone 181

Men, Sport, and Spinal Cord Injury: Identity Dilemmas, Embodied Time,
and the Construction of Coherence • *Brett Smith and Andrew C. Sparkes* 191

PART III: THE LARGER PICTURE

Introduction: Metanarrative Politics and Polemics • *The Editors* 203

Disability Income: Narratives of Women with Multiple Sclerosis
Lyn Jongbloed 209

Narratives of Trauma and Aboriginal Post-secondary Students • *Robert Procyk
and Christine Crowe* 217

Social Trauma and Serial Autobiography: Healing and Beyond
Bina Toledo Freiwald 227

Reports from the Psych Wars • *Richard Ingram* 237

Agoraphobia, Social Order, and Psychiatric Narrative • *Shelley Z. Reuter* 247

"They Say the Disease Is Responsible": Social Identity and the Disease Concept
of Drug Addiction • *Joanne Muzak* 255

Temporal Assumptions: Aging with Cystic Fibrosis • *J. Daniel Schubert* 265

Ableist Limits on Self-narration: The Concept of Post-personhood
James Overboe 275

NARRATIVE CONCLUSIONS: AN EXAMPLE OF
CROSS-DISCIPLINARY ANALYSIS

Margaret Edson's Play *Wit*: Death at the End or the End of Death?
Valerie Raoul, Connie Canam, Gloria Onyeoziri, Carla Paterson   285

Postscript: Un-fitting Stories, Un-disciplined Research • *Valerie Raoul*   297

References   307

Notes on Contributors   337

Index   349

Acknowledgements

This book is a product of the "Narratives of Disease, Disability, and Trauma" research project, funded by the Peter Wall Institute of Advanced Studies, undertaken at the University of British Columbia (Vancouver, Canada) from 1999 to 2004. The aim of the project was to bring together people from a range of disciplines and professions whose work involves an understanding of the functions of narrative in determining how disease, disability, and trauma are defined, experienced, and treated. The team from UBC was composed of researchers from the health sciences, the social sciences, and the humanities. It included ten faculty members and an equal number of postdoctoral fellows and graduate students. The editors wish to acknowledge the contribution to our debates of colleagues who were part of the project but are not represented in this book: they include Isabel Dyck (rehabilitation sciences), Susanna Egan (English), Janice Graham (medical anthropology), Susan Penfold (psychiatry), and Patricia Vertinsky (education/disability studies).

We also benefited from the input of inspiring visiting speakers at a series of events and workshops, among them Persimmon Blackridge, Howard Brody, Ross Chambers, John Eakin, Carolyn Ellis, Mary Gergen, Ann Kaplan, Hilde Lindemann Nelson, James Pennebaker, Bonnie Klein, and Susan Sherwin. Invited speakers at the "Narratives of Disease, Disability, and Trauma" conference held in May 2002, at which some of the papers in this collection were first presented, included Hilde Lindemann Nelson and Catherine Riessman, as well as several others who had already participated in our project in some way: Helen Buss, Thomas Couser, Arthur Frank, Barbara Havercroft, and Anne Hunsaker Hawkins.

Our thanks go to the Social Sciences and Humanities Research Council of Canada for funding the conference; to Pamela Brett-MacLean, Kate Collie, Karen Dias, Gabriele Helms, Marsha Henry, and Sue Mills for their role in its success; and to Colleen Derkatch and Roseann Larstone for invaluable assistance in preparing the manuscript. Above all, we are grateful to the Peter Wall Institute for Advanced Studies (UBC), as without their financial and moral support neither the project nor this book would have been possible.

The Editors

VALERIE RAOUL (Women's Studies and French, founding director of the SAGA Centre at UBC) was principal investigator for the Wall project. She is the author of two books on diary fiction in France and Quebec and co-editor of two other essay collections: *The Anatomy of Gender*, and *Women Filmmakers: Refocusing*. In her research and teaching, she brings feminist, poststructuralist, and psychoanalytic theory to bear on written, oral, and visual texts that raise issues of gendered identities and self-representation. Her current projects deal with diaries by nineteenth-century French women who were ill, and present-day diaries of illness by women.

CONNIE CANAM is a faculty member in the UBC School of Nursing and was a co-investigator on the Wall project. Her research focuses on chronic illness as experienced by individuals and their families, with a particular interest in the role of nurses in the primary health care of children with chronic health conditions. She has employed narrative methods in several studies, and has taught an interdisciplinary graduate course on illness narratives that brings together qualitative research methods and theories of narrative analysis.

ANGELA HENDERSON is a faculty member in the UBC School of Nursing and was a co-investigator on the Wall project. She primarily studies the role of health care professionals in addressing issues related to violence against women. Her research has dealt with women's needs during the immediate crisis period of leaving a violent relationship, social factors influencing the ability of women to access services for themselves and their children, and the provision of support groups. Her current interdisciplinary research focuses on workplace violence as it influences the ability of nurses to work effectively.

CARLA PATERSON was a postdoctoral fellow with the Wall project and is currently (2007) acting director of the SAGA Centre at UBC. She has taught in UBC's interdisciplinary Arts Foundations program and in the Faculty of Applied Science. Trained in the history of science and medicine, she has long been interested in bridging the gap between the arts and the sciences. Her research has focused on the shifting historical constructions of disease and the value of narrative in conceptualizing human and environmental well-being. She is a co-author of *Fundamental Competencies*, an introductory engineering textbook.

INTRODUCTION
Narrative Frames

THE EDITORS

Making Sense of Disease, Disability, and Trauma
Normative and Disruptive Stories

Whereas there were relatively few published stories of ill health or suffering twenty-five years ago, in English or other languages, a person visiting any library or bookstore today will discover a wide range of narratives that can be divided into several categories, including accounts of disease, disability, and trauma. These accounts have attracted attention from a wide range of professional and disciplinary perspectives. In the health sciences, such stories are used by practitioners and researchers who wish to go beyond biomedical perceptions of disease in order to understand the patient's experience of illness. Bioethicists invoke personal stories as an alternative to universal principles in their attempts to understand ethical dilemmas from the perspective of patients and their families. Adopting a broader focus, qualitative researchers in the social sciences solicit and analyze oral stories in order to document the social determinants of health, and to provide data that will influence policy making in the health care system. Therapists use storytelling as a healing tool in private, one-on-one encounters with patients. In the humanities, both written and visual representations of disease, disability, and trauma have been analyzed by literary scholars and historians, as well as by researchers in cultural studies and gender studies who are interested in how artistic expression and form relate to the body that produces those representations. "Narrative" is used as an object or means of inquiry, from political science to psychology, from social work to applied ethics,[1] yet the ways in which we receive, produce, analyze, and deploy the term, as well as the stories involved, vary considerably from one discipline to another. This is an area which demands multidisciplinary, cross-disciplinary, transdisciplinary, or interdisciplinary collaboration to enable a sharing of perspectives that can lead to new insights. Like experiences of disease, disability, and trauma, this type of inquiry challenges our assumptions about what can or should be studied, how, and by whom. It forces us, literally, to think of our research in new terms, and to assess where our approach is situated in relation to debates about research between and across the disciplines.

Such a dialogue (or "polylogue") takes place in this collection of essays, which brings together work by academics, health professionals, and authors of narratives of disease, disability, and trauma. Many of the individual contributions illustrate or question particular disciplinary approaches, and their juxtaposition with other contributions provides a collage of multi-, cross-, or trans-perspectives. A broader discussion of the issues raised by this juxtaposition provides a frame for these contributions, reflecting the debates that took place in the course of our collaboration. This book is a product of a self-consciously *inter*disciplinary research project, entitled An Interdisciplinary Inquiry into Narratives of Disease, Disability, and Trauma, often referred to as the Wall project, conducted at the University of British Columbia, and funded with a major thematic grant by the Peter Wall Institute for Advanced Studies. The initial team from UBC was composed of scholars from the health sciences, social sciences, and humanities, and our activities over five years included an international conference, at which some of these papers were first presented, held at UBC in May 2002. The entire project, which is still on-going in various forms, resulted in far more material than could be contained in one book. In order to convey the variety of approaches considered and issues raised, we have included a broad sample of essays, many in abbreviated form, that represent relevant research.

Research that crosses disciplinary boundaries is often assumed to be problem-based, occurring when specialists from different fields pool their resources to address a specific (often urgent) issue. In our case, however, what brought us together was not a specific problem but an interest in "narrative" as an object and means of inquiry, with different connotations, aims, and results, in various disciplinary and professional contexts. All the people engaged in this project shared a concern with the effects and implications of narratives in relation to experiences of ill health and health care delivery. Stories of illness and treatment emerge in very different contexts, and range from published autobiographies or novels to case notes and therapy sessions. In spite of these significant differences, they raise common issues regarding their status as sources of knowledge, and the ways in which we can or should analyze and interpret them.

"Illness" is a term that evokes experiences of disease from the perspective of the sick person or sufferer. While a number of works exist on illness narratives or "pathographies" (a term used by Anne Hunsaker Hawkins and Thomas Couser), this category of story related to disease overlaps with auto/biographies of disability and trauma. While it may at times be important to distinguish between these types of conditions, we found that most of the apparent distinctions are difficult to maintain. Many narrators emphasize that their experience combines elements of physical and mental suffering with acute and chronic effects, and involves visible and invisible factors. Whether the condition is life-threatening or not, congenital or acquired, it affects both self-definition and relationships with others. Whether they are dealing with disease, disability, or trauma, many narrators share common experiences of social barriers and stigma, shifts in their relationship to time and space, and problems in their interactions with medical institutions and health-care providers. We soon abandoned initial debates over diagnostic definitions and terminology, as we realized that conceptualizing disease, disability, and trauma as distinct categories was not useful, or even possible, where such stories are concerned. While the specific type of condition may be very significant in some cases, our focus as a group was on common elements that emerge from the stories narrated. Other types of questions, such as those concerning the gendered aspects of these experiences and the cultural differences that influence how experiences are constructed and interpreted, became central in our attempts to clarify the premises and implications of our diverse approaches to narrative analysis. Our own methods and attitudes were challenged by learning about those from other disciplines as we moved into an original interdisciplinary space that was new to us all.

Three assumptions held our group together, and provided common ground for discussion. The first is that disease, disability, and trauma, while often having physical or biological causes and effects, are socially and psychologically constructed and part of a life story which changes because of them. The second is that the exchange of stories is central to treatment, therapy, and advocacy for change. The third is that the stories exchanged (whether medical or personal, in the form of aesthetic or didactic accounts) are governed by cultural metanarratives that vary according to time, place, and socio-political context. Narrative constructions occur on multiple levels and can be seen from many perspectives, including the points of view of individuals or groups who experience disease, disability, or trauma; professionals and others who interact with them; researchers and policy makers; and those who produce art works from or about such experiences. Biomedical discourse tells a particular story about health and illness, based on distinct models and metaphors, that is conveyed through such texts as diagnostic manuals and training handbooks for health practitioners. That story can be confirmed or contested by accounts from individuals or groups about their own experience of disease, disability, or trauma. What is evident is that events or symptoms do not carry the same meanings when they are framed differently or viewed from different perspectives. Normative or disruptive stories can be used in various ways, fulfilling functions of which the teller may be more or less aware. They can also be analyzed from a range of methodological perspectives that raise academic and ethical issues regarding what can or should be done through or with personal narratives.

All the editors of this book have analyzed narratives of various kinds in the course of their own research. Two of us have worked mainly on published texts (Valerie Raoul as a specialist in women's autobiographical writing, Carla Paterson as a historian of medicine), while Connie Canam and Angela Henderson, who are both in nursing, deal with in-depth interviews and oral histories related to health care. One framework that enabled us and other project members to bring our perspectives together and see things differently was Roman Jakobson's model of the different functions of communication. Five of us first applied this model to a narrative of locked-in syndrome, Jean-Dominique Bauby's *The Diving Bell and the Butterfly* (Raoul et al. 2001), to show how each of our disciplinary approaches privileged one or more of the functions (the expressive, referential, conative, poetic, phatic, and metalinguistic) over the others. This discussion made us aware of the interconnections between the aesthetic, therapeutic, and polemical functions in narratives of ill health or suffering—three interlocking perspectives that serve to structure this volume.

Feminist bioethicist Hilde Lindemann Nelson, who gave the opening address at our 2002 conference, "Narratives of Disease, Disability, and Trauma," elaborated on the functions of narrative from the perspective of moral philosophy, and enumerated seven "things we do with stories": we construct and read them, invoke and counter them, analyze and compare them, and also may parody them.[2] These activities suggest ways in which the essays in this volume can be connected and compared across the three broad dimensions we have chosen to highlight. The book's tripartite division, based on the relative importance of the aesthetic, the therapeutic, and the polemical, parallels the distinctions made by Kristin Langellier (1989) in her analysis of perspectives on personal narratives. Langellier's overview is divided into five sections: the first two contain a discussion of personal narratives as "story-text" and "storytelling performance," emphasizing the aesthetic aspects; the next section addresses personal narratives as "conversational interaction," which corresponds to the less formal, often oral exchange of stories represented in Part II of this volume; and Langellier's last two categories deal with personal narratives as "social process" and "political praxis," the focus of our Part III. The writers in our Part I illustrate how meaning is constructed through narrative form, those in the second part show how the exchange of narratives affects the individual narrator, and the writers in Part III discuss how the individual narrative reverberates in a broader collective and socio-political context.

While narratives are always "framed" to the extent that they are produced and received by specific audiences, that framing is more self-consciously artistic in some than in others. The first section of this volume, entitled "Public Framing of Personal Narratives," deals with polished and published stories by authors who are consciously shaping their stories to appeal to a wide audience. The essays in this section look at what writers or film directors do with a personal, collective, or witnessed experience when they turn it into a book or film that depends on aesthetic value for a positive reception. How are the therapeutic and polemical aspects of storytelling integrated into works constructed and framed to produce a satisfying whole? How can distressing and painful experiences be converted into artifacts that audiences will want to read or see without trivializing or sensationalizing them? What difference does it make if the story is framed as truth or fiction? The authors of the papers in this section are all trained in the narratological or semiotic analysis of well-crafted stories; their discussions, emphasizing form and style, illustrate various methodological approaches to narrative that have developed in the humanities, but increasingly are being used in other disciplines.

Part II, "Representing the Subject," focuses on narrative therapeutics and emphasizes the transformative aspects of telling one's story, whether in a therapeutic setting or by the anonymous case-studies recorded in social science research. These papers discuss not so much the effect of the story on others as what telling the story does to and for the teller. Several of the contributors to this section have expertise in qualitative research and some are themselves personally engaged with disease or disability. These writers raise issues concerning the value of sharing stories as a way to build a mutually supportive community, as individual and collective stories can allow those who experience disease, disability, or trauma to reframe their identity and escape from the labels proposed by other stories about them. Such stories are usually less consciously constructed than many published accounts, and are often heard rather than read, which means that a different type of exchange takes place, requiring a different type of discourse analysis. Artistic merit is not often a conspicuous feature of stories such as these, which are invoked or countered in settings where too much attention to form may diminish the impression of authenticity and immediacy; yet the production of artwork may be part of the therapeutic process. The context of production and reception of such stories is less public, and they are often framed by someone other than the narrator before being shared with a wider audience. The role of the mediator as interpreter raises other issues regarding moral responsibility and "speaking for others."

The third section, "The Larger Picture," broadens the focus of the collection to include discussions of the narrative polemics that occur when competing collective frame narratives clash in the professional and political realms. The papers are by authors from a wide range of disciplines, who look beyond the stories themselves and those who tell them to consider the larger context of their production and reception. They analyze both individual and collective stories, and compare them from various perspectives to address metanarratives of identity that determine access to voice and audience. These contributions challenge us to rethink the ways in which public policy decisions are made, and how gender and race/ethnicity play a role in access to resources. Medical research frames disease, disability, or trauma in ways that define what stories about them are expected and, therefore, heeded. Ethical issues emerge as central in research that allows some people's stories to be disseminated, and those of others to be ignored or disregarded. The concluding essay in this section poses a challenge to narrative itself as a requirement for full "personhood," questioning the assumption common to many approaches to narrative that story-making and story-telling, or "making sense" of what happens in life, are essential to being human.

Each section begins with an introduction outlining the ways in which the issues addressed in the various papers can be linked. The introductions to Parts I and II incorporate material from two panel discussions held at the 2002 conference: narrative ethics (with Hilde Lindemann Nelson, Thomas Couser, and Susan Wendell) and narrative methods (with Anne Hunsaker Hawkins, Arthur Frank, and Catherine Riessman). Taken together, the contributions to this book constitute a story of research that is not confined within disciplinary and academic frames, and that deals with the personal, as well as with the professional and the political. They all raise questions about what "fits" into preconceived stories about health, disease, disability, or trauma, and what does not. They force us to see such stories within a different frame, one that challenges our perceptions of these experiences. While there are many existing works on narratives of illness, on bioethics, and on narrative theory (as reflected in the extensive bibliography), this volume is original in its attempt to break down barriers between the disciplines, between theory and practice, and between academic research and the community of those who live with the physical and social effects of disease, disability, and trauma. It is also unique and timely in its Canadian focus.

This introduction leads immediately into a discussion of the practical problems posed by interdisciplinary approaches in health research, with particular reference to the mandate of the Canadian Institutes of Health Research. Judy Segal, a specialist in the rhetoric of medical discourse and a member of the Wall project, outlines some of the challenges faced by humanities researchers, whose work relating to disease, disability, or trauma is too often ignored by health-care providers and medical researchers. Her discussion provides an overview of the obstacles to collaboration, and makes the case for narrative approaches as a bridge between otherwise incompatible discourses. At the end of this volume we have included a collective analysis of Margaret Edson's play *Wit*, about an academic woman dying of cancer, as an illustration of the type of exchange that took place throughout our project. This collective analysis demonstrates further the contributions that the humanities and the social sciences can make to a better understanding of what constitutes and impedes well-being. Finally, the postscript brings together the threads running through the collection, summing up the story of our exchange in relation to broader debates about cross/interdisciplinarity and "narrative."

We believe that our experience with this project confirms that a multidisciplinary team can provide richer insights than those produced by any one discipline, and that the attempt to communicate across substantial barriers in order to find new spaces in between conventional categories is well worth the effort. Our hope is that this collection will prove useful in courses for health-care practitioners, and for researchers and teachers focusing on the intersections of literature and medicine, as well as for other readers interested in narrative as a means to bridge divergent discourses about health and illness. The issues raised are certainly relevant to those of us working or living with people who experience pain, suffering, and exclusion, as well as to those who themselves have or have had such experiences.

The work of the original Wall project is being continued at UBC through SAGA, the Centre for Studies in Autobiography, Gender, and Age, established with and funded from the CFI/BCKDF. SAGA's mandate is to foster interdisciplinary research on narratives concerning life changes, as perceived by individuals from diverse backgrounds and framed by shifting socio-political contexts, and the work being done there follows up on the questions raised in this volume.[3]

Notes

1 The bibliography appended to this volume includes references to a range of works on the uses of narrative and methods of analysis in various disciplines. We found overviews by Kristin Langellier, Catherine Riessman, and Laurel Richardson particularly useful as points of departure for our initial cross-disciplinary discussions.
2 See her introduction to *Stories and Their Limits: Narrative Approaches to Bioethics* (1997) and development of these ideas elsewhere (Nelson 2001, 2002).
3 More information is available on our website, http://www.saga.ubc.ca.

JUDY Z. SEGAL

INTERDISCIPLINARITY AND POSTDISCIPLINARITY IN HEALTH RESEARCH IN CANADA

Many scholars have turned their attention to the definition of interdisciplinary studies, and to the advantages of interdisciplinary and multidisciplinary approaches to complex questions over strictly disciplinary ones.[1] However, feelings of ambivalence towards interdisciplinarity pose a special problem for health and medicine; even more than those that beset interdisciplinary studies in general. The word "interdisciplinarity" itself is a god-term in health research theory, and research administrators lavishly praise the idea of interdisciplinary health research. Yet, for often understandable reasons, the medical establishment still seems to like monodisciplinary, essentially biomedical research best.

In Canada, talk about interdisciplinary health research came to the fore especially during events leading up to the creation of the Canadian Institutes of Health Research in 2000. The purpose of the CIHR was to shift the Canadian research agenda away from more narrowly defined *medical* research, and in the direction of broader-based *health* research. CIHR's mandate was not only to take over biomedical and clinical research, supported to that point by the Medical Research Council, but also to fund health systems and services research, and populations and public health research—including research in the social sciences and humanities. Quite suddenly, Canadian researchers and research administrators were asking what counts as health research, who does it, and how it is done.[2]

CIHR marked its fifth anniversary in 2005, and it continues to operate, in principle, on the idea that interdisciplinary work, including the work of social scientists and humanists, is essential to improving the health of Canadians.[3] Central to the ideology of the CIHR is the notion that health problems are human problems, requiring study by more than traditional medical means. Pain may be a medical matter, for example, but suffering is a personal, and social, one. Death may frequently occur in hospitals, but dying is, first, a human experience. Medical researchers may study pathology, but humanists and social scientists illuminate the nature and meaning of pathology in everyday life. Even so, the CIHR was born into a research culture that made it very hard to know how to support truly interdisciplinary health research—beyond, say, the collaboration of a microbiologist, an epidemiologist, and a biostatistician.

I will argue here that interdisciplinary research (which I will reconfigure in part as postdisciplinary research) is difficult, but absolutely necessary to effect changes in matters of health. My discussion is in four parts. In the first, I explain what interdisciplinarity is, from the point of view of someone who has never been disciplinary. In the second, I enumerate some of the practical problems of doing interdisciplinary research. The third section suggests the contours of postdisciplinarity in health research, and the fourth focuses on narrative as a means of doing postdisciplinary health studies.

What Interdisciplinarity Is

A couple of years ago, I was invited to participate in a workshop at my university on *science envy*. The organizers were trying to understand why social scientists seek to emulate the methods and postures of scientists, humanists try to emulate social scientists, and other scientists try to emulate physicists. Personally, however, I was, and still am, coming to terms with the realization that for the past fifteen years, as a rhetorical theorist of health and medicine, I have been experiencing *discipline envy*.

Most of my colleagues in the English Department approach interdisciplinary work, if they do approach it, from secure places in the discipline; they are like contented singles ready to speed-date at scholarly gatherings. I come from a branch of English studies, however, that was not quite disciplinary to begin with. For one thing, rhetoric is always rhetoric *of* something (politics, advertising, science), so it always works in interstices. Also, studies in persuasion are almost always at least historical, cultural, and literary at the same time: in other words, interdisciplinary. My own situation has taught me that disciplinary studies have certain structural and institutional advantages over interdisciplinary ones.

Multidisciplinary studies are relatively straightforward, and are what many people mean when they talk about interdisciplinarity. In multidisciplinary research, disciplinary specialists work together. Complex health research on pain and suffering, for example, may require the cooperation of physicians, nurses, psychologists, historians, anthropologists, philosophers, and others, each ideally possessing some understanding of each other's approaches. In such a case, the researchers are disciplinary, while their project is multidisciplinary. A multidisciplinary treatment team in a hospital may include a physician, a nurse, a psychologist, and a social worker, who combine areas of expertise and work together to improve patient care. Multidisciplinary work is sometimes called *cross-disciplinary*; both prefixes suggest that disciplinary knowledges remain intact, while many disciplines are surveyed. *Transdisciplinary* is a term for describing some of what is common across disciplines, as in Louis Menand's observation that critical theory is a "transdisciplinary vocabulary" (1997, 212). Narrative research is transdisciplinary.

Interdisciplinarity includes the idea that some of the most exciting scholars working today work between and across disciplines as traditionally defined. For example, the person who knows the literatures and methods of both anthropology and history is in an unique position to study social and cultural elements in the history of infectious diseases (see King 2002); the person who knows both medicine and philosophy is well positioned to examine problems of human suffering (see Cassell 2004); and the person trained in both philosophy and history can bring theories of meaning to bear on the history of psychiatry in novel ways (see Hacking 1995). Moreover, new "interdisciplines," like science and technology studies, women's studies, cultural studies, and others, are themselves areas of specialization for researchers whose work is best described as problem- or inquiry-based, rather than discipline-based.

Cross-disciplinary collaborations and novel specializations—that is, the practice of both *multidisciplinarity* and *interdisciplinarity*—introduce a special complexity into research and are usually time-consuming, in part because most of us were educated in disciplinary cultures, with specialized languages, methodologies, and frames of mind. (Consider, for example, what the phrase "socio-economic status" means to a psychologist, a sociologist, and an economist, respectively; it's something different every time.) Interdisciplinary research is *necessarily* complex. Interdisciplinarity is not what you automatically have when you put a psychologist and a sociologist together on a single project, or when you recruit a humanist into a scientific research team because the conditions of funding require one. I was once invited to join a group of antibiotic-resistance researchers with a phone call from someone who said, "We were trolling for humanists and your name came up." That can't be good.

Problems of Doing Interdisciplinary Research

Partly because both we and our institutions have grown up with disciplinary thinking, interdisciplinary work is beset by practical problems. Here, under six headings, are some of them:

1. *Research funding.* Funding agencies want to see applications for collaborative projects involving teams of researchers, but these very agencies adjudicate on the basis of individual research records. To be competitive, individual research records need to show that applicants have been *sole* or *primary* authors and *principal* investigators on past projects. Stated research values are at odds, then, with operative research values. Notwithstanding their rhetoric of collaboration, funding agents remain loyal to a hierarchy of research values reflected in their criteria for assessing *curricula vitae*.

2. *Peer review.* Interdisciplinary work is often reviewed for funding and publication not by readers who are similarly interdisciplinary, but by readers from a range of disciplines who are part of a multidisciplinary collective. So, for example, a social scientist may be invited to review an application by a humanist. The result can be that the expertise which is meant to undergird the review system is simply absent, while reviewers understand interdisciplinary reviewing to be a matter of measuring work in one discipline by the standards of another discipline.[4] This sort of nonexpert review poses the very danger that those who oppose interdisciplinarity think interdisciplinarity itself poses: the danger that all research involved becomes a kind of lowest-common-denominator research.

3. *University appointment.* Scholars who identify themselves as interdisciplinary may find it difficult to find professorial work where institutional infrastructures have not caught up with the structure of interdisciplinary research. The person with a PhD in health studies, or science and technology studies, or women's studies, for example, may have difficulty finding employment inside departmental units organized by discipline. The person who began training as a sociologist, but then specialized in interdisciplinary health studies, may be less competitive than a health sociologist for a job in a sociology department. A historian of science with a PhD from a science and technology studies program may be less competitive for a job in a history department than someone with a PhD in history and a specialization in the history of science, because the second applicant will be seen to be a better bet for undergraduate history course coverage.

4. *Tenure and promotion.* The work that interdisciplinary researchers do may not be recognized as legitimate work in the departments or other

disciplinary units in which they do it. Tenure and promotion decisions tend to be based on disciplinary standards and measures. A dean of Arts may be wary of a health studies researcher who does not identify himself or herself as a historian or a sociologist or a geographer, but who does historical, sociological, and geographical research. A department head in English may not feel fully qualified to recommend enthusiastically for promotion a candidate who publishes not in familiar literature journals but in unfamiliar (to him or her) health or medical ones.

5. *Research dissemination.* Interdisciplinary researchers may have trouble finding the best venues for their work both in journals and at conferences. Sometimes the work is not considered properly inside a field because it crosses fields. At the same time, dedicated interdisciplinary journals have interdisciplinary editorial boards, and that means a scholar may face the same problem at review for publication as in applying for funding: the possibility that the work will be reviewed by someone with a discipline-based misunderstanding of it. Furthermore, for example, while some rhetorical theorists attend dedicated rhetoric conferences (say, the Canadian Society for the Study of Rhetoric), a rhetorical theorist with a specialization in health and medicine is more likely to attend meetings organized by theme: a conference on health values organized by bioethicists, or a conference on pharmaceuticals organized by researchers in the social studies of science. These theme venues may be excellent, but the rhetorical scholar is a transient participant, and community-building is difficult. Book publication would seem to pose the fewest special problems for the interdisciplinary scholar, who might, with a book, *create* an audience. Publishers, however, retain their disciplinary categories for books, as libraries do, and publishers' marketing boards may find interdisciplinary books simply ambiguous in terms of audience—and when publishers say they want interdisciplinary books, they often mean they want general ones.

6. *The work itself.* Interdisciplinary work requires a genuinely expansive expertise, often accompanied by researcher anxiety about entitlement to speak. In order to work in some areas of medical anthropology, for example, the anthropologist must know more than a little medicine, but will almost certainly know less medicine than his or her medically trained readers do. A job candidate at my university with advanced degrees in two disciplines, working across them, was looked at suspiciously by each of the two departments that met with her ("for a sociologist, she's not a bad philosopher"; "for a philosopher, she's not a bad sociologist").[5] Similarly, in a radio interview, one of his critics challenged David Healy's stature as a psychopharmacologist by saying, "he's an excellent historian."[6]

The student of a single discipline can be mentored more easily into a safe speaking position.

Indeed, any professor might be forgiven for advising graduate students to focus on disciplinary work. In disciplines, grant competitions are less fraught; appointment, tenure, and promotion processes are more predictable; publication and presentation venues are more obvious; mentoring is a more reliable initiation. The interdisciplinary researcher is frequently not a central member of a disciplinary department, and no member at all of a community of researchers with its own meetings and journals and secret handshakes. It is less stressful to be in a Department of English as a Shakespearean scholar, publishing in *Shakespeare Quarterly*, and attending annual meetings of the Shakespeare Society of America. Discipline envy.

Postdisciplinarity in Health Research

I will use the term "postdisciplinarity" to indicate the loosening of disciplines suggested by multi-, cross-, trans-, and interdisciplinarity, but characterized especially by the most radical of the constructs under discussion: interdisciplinarity. The term "postdisciplinarity" was coined, as far as I know, by Louis Menand, and takes disciplinarity as an important phase in the history of research. Postdisciplinarity recognizes, and preserves, the virtues of disciplinary research, while it refuses to enshrine disciplines in the form in which they were invented. Nineteenth-century universities in Europe and North America institutionalized specialization and departmentalization as modes of investigation and principles of the organization of instruction. The rise of English departments in North American universities, for example, was accomplished by a shift away from interdisciplinary studies of rhetoric and belles-lettres toward separate specializations in literature, composition, and speech communication—while many of the intellectual concerns of rhetoric were dispersed to disciplines such as psychology, linguistics, philosophy, and literary studies.

Postdisciplinarity is the next way of conceptualizing research. Disciplines persevere, but they may also be crossed, recombined, exploded, or disrupted to advantage. This is not to say that disciplinary restructuring is, in every one of its institutional forms, a desirable thing. Motive and purpose have a lot to do with whether initiatives against the separateness of disciplines are good for the people working or for inquiry itself. When departments are amalgamated, in order to save on administrative costs, for example, or when courses are cross-listed or team-taught primarily so that professorial salaries can be shared, some interesting things may happen, collaterally, but the acts themselves are not essentially postdisciplinary.

Conscious, and cautious, postdisciplinarity is called for in health research, where solely disciplinary research can leave too much uncovered and unthought. Research in "silos" (using the now common metaphor of vertical containment structures) is unable to answer, or even to pose, all of the best questions to the end of improved health. Three examples illustrate the point that research across, between, and beyond traditionally defined disciplines is required in health and medicine. In each of these examples, nontraditional research organization does not simply provide an added value; rather, it is constitutive of otherwise unavailable lines of inquiry.

1. In the spring of 2003, health professionals in Toronto, Canada, were responding to an outbreak of SARS (Severe Acute Respiratory Syndrome) that led to the death of over forty people and caused the World Health Organization to issue an advisory against unnecessary travel to the city. In such a case of emerging infectious disease, microbiologists and virologists are key experts for immediate response, as viruses are identified and mapped, and antiviral agents are sought. Other experts are needed as well: epidemiologists, to follow the spread of infection; experts in disease transmission, to advise on disease control; and public health officials, to keep people informed and to maximize necessary reporting and quarantine.

The problems that SARS posed, however, were not addressed sufficiently by traditional health disciplines, no matter how much specialists were in contact with each other (and retrospective accounts have suggested they were not in contact enough). Rather, an expert in disease transmission needs to know something about the strategies of persuasion most likely to move hospital workers to protect themselves adequately from infection, and to convince persons who have been exposed to enter and maintain quarantine. An expert in epidemiology needs to know something about race beliefs: in this case, to be able to speak intelligently on the relationship between being of Chinese origin and being at risk for spreading SARS. An expert in hospital management needs to know something about the human costs of institutional regulations that isolate patients who are *not* infected with SARS. An expert in disease control needs to know something about the ethics of personal surveillance and limiting a person's right to travel. An expert in public health needs to know something about international relations, and the economics and the politics of travel advisories.[7] An expert in emergency care needs to know something about the actual experience of illness felt by sufferers, and the figure of the patient as pariah.

Of course, some of these expert knowledges can be shared, but SARS is one of any number of diseases that is not only a medical problem, but also a wide-ranging health problem that requires researchers to think about things differently, and think about different things.[8]

2. Some questions that seem at first to be *essentially* medical turn out, on further examination, to be questions that medicine is not equipped to answer on its own. Recently, for example, some cancer specialists have reported that early detection, the very idea of which has driven policy on cancer diagnosis and treatment for decades, does not necessarily benefit patients, and may actually harm them.[9] The problem, they say, is that characteristically aggressive cancers will already have spread by the time they are detectable by current means, while very slow-growing cancers may best go undetected, obviating treatment more harmful than the cancer itself would ever have been. Should diagnostic screening routinely be performed, then, for cancers (prostate cancer is an example) about which the best time for intervention cannot be discerned by current tests? This ambivalence regarding early detection relegates medical information and the traditional evidence base to the status of a single element, or constellation of elements, in establishing protocols for best practice. The rest of the matter is the business of other researchers, humanists and social scientists, who deal with questions of quality of life, analysis of risk, trauma of diagnosis, distribution of health resources, management of doubt, and the composition of public messages. ("Always be tested," for example, is a better public message *rhetorically* than "sometimes be tested," but not necessarily a better message medically.)

Similarly, what are the questions of risks, rights, and medicine that should be asked when, for example, medical professionals are at odds with parents over the benefit of childhood immunization? Childhood immunization has become a matter of concern recently, especially in Great Britain. Many parents are convinced, despite medical evidence to the contrary, that the measles-mumps-rubella vaccine exposes their children to significant risk of developing autism. As a result, some parents are refusing to immunize their children, against their physicians' advice, thereby creating the possibility of a resurgence of diseases statistically more likely than immunization itself to cause brain damage. These are proxy-patients whose participation in decision making is, according to the current state of knowledge, to the detriment of their children and the community at large. The solution to the problem is not to be found (as might be thought) in the mix of the skills of an internist, an epidemiologist, and an ethicist. Rather, postdisciplinary researchers can help to formulate questions for public debate about communicable disease, the management of risk, and the management of uncertainty: critical thinking on a large scale.

3. Cosmetic surgery is one means by which unattractiveness, under some description, is absorbed into the medical realm, and made a treatable condition. On two American reality television series, *Extreme Makeover* and *The Swan* (both cancelled after impressive multi-season runs), contestants desiring a cure for unattractiveness were subjected to surgeries on the eyes, nose, ears, chin, stomach, and breasts, for example. The operations radically conventionalized them, engraving on them an aesthetic norm that itself is assumed to be a sign of health. As contestants were transformed into patients, the plastic surgeon became one member of a makeover team that included, among others, a personal trainer, a hair stylist, and a fashion consultant. Surgery was not, by that association, de-medicalized; instead, the haircut became a kind of surgery; dressing the patient, a fashion cure.

The questions raised by cosmetic surgery are not only about how to do it better or faster or more economically—or even whether to do it at all. The research involved not only questions whether cosmetic surgery should be an insurable procedure, or under what conditions it might be one, but also concerns critical studies of health and medicine, already underway, including historical studies about what the desire for cosmetic surgery means. *Extreme Makeover* and *The Swan* are phenomena of their times, but they are also twenty-first-century versions of the 1924 *New York Daily Mirror* "Homely Girl Contest," in which, according to historian Elizabeth Haiken, a contestant won the opportunity to be operated upon by a plastic surgeon who (Haiken cites the *Mirror*) "offered to take the homeliest girl in the biggest city in the country and to make a beauty of her" (1997, 98). Haiken also documents the deployment in the 1930s of the "inferiority complex" as the medical/psychiatric rationale for surgery aimed at beautification. Recently, sociologists Peter Conrad and Heather Jacobson (2003) have written about breast augmentation as biomedical enhancement. Each age seems to have its own aesthetic hypochondria, the often unaccountable sense of having an ill appearance. The relation between appearance and diagnosis is a topic for postdisciplinary study.

Narrative as a Means of Postdisciplinary Research

Narrative research is an interesting subset of nontraditional health research. When, as a humanities researcher, I talk to medical researchers about a role for the humanities in health studies, they often seem a little bewildered. ("What would a humanist in health studies do?") But, when I say the word "narrative," they look at me appreciatively—almost as if I had said "ethics." Across disciplines, researchers have begun to take note of the value of stories.

Earlier, in talking about the range of research necessary for responding to SARS, I said that an expert in emergency care ought to know something about the experience of illness as felt by sufferers and, especially in the case of communicable diseases, the figure of the patient as pariah. Students of narrative will not be surprised that SARS took on a particular, and necessary, poignancy and humanity when the Canadian Broadcasting Corporation (CBC) aired a long interview with a woman called "Patient Three," the adult daughter of the woman believed to be the index case of the disease in Toronto. Because "Patient Three" told a story—the story of her mother's illness and death, her brother's illness and death, and her own efforts, in the course of her grieving and her own grave illness, to protect others from exposure to infection—the anonymous, always racially identified, and often vilified person, known only for being the body in which the virus was imported from Hong Kong, became an innocent individual—someone's mother—who suffered and died.

Narrative, as will be seen over and over again in the pages of this volume, gives meaning and texture and humanity to what might otherwise be just cases; the embodiments of disease, disability, and trauma. Narrative is the corrective to biomedical discourse, which is, conventionally at least, characterized by a thinness in descriptions of patient experience, a tendency to measurement and quantification, and an embrace of the mores of Foucault's clinic, where the "individual in question was not so much a sick person as the endlessly reproducible pathological fact to be found in all patients suffering in a similar way" (Foucault 1973, 97). Narrative, as Anne Hunsaker Hawkins says, speaking of pathography, "returns the voice of the patient to the world of medicine, a world where that voice is too rarely heard, and it does so in such a way as to assert the phenomenological, the subjective, and the experiential side of illness" (1999, 12). Narrative "restores the person ignored or canceled out in the medical enterprise, and it places that person at the very center" (12).

Narrative facilitates transdisciplinary study as a focus and a means of research across disciplines deployed by a range of scholars, some of whom have contributed to this volume. Sociologist Arthur Frank (1995; 2004) studies the variety of genres of narrations of illness experience; philosopher Susan Wendell (1996) uses narrative to illuminate the phenomenology of disability; Kathryn Montgomery Hunter (1991), a literature specialist working as an epistemologist, describes the narrative structure of knowledge-making in medicine; James Pennebaker (1990; 2000), a psychologist, explores narrative as a means of psychotherapy; Hilde Lindemann Nelson (1997; 2001), a philosopher, explores the reaches of narrative ethics. Narrative study profits from the specific knowledges of disciplines—but because it frequently resists classification, narrative study is also postdisciplinary. Narrative study includes research on, with, about, and through stories. The prepositions themselves are a sign of the postdisciplinary nature of the enterprise.

Disciplines exist partly to constrain and authorize research, and disciplines have canonical literatures, histories, and stellar exemplars. Postdisciplinary researchers, then, face particular challenges for doing their work well, for knowing when they have done it well, and for persuading others that it has been done well. Postdisciplinary researchers in health studies face these challenges especially. When money is in short supply, and it almost always is, health funders would rather sponsor cancer research than cancer narrative research; funding councils focus on the structure of the SARS virus before they focus on the social suffering of SARS patients. These priorities are not really controversial, but they are evidence that health researchers from the humanities and social sciences, including narrative researchers, need to conduct their research and represent it with particular self-consciousness and diligence, for the usual categories of disciplinary health research, designating it as basic or applied, do not necessarily apply here. Narrative scholarship is often neither basic nor applied but it is *useful*, and the special task of postdisciplinary health researchers is to demonstrate how this is true.

Susan Sontag was a particularly interdisciplinary cultural critic, ranging across literature, language, history, philosophy, and anthropology in her work. Commenting in *AIDS and its Metaphors* (1990) on her decision to write her earlier essay, "Illness as Metaphor" (1977) on the cultural meanings invested in illnesses, Sontag, referring to her own experience of breast cancer, wrote:

> I didn't think it would be useful—and I wanted to be useful—to tell yet one more story in the first person of how someone learned that she or he had cancer, wept, struggled, was comforted, suffered, took courage ... though mine was also that story. A narrative, it seemed to me, would be less useful than an idea. (1990, 101)

Sontag's reluctance to tell a story, only a story, is important to acknowledge, as is the extraordinary contribution Sontag made in humanist, interdisciplinary studies of health. One goal of narrative research is to find the place where the idea and the story meet, or are the same—and to make stories useful. Narrative research is one sort of study that, in its best examples, repays new interest in inter- and postdisciplinary work in health studies.

Notes

1 Useful sources on rationales for interdisciplinarity are Sander Gilman (2000) and Mieke Bal (2002).
2 There followed, on the heels of the CIHR mandate, a kind of Canadian national project in health meta-research. One result is a 2005 report of the Atlantic Health Promotion Research Centre (with funding from CIHR and SSHRC [Social Science and Humanities Research Council of Canada]): *The Social Sciences and Humanities in Health Research*—largely a disciplinary, sometimes interdisciplinary, encyclopedia, with entries on health research under headings like "Philosophy," "Narrative Studies," and "Comparative Literature."
3 From the start, much of the health research community understood that there has to be a place for social scientists at the table. Clearly, research on social determinants of health, for example, is indispensable. The case for humanities research on health has been more difficult to make. In a country not known for its medical humanities programs, that a person in an English department would do or does health research remains an idea of some curiosity. The default notion of "medical humanities" is still of a project to get medical students to read novels and poems.
4 Here is an excerpt from a peer review by a social scientist of a humanities grant application in a CIHR competition: "As a social scientist," the reviewer writes, "I find it surprising that so few details are spelled out about study designs, samples, analytical tools, and statistical analyses, even allowing for the fact that the proposal does not call for detail about these research elements."
5 I have made changes to preserve the candidate's anonymity.
6 Paul Garfinkel, interviewed by Michael Enright on the CBC (Canadian Broadcasting Corporation) Radio.
7 Responding to the WHO travel advisory, Margaret Wente, a regular columnist in the national newspaper *The Globe and Mail* (24 April 2003), saw fit to write, "Toronto is now assumed to be as perilous as any pestilential Third World cesspit." Health advisories and the responses to them are not only about health.
8 In June, 2003, the Peter Wall Institute for Advanced Studies at the University of British Columbia (the institute which also supplied the major grant for the Narratives of Disease, Disability, and Trauma project) sponsored a forum called "SARS: An Interdisciplinary Disease." The forum brought together researchers from the biological sciences, the health sciences, the social sciences, and the humanities to discuss how SARS had affected their research and/or that of their fields.
9 Cancer experts Barron Lerner and Barry Kramer have been featured with biostatistician Don Berry in discussions of the myth of early detection.

PART I

Public Framing of Personal Narratives

THE EDITORS

Introduction
Aesthetics, Authenticity, and Audience

Recently, there has been a new wave of interest in narratives of ill health or suffering, texts that Anne Hunsaker Hawkins first termed "pathographies" and G. Thomas Couser calls "autopathographies." It began as a reaction to the growing number of written accounts of disease, disability, and trauma being published in a variety of forms, and representing both a wide range of motivations and various degrees of literary or artistic accomplishment. Hilde Lindemann Nelson's list of "things to do with stories" (discussed in the introduction to this volume) begins with "constructing and reading" narratives, assuming a crafted written account destined for an audience. This section of our book groups together six analyses of published autobiographical or fictional accounts, presented by readers trained in literary analysis. They are followed by two responses to film narratives by academics with a literary background, who are interested in the particular possibilities provided by a different medium of narration. While the topics covered vary considerably, all focus on how rhetoric and aesthetic shaping are consciously deployed to frame and determine the meaning assigned to the story and the receiver's response. These works of art also illustrate to some extent how telling the story affects the author/narrator in significant ways, as discussed in Part II of this volume. When the account is autobiographical and makes a direct appeal to the audience for it to revise its perceptions of the writer's experience, that experience may be redefined through being shared, and the aesthetic and therapeutic functions are effectively linked. The narrative may also ultimately constitute a call for solidarity or action, implying a political or pragmatic agenda, as discussed in Part III.

The receiver's response is dependent on trust in the authenticity of the account presented, and belief that the narrator has some authority to speak on the subject. The authority here is not usually based on medical expertise, but rather on personal experience. Helen Buss, a specialist in Canadian women's life writing who has written her own memoir of growing up in Newfoundland, examines how the issues of authority and authenticity are illustrated and problematized in Lauren Slater's serial memoirs of mental illness, particularly in the volume entitled, significantly, *Lying*. Slater is both a therapist dealing with clients with mental illness and a patient with symptoms that may include lying. She challenges us to consider how illnesses are diagnosed, by reading symptoms that may be interpreted to form different stories. Her refusal to speak authoritatively about her illness is in contrast to medical assumptions that disease follows well-defined paths that clearly indicate certain treatments. The skill with which she constructs her ambivalent account underlines how stories of "experience" are constructed, both by the individual involved and by the sociocultural and professional discourses that surround them. "Truth" may be found in fiction or fantasy, as much as in medical files.

The two texts examined by Hilary Clark, like Slater's, deal with the new identity a writer has been forced to assume because of a medical diagnosis. The stories told by Nancy Mairs (1986) and Susanna Kaysen (1993) bring out specific aspects of how a diagnosis of "borderline personality disorder" disrupted their lives as women, imposing a traumatic experience of hospitalization. Subsequently, living with the stigma of mental illness is comparable to experiencing a chronic disability. In each of these texts, the writer tries to "make sense" of events by turning an incomprehensible experience into a communicable story, especially through the use of humour and satire. The narrative serves as both a personal therapy and a witnessing to others—a warning to those who may become trapped by the system, and an example of how writing about the experience and imposing a form on it can be one way of escaping from prescribed patterns. Clark's contribution illustrates the possibilities of comparing texts with common elements to illustrate both similarities of experience and the unique aspects of each situation. The Kaysen account, when juxtaposed with the film based on it *(Girl, Interrupted*, 1999), can also serve to compare the results produced by a different medium of telling or showing the story.

While Slater's serial memoirs show change over time within an individual life, American poet Paul Monette produced a number of writings in different genres that convey a broader picture of change that occurred over a ten-year period throughout the AIDS crisis in the American gay community. Lisa Diedrich discusses Monette's elegy for his lover, who died before him, as well as his memoir entitled *Borrowed Time* (1988), which recounts how his lover's experience literally became his own. Unlike mental illness, AIDS at that time was deemed to be a terminal disease, and, beyond the loss of their loved ones, patients were anticipating their own death. Individual drama becomes part of a collective drama, and personal suffering is transformed into a political act aimed at raising awareness, becoming part of a social movement (as discussed in Part III of this volume). Diedrich uses some concepts from psychoanalytic theory in her essay to look more closely at issues of time in stories that centre on death—that of the significant other or/and the self.

Time, in fact, transforms the individual, who may be able to look back on an experience of illness from some distance: enough distance, in the case of Geneviève Brisac's autobiographical novel *Petite* (1994), to treat the youthful, anorexic self of the past as another person, with a different name. Barbara Havercroft introduces this French text to an anglophone audience, showing how its structure and language reflect and construct an experience of shrinking, both physically and mentally. The narrative form conveys the experience of anorexia as a threat to the very existence of a self that literally risks disappearing. Yet, the production of a fiction based on that experience provides an amplification: a story of recovery that manages to fulfill the need for control represented by anorexia, by controlling the language that speaks of it. The text becomes an extension of the body: one that enables the body to survive.

In some cases, however, the text may be in competition with the body, or betray it. Ulrich Teucher, who is both an academic specialist in comparative literature and psychology and a nurse who has cared for cancer patients, uses an autobiographical novel by German writer Maja Beutler to illustrate the benefits and dangers of aestheticizing the experience of cancer. This example, he suggests, shows that a self-consciously literary representation may serve to come to terms with an overwhelming experience more effectively than a factual personal account. The distance achieved counters the anxiety experienced by many cancer patients who find talking or writing about their experience threatening and not necessarily helpful. Should the unspeakable sometimes remain unspoken? Like mental illness or AIDS, cancer might justifiably be classified as "traumatic"; it also entails an on-going stigma, and provides stories with uncertain ends.

To what extent is the experience of these illnesses comparable to living with a non-life-threatening disability that, nevertheless, determines how a life can be lived, and whether it can become a publishable story?

Heidi Janz and Julie Rak juxtapose the autobiographical narratives of Ruth Sienkiewicz-Mercer and Christopher Nolan, both of whom have severe disabilities, and focus on the ways in which their stories have been marketed as triumphs over circumstances with "universal" value. This assessment may be seen as "disabling" their attempts to challenge the conceptions of disability that dominate TAB (temporarily able-bodied) discourse. Here, their stories are read as narratives of resistance illustrating the political dimension of *testimonio*. These texts also raise questions of mediation and translation, when the "speaker" is unable to produce the story unaided. Janz, who experiences some barriers to communication because of a disability, spoke for herself when this paper was presented at our conference. The way in which Rak facilitated her talk provided an embodied example of the issues raised in the narratives they discussed.

All these papers on literary works, produced by specialists in narrative analysis, emphasize the importance of the account's form to the story told: in fact, the two are inseparable, as the shape, style, and central metaphors of the narrative govern its interpretation. The storyteller is constructed as a persona, and the implied reader is encoded as an ultimately sympathetic audience. The imposition of artistic form may provide coherence, re-establishing a wholeness or healing lacking in life, but this is not always the case. An existence interrupted or disrupted by disease, disability, or trauma may be conveyed narratively by an aesthetic structure that reflects the fragmentation and patching together of a broken life, or through a story which presents an enigma rather than a "remedy" or solution. Speaking of the unspeakable, paradoxically, also raises issues of the communicability of "exceptional" experiences, and the extent to which they must be modified to be made comprehensible.

The sharing of such stories sometimes becomes the focus of the account, as illustrated in the last two papers in this section. Both deal with cinematic representations of shared trauma—one a family trauma, and the other the collective, intergenerational experience of the aftermath of the atomic bomb. Gail Finney compares an American film, *A Thousand Acres*, with a British one, *The War Zone*, to look at how the drama of incest is conveyed through both speech and visual images. Whereas speech dominates in the first film, the second shows a shift to a scenic mode that evokes immediacy rather than self-conscious reflection. Both techniques can prove to be powerful tools for catharsis. Finney's discussion builds on concepts from Freudian theory that, in turn, draw from Greek legends, to show how aestheticized stories of family trauma that reflect actual social pathology serve as collective consciousness-raising mechanisms.

Sally Chivers turns our attention to *Rhapsody in August*, a film by Japanese director Akira Kurosawa that commemorates the bombing of Nagasaki. Here, the family drama centers on a grandmother who lost her husband in that event and suffers herself from the effects of radiation. The trigger for memory is the impending death of a lost brother, who became mad as a result of the bombing. In the absence of her children, Kane tells a confused story to her grandchildren, becoming herself the embodiment of a collective cultural trauma. What can be transmitted across two generations, before it is too late? The need to hold on to the repressed experience, as it recedes into the irretrievable past, is conveyed at the level of the family and also of the nation, since this is a film addressed to a wide audience. Private loss and suffering are interwoven with the politics of war and reconciliation in a narrative that brings out the role of age and aging in the passing on of experience.

All these papers raise issues about the documentary value that should be accorded to texts that may or may not claim to be factual accounts. Several provide examples of the complexity of self–other relations, whether the author distanced from a former self or identifies with a significant other. They imply a commonality of experience among those with certain illnesses or disabilities, while also highlighting those experiences as solitary and, in some ways, unsharable. They force us to recognize the ethical issues involved in telling and interpreting stories of disease, disability, and trauma. These very issues were the focus at the 2002 Wall project conference of a panel discussion entitled "Narrative Ethics," during which Thomas Couser, Hilde Lindemann Nelson, and Susan Wendell engaged in a lively debate as they shared their current concerns, bringing literary theories of autobiography and gender to bear on bioethical debates on personhood and pain.

Couser spoke of his elaboration of the concept of "vulnerable subjects" as explained in his 2003 book of the same name, a term he uses to refer to "second-person subjects" of auto/biography: those who are spoken about or for, since they cannot speak directly for themselves. They may be dead (as was Monette's lover) or incapacitated by a disease, disability, or age (as in John Bayley's account of Iris Murdoch's fight against Alzheimer's disease, or in Morton Kondracke's *Saving Milly*, which may be read as a lobbying effort to raise funds for Parkinson's disease research).[1] When does life-writing become a commodity, and is it ethically permissible to market someone else's life rather than one's own? Pursuing issues related to "speaking for others," raised some time ago by Linda Alcoff (1991; 1993), Couser argued for "transactional transparencies." This term evokes an ethical code that would force writers to recognize the rights of those who, though close to them, might not agree with the interpretation offered of their "suffering."

The biomedical assumption that pain and suffering are necessarily always bad and must be relieved by any means available was questioned by both Hilde Lindemann Nelson and Susan Wendall.[2] The cultural and religious beliefs of some individuals may lead them to see consciousness as more valuable than pain relief (Nelson cited a Jewish example), or pain itself as a gift from God (as was the case for some Catholic mystics). Wendell reminded us that someone with a disability may be assumed to be in unbearable pain when that is far from proven, and this presupposition based on ignorance can serve as a pretext for euthanasia. Nelson used the expression "holding someone in personhood," introducing the issue of what defines a person (one that became central to discussions throughout our project, as described in James Overboe's contribution to Part III of this volume). Helen Buss pointed out, in response to the panel discussion, that writing one's own life always affects other people who have played a part in it. She described how, as a mother, she finds it difficult to write critically about that experience without damaging her children. The ensuing discussion addressed the view that women, who have traditionally been assumed to live through and for others, may be able to speak of themselves only obliquely. Yet everyone, in fact, has a "relational self," a term coined by autobiography specialist John Eakin (1999). Where are the limits of self and other, and in what ways do disease, disability, and trauma force us to recognize "otherness" in ourselves (as in Lauren Slater's case)?

Balancing the right to freedom of expression and the ethical imperative to do no harm to others is a precarious undertaking. Public criticism of medical treatments or practitioners also raises the possibility of lawsuits (against medical professionals or authors). Should there be ethical review boards for literary accounts, as there are for qualitative research projects? So far, such accounts are not considered "documents" making truth claims of the same order as "scientific" studies. They may stand accused, from another perspective, of transforming a painful and difficult experience into a fictional triumph of overcoming, if only by imposing an aesthetic form on it. Published accounts convey the process as cathartic or therapeutic, or valuable because they leave a "useful" message behind. Yet these are selected accounts by authors for whom "writing it out" is an option, and they may not represent a majority of those with the same condition. The stories evoked in Part II of this volume will allow comparisons to be made with less literary exchanges of stories in health-related contexts.

NOTES

1 Couser, *Recovering Bodies* (1997) and *Vulnerable Subjects* (2003); Bayley, *Elegy for Iris* (1999) and *Iris and Her Friends: A Memoir of Memory and Desire* (2000); Kondracke, *Saving Milly: Love, Politics, and Parkinson's Disease* (2001).
2 Nelson, *Damaged Identities, Narrative Repair* (2001) and ed., *Stories and Their Limits: Narrative Approaches to Bioethics* (1997); Wendell, *The Rejected Body: Feminist Philosophical Reflections on Disability* (1996).

HELEN M. BUSS

Authorizing the Memoir Form
Lauren Slater's Three Memoirs of Mental Illness

Dr. Lauren Slater is a practising psychologist with degrees from Harvard and Boston University, as well as an award-winning creative writer, having won the New Letters Literary Award in Creative Nonfiction in 1993. In her first memoir, *Welcome to My Country: A Therapist's Memoir of Madness* (1996), she writes a series of short sketches of patients she has treated in her career as a psychologist. *Welcome to My Country* exemplifies an important feature of the traditional writing mandate of the memoir—the concentration on the other—yet it uses that concentration to authorize a story of the self. In the last pages of the text, as Slater constructs an anecdote in which she visits a psychiatric hospital ward to see a patient, she confesses that "from [ages] fourteen to twenty-four, I spent considerable portions of my life inside th[is] very hospital ... and even today, at thirty-one years old, with all of that supposedly behind me, with chunks of time in which to construct and explain the problems that led me to lockup, I find myself at a loss for words" (181).

Yet Lauren Slater is not long "at a loss for words," in a publication sense, as two memoirs swiftly follow *Welcome to My Country*. Slater's confession at the end of *Welcome* authorizes her to tell a more personal story in *Prozac Diary* (1998), which gives an account of her mental illness and the drug therapies that allow her to function, and this more personal document leads to *Lying: A Metaphorical Memoir* (2001), where she searches backward in time in a coming of age story which becomes a meditation on the nature of truth in writing. Thus, the personal life further authorizes a therapeutic and spiritual journey that does not depend on traditional modes of external authorization by way of a historically verifiable

33

fact base. I propose that Slater's three books represent not only a patient/therapist's autobiographical account of mental illness in contemporary times, but also a writer's exploration of how form shapes truth, and how fact and fiction, self and other, history and literature, science and art can be aesthetically shaped to authorize the changing nature of one's self-knowledge. In constructing these steps in authorization of the autobiographical story, a serial autobiographical practice leads beyond self-accounting to self-creation, the authorization of the self through the special writing advantages of the memoir form.

"Authority," as G. Thomas Couser reminds us, has been located in an "extratextual reality" in traditional formulation and in the "self-determining agency of language" in postmodern terms. Couser proposes that, in autobiography, authority is contested and negotiated between "autobiographers and others—collaborators, editors, critics, biographers, historians, and lay readers" (75). I find the authorization of memoir to be located in all three of these areas: external reality, the agency of language, and the negotiation of the text between interested parties. However, I would like to bring attention to the authorization that takes place as the result of the negotiation between the writer and the typical, formal elements of the memoir form. In making my case for these books as experiments in authorizing the memoir form as a vehicle for public discourse as well as for private healing and self-revision, I will first take up the function of the significant other as a hallmark of memoir in Slater's first memoir; secondly, I will deal with the strategic function of the "diary" and "letter" formats as part of memoir writing in *Prozac Diary*; and thirdly, I will take up the implications for the authorization process in "memoir" implied in the title of Slater's most recent text, *Lying*. In treating the three texts as serial in nature, rather than as quite different, even contradictory stories of the self, I will also be proposing that these various pieces are necessary to the fuller performance of Slater's subject positions.

These concerns reflect my continuing interest in the memoir as a literary discourse, as I explored in my book *Repossessing the World: Reading Memoirs by Contemporary Women*, where I propose that the memoirist whose text uses identification through the other as its primary strategy of self-performance is particularly "useful to a provisional and contingent subjectivity unable to buy into traditional constructions of the self.... The narrator finds her own self-performance through the exploration of the biography of significant others who occupy the text as fully as she does" (Buss 2002, 37). Slater's provisional and contingent position as a subject derives from the irony and instability of being both a former mental patient and a mental health professional, a conflation of subject positions not often admitted to openly in Slater's professional world. Part of her therapeutic goal is to understand herself through understanding her patients. In *Welcome to My Country*, she writes of several of her patients, subtly interweaving insights gained from her personal struggles. Most important of these, for the purpose of talking about form, is her chapter on Joseph, a schizophrenic patient who suffers from "overinclusion," which means he "lacks the capacity to put information into appropriate categories" (1996, 73). Although once a brilliant student at Princeton, after his illness Joseph's writing becomes "hypergraphic," or compulsive, and Slater asks how Joseph can "become what he once was, a storyteller, a social participant whose words would break the barrier of isolation and thrust him into community?" (89). As a writer herself, Slater takes an aggressive stance as she "plucked up the pencil, and scrawled my way right into his page" (90), picking up on his partial phrases and thoughts and writing them into short, sentence-long plot lines. This amazes Joseph, who actually strokes the words, pats the sentences she writes, and murmurs over and over, "I once could" and "I, too," sadly expressing both his history and his hope. Slater realizes that "my letters next to Joseph's ... were jewels to him, crafted shapes that gleamed with sense" (91). After some time has passed, Joseph is able to assert "I want to stop failing" (100). Although Joseph's progress is by necessity very limited, considering the nature of his disease, he is able, with Slater's editing help, to take a creative writing course and pass.

What is important to the formal arrangement of this memoir is that after Slater discovers the centrality of written words to Joseph's more positive functioning on a daily basis, the therapist's and the patient's story travel side by side. In helping Joseph to edit the story of his relationship with his mother, Slater begins to feel memories of her own mother return to her—not in the plot that she and Joseph have carved out from his jumble of words, but in "the rising rhythm in the language" (109). The sense that the language of Joseph's story is their shared creation, that all stories are, in ethnographer Elliot Mishler's words, a "joint construction of meaning" (Slater 1996, 109) leads Slater to conclude tentatively that "perhaps narratives are the one realm that cannot ever—despite the consumerism and capitalism in the publishing industry—be confidently claimed by any individual" (110). The memoir form's typically dialogic mode—indeed, in the Bahktinian sense, its heteroglossia of texts and intertexts—expresses this communality of linguistic acts in the strategy of self-performance through the vivid recreation of the other. In each of the portraits of patients subsequent to Joseph's—Marie, a depressive, Oscar, a catatonic schizophrenic and, in the culminating portrait, Linda, a bulimic with a terrifying range of self-destructive behaviors—Slater uses her empathy with her patients and her detailed construction of her work with them to gain authority in terms of her insight into mental illness, and to use that authority to move towards her own story.

However, when she confesses, in the final pages of the book, that she has been a patient in the very hospital where she meets Linda, she is reluctant to take up her own story except to emphasize the factors in her life that saved her from the ultimate fate of most of her patients. This is where she says she is "at a loss for words," and she frames her silence this way: "American culture abounds with marketplace confessions. I know this. And I know the criticisms levied against this trend, how such open testifying trivializes suffering and contributes to the narcissism polluting our country's character." I agree with some of what the critics of the confessional claim, and the phenomenon is especially de-authorizing to women such as Slater. She is particularly damning of the television show *The Oprah Winfrey Show*, which "extracts admissions from the soul like a dentist pulls teeth, gleefully waving the bloodied root and probing the hole in the abscessed gum while all look, without shame, into the mouth of pain made ridiculously public" (179). I would give some exemption to the host and producers of *Oprah* based on my viewing of a variety of these shows over many years, finding that while most shows certainly do demean their confessional guests, the Harpo production team seems to have learned how to be respectful of their subjects over the years. However, the dental metaphor indicates the intensity of fear and loathing Slater had for the public confession at the time of her first book and how de-authorized she felt to tell a personal story, and also helps to explain why this text makes consistent use of the strategy of othering the self in a series of anonymous others to avoid the trivialization of suffering and the narcissism that Slater finds so distasteful. The strategy of othering authorizes Slater to speak of mental health problems, and it also avoids the de-authorization that women suffer from when they write of their own emotional and psychological problems.

Then why would Slater go on to write *Prozac Diary* (1998), a text which is nothing if not confessional? As its book blurb indicates, this text is her personal story of how by the age of twenty-six, "depressed, suicidal, and unemployed ... she became one of the first users of a brand-new drug, called Prozac." Not only would it seem that Slater has entered the "marketplace confessions" business she once abhorred, but she has become an advertisement for the drug industry and shaped her story into the required happy ending, as the blurb goes on to speak of her "life restored to productivity, creativity, and love." Yet this book is not, or not only, a stereotypical "marketplace confession": rather, it is an exercise in using the confessional form while skirting some of its risks through various authorizing formal moves.

In her introduction to *Confessional Politics*, Irene Gammel formulates the problem of revelatory confession this way:

> The female voice relating personal experience, like the sinner's and the patient's, belongs not to the realm of abstract and official langue but to parole, to familiar and intimate speech, and is thus characterized by a low degree of formality and authority, as it is perceived as ephemeral or trivial. Women's personal ... stories in life writing and popular media tend to make a dramatic splash when they first appear; they descend into the subconscious realm of memory only to surface later in more authoritative frames in appropriated and tamed forms. Generally the traces of women's voices survive but under the name of a different author/ity." (1999, 4)

The authority, according to the essayists in *Confessional Politics*, can be any mode from patriarchal psychiatric discourse through exploitive talk show formats, to the disempowering and sadistic pornographic gaze. What Lauren Slater works at in *Prozac Diary* is finding a professional and public "langue" to authorize her own "parole."

Her purpose in the text is to talk about Prozac as both a miracle drug—it has indeed tamed her various obsessive compulsive behaviors and made a dysfunctional life into an astoundingly accomplished one—and Prozac as a continuing and dangerous trade-off in terms of psychic function versus physical well-being. Slater, like 40 to 60 per cent of long-time Prozac users, suffers sexual dysfunction and memory problems, and has had to increase her dosage to more than recommended amounts to maintain her psychic equilibrium over ten years. In this memoir, she needs to be able to write about Prozac both as a consumer of the drug (and therefore confess the symptoms and behaviors that make Prozac essential to her functioning) and as an expert in mental heath. Obviously she does have an expertise; as a PhD in psychology and an experienced counselor, she can speak as an equal with the medical doctors and scientists whose concerns are primarily with the biochemical miracle that the drug creates. This expertise authorizes her to speak. However, Slater as patient has another expertise: She knows that the "cure" is as complex as the illness. As she says, "Cure is complex, disorientating, a revisioning of self, either subtle or stark. Cure is the new, strange planet, pressing in. The doctor could not have known. And that made me, as it does every patient, only more alone" (9). Her challenge in this memoir is to authorize her personal story as a patient "alone," the figurative parole of this text. To do that she must not only use the langue of the psychologist to convince us of her equal authority in terms of mental illness, but use the langue of the creative nonfiction writer—the tropes of literature—to shape the memoir form.

In *Prozac Diary*, Slater puts the everyday formats of the letter and the diary into subtle interplay with the forms of the medical report and the scientific language of the biochemists. Most of the chapters of the memoir bear the heading "Letter to my Doctor." In these chapters, Slater sets up a medical report in the kind of typeface one sees on such official documents. The first one, an "evaluation and treatment" plan, reads in part:

> Patient currently presents with symptoms that meet the criteria for Obsessive-Compulsive Disorder. However this diagnosis can be seen as secondary as opposed to primary. Patient reports OCD, with its attendant compulsions to count, check, and wash, emerged rather suddenly and unexpectedly w/in last few months. However, patient does have a long history of psychopathology prior to the manifestation of her present complaint. Has in the past attempted suicide, and engaged in self-mutilating behaviors, including anorexia, that resulted in psychiatric hospitalizations: dates 1977, 1979, 1984, 1985. Record indicates patient has carried a diagnosis of Borderline Personality Disorder since 19 years of age, and a diagnosis of major depression, severe and recurrent, beginning in her early ... (1998, 15–16)

At this point Slater breaks off the report, and, in an italic typeface conventionally used to indicate a diary or letter entry, she writes: "How do you describe emptiness? Is it the air inside a bubble, the darkness in a pocket, snow? I think, yes, I was six or seven when I first felt it, the dwindling that is depression" (16). These words begin a four-page account of an incident from her childhood which allows Slater to be both reflective on her active, energetic, child self—"I have yet to understand how energy can so easily coexist with what is hollow" (17)—and reflexive about its meaning as she observes that the result of the childhood incident was that "I had moved into metaphor, a significant developmental stage" (19). The formal effect of this short chapter is multifold. The use of the medical report allows her to authoritatively assert her position as mentally ill person, without the attendant risks of a more confessional format. The doctor voice summarizes her condition and her history crisply, unemotionally. Normally the confession comes first, then the langue of whatever authority will make use of the confessional parole. Here the langue is used, ironically, to authorize the parole that follows, the italicized words becoming more powerfully authorizing because they create a metaphorical depth that the langue of the medical report cannot. Slater authorizes herself as both analyzing psychologist in her word choice—speaking of a "developmental step," advising her reader at one point to take "note" as she observes her childhood self—and also as life writer, authorizing the metaphorical language she will use throughout the text to deepen and broaden our concept of the disorders of "emptiness," of "air inside a bubble," of "darkness in a pocket," of the muffle and chill of "snow," that bring us imaginatively closer to her experience of depression. As philosopher, poet, and life writer, as well as in her role of psychologist and patient, Slater authorizes her own discourse.

She sets up her opening like a good novelistic script, with herself the doubtful patient set against the confident but impersonal "Prozac Doctor," set in contrast to the life-saving healer who should comprehend "what even many a surgeon knows: that you must smooth the skin, that you must stop by the bedside in your blue scrub suit, that language is the kiss of life" (11). While playing the patient, she slyly inserts herself as the psychologist, being herself an expert in talk therapy and authorized to be critical of the "Prozac Doctor." In the chapter on sexual dysfunction, she defuses the potentially other- and self-damaging confessional aspect of such a subject, first by including her lover as a speaking character in the text (and making it obvious he has had a part in constructing the chapter) and framing the sadness of her reduced sexual response within the comedy of their search for aphrodisiacs. Humour in confessions, although rare, is a wonderful saving grace for both author and reader and a subtly effective authorizing factor. The text of *Prozac Diary* is followed by "A Conversation with Lauren Slater," one of those question and answer pieces that authors often do to help publicize their books. I have no idea if this is the kind of mock interview that many of us do in which we get to ask ourselves our own questions, or if Slater was actually interviewed. I suspect the former. At any rate, the interview works to further point to her authority as mental health professional, and Prozac consumer, as well as self-conscious creative writer.

In *Lying: A Metaphorical Memoir* (2001), Slater tangles with an important aspect of the memoir form: its location on the borderline between fact and fiction, a location that is often used to de-authorize memoir writing. Timothy Dow Adams outlines in his book, *Telling Lies in Modern American Autobiography* (1990), the centrality of lying to the art of autobiography, proposing that lying is as important a consideration to understanding how autobiography works as are the two essentials outlined by Roy Pascal in his foundational work, *Design and Truth in Autobiography* (1960).

For Adams, part of the autobiographical act includes trying "to keep the reader off balance" (8), a legitimate writing strategy for a creative writer. In *Repossessing* (2002), I discuss the changing nature of memory over time, of how memory is as much a function of imagination (especially in its scenic quality) as it is a function of recall. As well, I emphasize the importance—for women, in particular, who lack originating myths in the broader culture—of using fantasy to effect a change in subjectivity, but I am not entirely comfortable with either Dow's proposal of the literary necessity of lying, or my own proposal of its importance to women's subject formation. Because of memoir's claims to truth, that it does indeed have a historical reality base in personal lives that novels do not claim, memoir writers and critics need to have reference to a mediating ethics of lying. Adams surveys Sissela Bok's (1979) work on the ethics of lying and I agree with his analysis of Bok's work (Adams, chapter 5), in that not just the truth or falsity of your statements are important in autobiography, but the intention of your lie must be determined as well.

As a literary critic, I am aware of the dangers in entering the swampy ground of authorial intentions on which postmodernism has staked a no trespass sign, but I still think that critics and theorists of life writing, in their task of analyzing texts that do not claim the fictional authority of novels, have to deal with authorial intention. They have to because they are working with a genre in which the supposed distance between narrator and writer, assumed and allowed by fiction, has been put into profound question by the contemporary explosion of the creative non-fiction memoir form. It is fine for a memoir writer to include fantasy in her work as a means of self-invention, and keeping the reader "off balance" may well be an acceptable aesthetic practice. However, I think the contract of memoir (as opposed to novel and short story) requires that the reader be given fair warning, either through the declarations typically found in prefaces (about composite characters, telescoping of time, etc.) or through narrative commentary within the text, that the writer is using her life in a particular manner that seeks truth through various fictive devices. I think that this is essential in the writing and critiquing of a genre in which the truth is found, as Adams puts it, "in the relational space between the story and its reader" (1990, 12).

Slater begins *Lying: A Metaphorical Memoir* with a chapter that has only two words: "I exaggerate." This blatant declaration of her text's precarious position on the borderline between fact and fiction is also a statement of intention; a fair warning to readers. We are never sure in this book when she is merely exaggerating through the device of intensifying though literary trope, and when she is lying. Her book makes me realize how utterly reliant the memoir form is on the reader's acceptance of the authenticity of the narrative voice, and I marvel at Slater's willingness to risk so much of the authority that the intimate narrative voice can give a memoir. What she does is attempt to authorize her text by de-authorizing her own narrative voice. She invites us to suspect her honesty as a narrator in order to reinforce her authenticity and sincerity. Why this strategy? Because the "real" Lauren Slater has suffered from several psychiatric complaints and one of them is Munchausen syndrome, in which the patient fakes illnesses to gain attention. The text constantly plays with our sense of narrator reliability. Is Slater a victim of epilepsy, the symptoms of which she plots with such imagination and rigour throughout the text? Or is she faking it?

At the beginning of the text she states equivocally, "I have epilepsy. Or I feel I have epilepsy. Or I wish I had epilepsy, so I could find a way of explaining the dirty, spastic, glittering place I had in my mother's heart. Epilepsy is a fascinating disease because some epileptics are liars, exaggerators, makers of myths and high-flying stories" (6). In the middle of the text, after making this reader forget that she ever placed her diagnosis of epilepsy in doubt, she confesses:

> Now we get to the little hoary truth in this tricky tale. The summer I was thirteen I developed Munchausen's, on top of my epilepsy, or—and you must consider this, I ask you please to consider this—perhaps Munchausen's is all I ever had. Perhaps I was, and still am, a pretender, a person who creates illness because she needs time, attention, touch, because she knows no other way of telling her life's tale. Munchausen's is a fascinating psychiatric disorder, its sufferers makers of myths that are still somehow true, the illness a conduit to convey real pain. (89)

Munchausen syndrome, in this book, is a metaphor for writing memoir, in which the writer creates tales on the edge of truth and fiction that can translate her pain into language and receive the attention she desires and the healing she seeks. At the end of her text, Slater says that she feels that "although [the memoir] is not always factually correct," she has "finally been able to tell a tale eluding me for years, a tale I have tried over and over again to utter, the story of my past, of my mother and me, the story of the strange and fitful illnesses claiming most of my moments, the humiliating birth of sexuality, my love of myths and proclivities toward deceit. I have told it all and it is a relief. A relief to put it to rest" (220). Yet she knows she has not given the reader rest, for she ends by asserting that "despite the huge proliferation of authoritative illness memoirs …

something is amiss. For me the authority is illusionary, the etiologies constructed. When all is said and done, there is only one kind of illness memoir I can see to write, and that's a slippery, playful, impish, exasperating text, shaped, if it could be, like a question mark?" (221). The sense that an autobiographical narrative of an ongoing mental illness is a "slippery … exasperating" activity, one characterized by questions, playfulness, even an impish tendency to question the usual modes of authorization of the self, implies an important shift in our ideas of autobiographical practice.

While I write of a generic change and a stylistic change in autobiographical practice, another writer in this collection, Anne Hunsaker Hawkins, has observed that there has been a "paradigm" shift in the kinds of illness narratives written by contemporary trauma memoirists from a social science perspective.

> It seemed as though pathography had undergone a kind of paradigm shift, with acute illness displaced by chronic illnesses. I also found that people were writing much more about disabilities, both major and minor—conditions that one tends neither to recover from or die from.

I propose that it is not coincidental that, as our cultural interest in illness narratives changes from a desire for narratives of acute illnesses cured to an interest in chronic illnesses tolerated, that the memoir form, with what I have called its "provisional and contingent" subjectivity formations, should become the generic shape that best expresses the human subject as survivor: one who can never overcome but can invent and reinvent tactics of survival, and indeed, express those reinventions in serial form. So it is with Slater's experience of mental illness, a condition "one tends neither to recover from or die from," but which one needs to find a continuing or staged linguistic reconfiguration as one does in a series of autobiographical performances.

What Hawkins calls a "paradigm shift" in subject matter is a signal to literary critics of a need to study the ways in which the form and shape of autobiographical practices are being changed by specific interests of a given cultural moment, and by the different subject positions of writers in that moment. Such subjects and such moments shape their truths through the use of various fictive devices, as well as being shaped by the narrative permissions and taboos of the culture. In doing this, a writer must seek a new authorization for testifying to her life, a survivor's authorization, that lacks certainty and "authority" in the traditional sense but reflects the contingency of a subjectivity more typical of our cultural times.

Jane Lazarre, in one of her memoirs, writes of how she shapes her life story like a piece of art, "rubbing it, slowly scraping away at it, polishing it" (1998, 9), so that eventually she can have the "exhilarating" experience of being "saved by form." I have proposed, in *Repossessing*, that such acts of writing work not only to translate to the reader the experience of the memoirist, but are part of the continuing process of surviving difficult circumstances for the memoirist, and, by implication, the reader who faces similar uncertain times. What is being healed is not only some personal disorder, but also a cultural disease that has divided and dichotomized so many aspects of our human natures, and robbed us of a psycho-social integrity we need to be effective actors in the world. Memoirs like Slater's violate our sense of the clear binaries of disease and health, and violate too our cultural separation of personal confession, the unauthorized parole of the suffering individual, and the discourses of public discourse, the authorized langue of fact making. Memoir is, at its heart, this kind of violation, a violation of linguistic separations, and in being so it is creating a new discourse that addresses the artificial and repressive separations our culture perpetuates.

What memoirs such as *Lying* and, reflectively, its predecessors *Welcome* and *Prozac* do, is ask us to take up a study of formal construction—not merely the identification of certain story lines and content themes, but the nuts and bolts of the build-up and selection of language in the text—in order to understand how this new discourse of contemporary memoir authorizes itself. Such a series of memoirs invites us, as well, to consider the process of healing as ongoing; not a cure that can be told in one book, but a coping, adjusting, creative survivorship that continues through a series of literary expressions. Indeed, in Slater's most recently published memoir, *Love Works Like This*, an account of her pregnancy, birthing experience, and the first year of her daughter's life, Slater continues the typical strategies I have outlined here, especially in her poetic renderings of scientific information on hormonal production and other topics germane to pregnancy, and continues her creative survivorship. In reading a series of memoir texts like this for what it exhibits of a particular discourse of memoir, I think we will come to understand the way the contemporary memoir builds itself on the dynamic dialogic between binaries that have been traditionally dichotomized, to understand the joined nature of fact and fiction, literature and history, self and other, form and content, and illness and wellness.

HILARY CLARK

Telling Trauma
Two Narratives of Psychiatric Hospitalization

We do not fully choose our research, I believe. My interest in narratives of mental illness derives from my experience, as a twelve-year-old girl, of going with my father and younger sister to visit my mother in the psychiatric unit of the local hospital. Suffering from "a nervous breakdown," she was admitted several times. I've forgotten (or blocked out) some memories of those visits, but will never forget the smoke—everyone smoked. Even my mother, who didn't smoke, would puff away. Patients shuffled around in slippers, holding on tightly to their cigarettes and lighters. They played cards or watched TV or made instant coffee in the ward kitchenette; when visitors came they would all sit around tables and smoke. Some patients didn't come out of their rooms at all. As I left the ward, I could see them lying silently on their beds as I walked past, turned away from the open doors. This paper bears witness to my mother's experience.

Within narratives of illness, hospitalization is often a central episode, one closely associated with the experience of receiving a diagnosis and hence a new identity of illness. In narratives of mental illness, it can be an especially crucial episode. Indeed, given the stigma still attached to a psychiatric diagnosis and, particularly, to admission to hospital for a psychiatric crisis, this critical stage in a mental illness "career" (Karp 1996, 55–57), when worked into a narrative, has the potential to repel a general reader.

In this paper I focus on two such narratives of psychiatric hospitalization: Nancy Mairs' essay "On Living Behind Bars" (from *Plaintext*, 1986), which recounts a hospital episode and reflects on the place of depression in the author's life so far; and Susanna Kaysen's book-length hospital narrative *Girl, Interrupted* (1993). Although men have written hospital narratives, too—most notably William Styron in his *Darkness Visible: A Memoir of Madness* (1990)[1]—I am focusing on women's narratives because depression and borderline disorder (Kaysen's diagnosis) are more commonly diagnosed in women, and because both writers analyze their diagnoses and experiences of hospitalization within the context of their lives *as women* in a sexist society. (An earlier example of such analysis, although somewhat more fictionalized, is Sylvia Plath's *The Bell Jar* [1963].) Both Kaysen and Mairs look back on themselves as young women who signed themselves into a mental hospital for reasons they were unsure of and for a length of time they did not foresee. Both entered hospital in 1967, and both in Massachusetts—Kaysen signing herself into McLean Hospital (alma mater of poets Robert Lowell and Sylvia Plath), and Mairs into McLean's poor cousin, Metropolitan State. I will compare the rhetorical strategies in their narratives, looking at the means each writer uses to present the episode to her readers and move them to sympathy. Also of interest is how each writer sees the episode as relating to the ongoing story of her life. I will suggest that each presents her time in a psychiatric hospital as an inevitable consequence of the way her illness and her life were developing, yet also as a major disruption in her life—a traumatic hole she fell into, whose meaning she cannot completely discern. Both authors hedge on closure; the episode may be over, but there is no forgetting. Identity has been irretrievably changed; neither can reclaim what she has lost.

Each author tells her own hospital story as a way of reclaiming the illness experience (Frank 1995) from the institutional discourse of doctors' case notes and hospital reports. As well, each bears witness, offering a critique of the hospital experience and of biomedical accounts of mental suffering that would reduce it to a neurobiological disorder treatable by medication alone. In referring to the "rhetoric" of these hospital narratives, then, I am situating them as instances of therapeutic expression (catharsis), but also more importantly as testimonies aiming to affect and persuade, and to find or create a receptive audience for their narrative of a highly stigmatized experience. They adopt certain strategies to achieve this end—often the use of humour or satire, with recognizable (sometimes almost stereotypical) situations and characters, along with references to the myth of the descent into hell and ascent back into the purgatory of everyday life—into a recovery both authors make quite clear is provisional and maintained with some difficulty, inasmuch as the struggle with mental illness is often a chronic one. This myth, taken up quite explicitly in William

Styron's *Darkness Visible* with references to Dante's *Inferno*, seems for both author and reader to be an inevitable cultural mode of "re-formulating" the experience of mental suffering (Hawkins 1999, 24). The shared cultural narrative makes some sense of the experience and provides a dam against trauma.

Kaysen's *Girl, Interrupted* takes its title from a painting by Vermeer, "Girl Interrupted at Her Music" (c.1660). Kaysen describes the girl in the painting, thus: "[S]he was sad. She was young and distracted, and her teacher was bearing down on her, trying to get her to pay attention. But she was looking out, looking for someone who would see her" (1993, 167). She alludes to this painting at points throughout her narrative, comparing her experience as a girl in a psychiatric hospital with this girl's situation under the control of a "beefy music teacher" (165). She frequently returns to the idea of interruption, and of lost or stolen time: "Interrupted at her music: as my life had been, interrupted in the music of being seventeen ... What life can recover from that?" (167). Kaysen thus frames her narrative with an act of aesthetic identification. As well, she incorporates psychiatric and hospital documents (her own admission record, case records, memos, progress reports, and discharge record), and these form another frame, ironic and alienating, for her story. Whatever the status of these documents (fictive or real), they *look* authoritative. Their inclusion invites us rather pointedly to compare the psychiatric model of onset, diagnosis, medication, and assessment of progress to recovery with the author's own experience of mental suffering, which has a much less clear-cut beginning and end.

For Kaysen, while the hospital sometimes seems a refuge from the expectations of others, it represents most of all a break or crisis—a catastrophic turning-point. She is admitted on the basis of a short interview with a doctor she has never met before and, it appears, because she has picked at a pimple:

> "Picking at yourself," [the doctor] repeated. He popped out from behind his desk and lunged toward me. He was a taut, fat man, tight-bellied and dark.
>
> "You need a rest," he announced. (7)

Described as bulging like a pimple himself, the doctor proceeds to book her into the adolescent women's ward at McLean for two weeks, a stay which expands, unaccountably, into almost two years. She signs herself in under the mistaken impression that, if she doesn't do so, she could be committed against her will, and she is not enlightened otherwise. The older Kaysen knows better, looking back on the doctor as an incompetent fraud. This characterization of doctors is typical of *Girl, Interrupted*, and is not unusual in other narratives of mental illness.

Is she being committed for two years for picking at a pimple? As it happens, not quite. As the story proceeds, we learn through flashbacks that the author overdosed on aspirin and had her stomach pumped two years earlier. As well, we learn that in the past she has engaged in self-mutilating behaviours (wrist-banging and facial scratching) and that she has spells of frighteningly vivid, obsessive thinking. However, her "borderline" diagnosis seems to be based as much on her general "social contrariness" and "pessimistic outlook" (phrases from her patient report)—her resistance to adult expectations of a nice, well-off, seventeen-year-old girl—as it is on her self-injuring and suicidal behaviour. She flunked her senior year in high school, handing in poems instead of essays; she has never had a regular job and has had "boyfriends by the barrelful" (155). She only learns of her diagnosis—"borderline personality disorder"—twenty-five years later when, with the help of a lawyer, she obtains her hospital records. This diagnosis, more often applied to women than to men, is to her an alien construction imposed on a unique life story. In part, she copes with this diagnosis by representing doctors as incompetent; even more effectively, she rewrites it, adding her own "particulars" and comments to create (in a chapter entitled "My Diagnosis") "an annotated diagnosis" (150).

In a defensive move that is fairly common in illness narratives, Kaysen subjects doctors and hospital staff to satirical treatment. Besides the initial pimple-shrink (later charged by a patient with sexual harassment), she offers us the following suspects, all guilty of violating personal boundaries and privacy: a female ward doctor who looks like "the ghost of a horse" (84), who diagnoses her with "compulsive promiscuity" and then prods her to reveal all the juicy details; a male resident who questions her relentlessly about her bowel movements; and therapists who are "addicted to" prescribing "Thorazine, Stelazine, Mellaril, Librium, Valium" in knock-out combinations (87). There are nurses who do half-hour, fifteen-minute, or five-minute checks, appearing and disappearing with the word "Checks," and a rather frightening matron named Mrs. McWeeney whom the inmates judge to be "nuts": "We were locked up for eight hours a day with a crazy woman who hated us" (89). Life on the ward is represented as a kind of guerrilla warfare in which the patients, enduring constant surveillance, learn to exploit the hospital's "byzantine" systems of privileges and punishments. Like prisoners in jail, the patient-inmates learn to survive by knowing the enemy and looking for breaks in its cover. Most importantly, they survive by banding together in solidarity. Their main goal is less to get out of hospital than to avoid being sent into solitary confinement—or, worse, to the maximum-security ward, where patients sit in cells smeared with their own excrement. This is a line of abjection they are terrified to cross. At one point, the narrator almost does cross this line: in an acute episode of self-mutilation, she scratches and bites at her hand, convinced she must look for her own bones. She is brought back from this deepest of pits with a stiff drink of Thorazine. From this point on, Kaysen recounts a slow (and not very enthusiastic) climb back to "normality."

Kaysen's story, then, attempts to integrate the hospital "interruption" into her life story while, at the same time, bearing witness to a Kafkaesque institution that operates by lying, applying mystifying diagnoses, and probing patients with questions while evading the patient's own questions, and withholding information from them. It is another comment on the system and its sexist norms at the time (the late 1960s) that the young woman is considered to have recovered, and is allowed to leave, when she accepts a rather hasty marriage proposal. Her recovery, if it is that, seems flat and unredemptive; she is unclear as to why she is marrying and is still unwilling to do "useful" work. Eventually, however, she becomes a writer and attempts to make sense of the traumatic two-year interruption of her life, in order to ensure that she may never again lose time so unaccountably, never again cross that "shimmering, ever-shifting borderline" (159) into the "parallel universe" of the mad (5). Her narrative is also a witnessing to self and others, a warning to readers of how easily one's life can be interrupted by trauma.

Nancy Mairs has written a number of personal essay collections that are smart, moving, and often very funny. In her long essay "On Living Behind Bars," Mairs recounts one particular period of hospitalization for depression and agoraphobia while exploring the larger context of this episode: a life of depression marked by fears of loss and change; a sense of never measuring up to the norms of femininity. Like Kaysen, she represents the hospitalization as an extended break in the story of her life—a hiatus that certainly followed from a crisis (agoraphobic panic attacks, an inability to eat or look after her young child), yet ultimately resists full explanation or even recollection:

> I lived for more than six months there, at Metropolitan State Hospital in Waltham, Massachusetts ... [D]uring the latter part of my stay my brain was zapped twenty-one times ... What I have left are mostly random images, some in remarkable detail and clarity, but few embedded in any logically continuous context. (1986, 125)

In this essay, Mairs takes her narrative back into her childhood and adolescence in an attempt to provide such a context; however, she realizes that a portion of her life has been lost and "barred" from her, simply erased between those "zaps." She uses a broken necklace to symbolize this loss, a "string of black clay Mexican beads" of hers that "snapped suddenly" in class once, scattering beads everywhere. Most were retrieved by her students and strung back together by one of her children, but "in a new pattern necessitated by the missing pieces, into a shorter necklace." Some of the beads, she realizes, "are gone for good" (125–26).

Like Kaysen's hospital stay, Mairs' is supposed to be short (ten days) and ends up much longer; and, like Kaysen, Mairs suspects her psychiatrist of lying or at least of incompetence: "He can't have been many years older than I was, still in training as a psychiatrist ... and I think *he* panicked. He knew that he couldn't cope with me ... so he turned me over to the keepers of madwomen where whatever trouble I might cause could be closely contained" (126). One way to deflate psychiatrists as authority figures is to apply one's own diagnosis to them; here, Mairs reads her own anxiety and panic attacks into the young doctor's behaviour. The session with the admitting psychiatrist is also presented as farce as the doctor, newly arrived from India, and the inarticulate, weeping patient struggle to communicate. Once settled in, Mairs is assigned to a woman psychiatrist whom she eventually comes to respect, but she also recounts run-ins with dangerous incompetents, like the doctor who, under the impression she is a schizophrenic, almost puts her on a course of insulin-shock therapy.

Like Kaysen, then, Mairs provides a satirical critique of the psychiatric establishment. She conveys an unforgiving view of a daily hospital routine centred on meds ("three tablets—one yellow, one blue, one white—and a little translucent green football" four times a day [127]) and characterized by constant mystification and lack of privacy: "No one ever explained any aspect of my condition to me," she notes (135). While Mairs does not try to get around authority in the supportive company of noisy and colourful women friends, as Kaysen does, she has her own ways of evading it, especially by means of a not-so-discreet sexual intrigue with a male patient.

And yet, despite all the tricks and guerrilla moves required to survive in the culture of the mental hospital without going "nuts," Mairs finds her prison to be a refuge, just as Kaysen does—a refuge from those who are patiently waiting for her at home, an "intelligent, loving" husband and a "healthy and charming daughter" (127). These would seem to be the terms of a successful woman's life, at least in the norms of the time. Yet Mairs rejects this life, even while she is sure she must be mad for doing so, just as Kaysen rejects college, the expected narrative of a daughter of well-off academics. In her journals from the time, Mairs complains of having feminine norms "cramm[ed] ... down [her] throat" (137). Like Bartleby the Scrivener in Melville's story of the same name, Mairs "would prefer not to." She refuses to eat, thereby enacting her resistance to the feminine norms she feels are being force-fed to her: "No wonder my throat tightened and my stomach heaved in the face of food" (137). This is the crux of her status as "a sort of cultural prisoner" (134) at Met State: she doesn't want to do what a woman "must" do, even to the point of attempting suicide to avoid going back to a life she deems herself mad not to want. However, she is also terrified of hitting bottom, finally consenting to ECT after her doctor "scare[s] the wits out of her" by having her spend a week on the chronic ward in all its abjection: "Everywhere grime and the sour stench of sweat and urine" (139). Like Kaysen, Mairs is finally declared recovered when she is ready to resume her expected feminine vocation: mothering her child and being a faithful wife to her husband.

For Mairs, looking back, the diagnosis of depression was a confirmation not only of her own personal "terms of ... existence: sickness, isolation, timidity, desire for death ... [lying] black as bars" across her life (151), but also of her cultural incarceration as a woman, a "dis-ease" (150) that is rarely recognized by a patriarchal medical establishment. Her hospital narrative, like Kaysen's, is a witness to the lack of fit between women sufferers and the patriarchal regime that would cure them. It is all the more effective for being embedded in a very personal memoir undertaken as a means of coming to terms with a life of chronic depression.

Mairs, like Kaysen, presents narrative as both a form of personal therapy (stringing the beads, the life, back together) and a witnessing to the "dis-ease," both personal and political, of mental illness. While Kaysen writes so that she may never go back behind bars, Mairs writes in order to make sense of a life that she knows will *always* be behind bars, and to create the sympathetic reader who will ensure a healing testimony (Laub 1995). Indeed, she addresses this ideal reader in her final words: "This place is real. I can live here. Come by, and I'll make you a cup of almond tea" (154). In this closing metaphor of imprisonment, which frames the essay as much as the image of the broken and restrung necklace does, Mairs situates herself in another prison—but one she has remade to fit herself (rather as Kaysen annotates and personalizes her own official diagnosis). This "prison" is the study of the melancholy writer: it has bars on its window but also a desk, pen, and lined paper at its centre, paper already "inscribed with [her] round black hand" (154).

For Kaysen and Mairs, the act of recounting their term in a psychiatric hospital is an attempt to integrate this episode into the larger story of a life, to find meaning in this traumatic interruption in the context of a life's continuities or ongoing "terms of existence" (Mairs 1986, 151)—including, for both Kaysen and Mairs, the vocation of writing. Their strategies of satire and mythmaking are used to the end of bearing witness to the traumatizing and shaming effects of psychiatric regimes. Like any "narrative organization of pain" (Gilmore 2001, 22), however, their narratives are fraught with ambivalence. Ultimately, traumatic interruption can never be entirely recounted or accounted for. In each case the hospital episode represents, to some extent, the logical outcome of a distress intensifying to crisis—for these women authors, a distress stemming as much from their inability to easily assume conventional feminine roles as from neurobiological factors. However, the episode also represents a traumatic break exceeding the narrative closure of crisis and recovery, descent and re-ascent. The lost time of hospitalization, like that of chronic depression itself, in the end exceeds all telling.

Note

1 Besides Styron's *Darkness Visible*, other recent depression memoirs by male authors include the following: John Bentley Mays' *In the Jaws of the Black Dogs* (Toronto: Penguin, 1995); Jeffery Smith's *Where the Roots Reach for Water* (New York: North Point Press, 1999); and Andrew Solomon's *The Noonday Demon* (New York: Scribner, 2001). Recent depression memoirs by female authors include Martha Manning's *Undercurrents* (San Francisco: HarperCollins, 1994); Tracy Thompson's *The Beast* (New York: Plume Books, 1995); Kay Redfield Jamison's *An Unquiet Mind* (New York: Vintage Books, 1995); Lauren Slater's *Prozac Diary* (New York: Penguin, 1998); and Meri Danquah's *Willow Weep for Me* (New York: Ballantine, 1998).

LISA DIEDRICH

BETWEEN TWO DEATHS
AIDS, Trauma, and Temporality in the Work of Paul Monette

In this essay, I explore Paul Monette's attempts in and through various forms of writing to bear witness to the early years of the AIDS crisis in the United States.[1] In his work, including *Borrowed Time*, an AIDS memoir, and *Love Alone*, a collection of elegies for his lover Roger Horwitz, who died of AIDS on October 22, 1986, Monette offers an account of the heroic struggles in the early days of the epidemic, not only against the virus, but also against the general sense that death was the inevitable outcome of having AIDS. The heroes of Monette's account are the "men of '85," the countless gay men afflicted in the first years of the plague in the U.S. The "men of '85" include Roger, who, Monette shows us, faced his illness bravely and with *sōphrosynē*, a classical Greek idea that defines virtue as "an inner harmony of the soul, a reasonableness which reveals itself in every action and attitude" (1988b, 65). If Roger is the epitome of restraint and reasonableness in virtually every situation, Monette is the opposite: a whirlwind of nervous, unfocused energy that only finds its focus in caring for Roger, and after his death, in writing about him. But, as Monette recognizes in the first weeks after Roger's diagnosis, "[w]hatever happened to Roger happened to me" (65), and this recognition of *shared experience in the present but also in the future* both fuels and haunts Monette's account. Although Monette is telling of the death of Roger and the deaths of countless others in the present, he is also in many ways describing his own death in the future. The borrowed time of his title refers both to the desperate attempts to extend Roger's life in the face of almost certain death, and Monette's own HIV+ status at the time of his writing, which places him in some sense ahead of time, or outside of time, awaiting death.

His own death will come both too late—Roger will die first, leaving Monette as survivor and witness—and too soon, as Monette will die in 1995 just as protease inhibitors come onto the AIDS treatment scene. Monette's writing is a symptom of this death that is both too soon and too late.

I also am interested in Monette's position as witness in relation to what I call *the time of AIDS*, which refers on the one hand to the historical time of the emergence of the AIDS epidemic, and on the other hand to a particular temporality that the diagnosis of HIV/AIDS brings into being. In my examination, I will introduce briefly Freud's theory of latency and trauma as well as Lacan's theory of being between two deaths in order to look at the temporal structure of HIV/AIDS as described in Monette's writing, before considering Monette's politicization as he quests for a magic bullet to save Roger, himself, and others. The political, for Monette and other AIDS activists, becomes a means to a future time, but whether that future time is a time after AIDS is a question I consider in the conclusion to this essay. Are we still in the time of AIDS? Can we begin to imagine a time after AIDS, and how does such imagining transform the time of AIDS and those still in it?

Past and Future Repetitions

In *Moses and Monotheism*, Freud says that latency is a feature of not only infectious disease but of trauma as well. In other words, there is a gap between the traumatic event and the appearance of symptoms (1939, 84). To take Freud's analogy full circle, HIV/AIDS is an infectious disease that also has the temporal structure of a trauma. While latency is a characteristic of all infectious diseases, HIV/AIDS has added a peculiar twist to the phenomenon of latency, partly because latency in HIV/AIDS is such an unknown quantity; there is no standard amount of time from the point that one becomes infected with the HIV virus to the point that one becomes ill. As Monette writes on the first page of *Borrowed Time*, "No one has solved the puzzle of its timing" (1988b, 1). In *AIDS and Its Metaphors*, Susan Sontag also seeks to understand AIDS in temporal terms, noting that "with the most up-to-date biomedical testing, it is possible to create a new class of lifetime pariahs, the future ill" (1989, 33–34).

As I hope to show in the conclusion to this essay, the experience of AIDS, in some places at least, is now changing with the advent of new treatment options. Nonetheless, I want to focus here briefly on the traumatic structure of AIDS, which has had individual as well as social effects. "Has anything ever been quite like this?" Monette wonders. "Bad enough to be stricken in the middle of life, but then to fear your best and dearest will suffer exactly the same. Cancer and the heart don't sicken a man two ways like that" (1988b, 83). Furthermore, prior to becoming sick, the person who is HIV+ often experiences—as friend, lover, and/or caretaker—the illness and death that awaits him or her. "Added to the caretaking and loss of others," Douglas Crimp notes, "is often the need to monitor and make treatment decisions about our own HIV illness, or face anxiety about our own health status" (1990, 241; see also Kayal 1993, 9).

In his seminar on ethics in general, and with regards to his reading of the figure and story of Antigone in particular, Lacan speaks of the ethical possibility of being *between two deaths*.[2] Antigone opposes the laws of the city—which are, of course, also the laws of her uncle, Creon—when she attempts to bury her brother, Polyneices, who has died opposing Creon. By her action, Antigone exiles herself from the law—the law of the father, the symbolic order—and, as a result and as punishment, she is buried alive in a tomb. Her transgression places her in the impossible position that is, according to Lacan, the position of being *between two deaths*. In an explication of Lacan's concept of two deaths, Zizek writes that "Lacan conceives this difference between two deaths as the difference between real (biological) death and its symbolization ... in Antigone's case, her symbolic death, her exclusion from the symbolic community of the city, precedes her actual death and imbues her character with sublime beauty" (1989, 135). Antigone is neither of the living nor of the dead; she is in between, and it is this inbetweenness that language cannot describe. Her entombment signifies an experience that is liminal to both the living and the dead. It is this inbetweenness that is outside of symbolization, beyond symbolization: indeed, is the death of symbolization. In all of his writing on AIDS, Monette attempts to articulate this inbetweenness, this gap between a first, witnessed death and a second, absolute death. For him, the first death is the death of an other, but because Monette, in a sense, will die the "very same" death, it is both the death of the other and the death of the self. There is, in other words, an echo of Monette's own future death that reverberates beyond Roger's death and throughout Monette's writing.

In the poem "Current Status 1/22/87," Monette explores the ways in which the present is a repetition of not only the past (1/22/87 is three months to the date after Roger's death) but also a rehearsal of the future. Monette's poem describes his current *physical* status as of 1/22/87, including his latest T-cell count and the endless drug regimen to maintain that count. Monette's doctors declare him *physically* fine, healthy, and asymptomatic; but *metaphysically* he is a wreck, just a symptom of Roger's death and, in many ways, dead himself. The crisis of Roger's death is the crisis of Monette's survival of Roger's death *and* the crisis of a future repetition: "my condition is just a prefix," according to Monette (1988a, 34).[3] For him, the set of printouts that declare him "clinically healthy" in fact "sound like a qualification," and he wonders, "is this how/ being a hero starts or just dying?" (36). Lawrence Langer's rendering of the Holocaust survivor as a "diminished self" captures best, it seems to me, Monette's "current status." "Rejecting nihilism *and* heroism," Langer writes, "the diminished self lapses into a bifocal vision, as its past invades its present and casts a long, pervasive shadow over its future, obscuring traditional vocabulary and summoning us to invent a still more complex version of memory and self" (1991, 172).

Monette reveals over and over—and such repetition is inherent to the trauma as an essentially missed encounter with the real, according to Lacan—that the trauma of Roger's death is also always the trauma of his own survival, and the ethical imperative that is inherent to that survival. In the poem "Readiness," Monette considers suicide—"a cocked .32 will do in a pinch"—but admits "I'm not half ready to leave us here without us all told" (1988a, 14). The odd locution of this sentence—"I'm not half ready to leave us here without us all told"—points to a death that is missed, yet still somehow must be told. In the poem "The Very Same," as well as in *Borrowed Time*, Monette describes a moment just before Roger's death in which Roger, mostly blind, "sees" Monette come into his hospital room, and says, "*But we're the same person when did that happen*" (1988a, 20; emphasis in original). Roger's uncanny statement "unknowingly and knowing full well" acknowledges the "Other within the Same, death in life,"[4] and interpellates Monette into writing about Roger's death as always being his own as well: "I had a self myself once but he died," Monette declares in the poem "Manifesto" (1988a, 41). This doubling—this death in life—is apparent as well in the poem "Half Life,"[5] in which Monette grieves:

> I get up and half of me doesn't
> work I drag me like a broken wing my good
> eye sees flesh and green the dead eye an X-
> ray gaping at skeletons ... (1988a, 16)

When Monette is told after Roger's death that it is *"time to turn the page"*—to move past Roger's death—he retorts "BUT THIS IS MY PAGE IT CANNOT BE TURNED" (1988a, 20; emphasis in original). The pages and pages of Monette's work can be distilled into a single page that cannot be turned—one that is outside the linear temporality implied in the act of turning pages—and must be filled edge to edge with Roger and Paul's "growing interchangeability," until they are both "all told."

THE FUTURE TIME OF THE POLITICAL

As feminist philosopher Linda Singer has noted, the AIDS epidemic in the U.S. inspired "the politicization of patienthood" (1993, 105), but the politicized patient was not spawned, fully-formed, at the moment of ACT UP's first zap; rather, as we see in *Borrowed Time*, the politicized patient was emerging even in the early 1980s, as PWAs (People With AIDS) and their loved ones realized that they weren't going to get the treatment they needed unless they sought it.[6] "*Living with AIDS* is a rallying cry now," Monette tells us, "and the men of '85 were the first division to hum a few bars" (1988b, 142; emphasis in original). What Lawrence Langer has called "the grammar of heroism and martyrdom" pervades Monette's work, as he describes the pursuit of new knowledge, better drugs, and just a bit more time.

We see this grammar most strikingly when Monette describes his own ceaseless pursuit of the "magic bullet," the elixir that will restore Roger's (and, of course, Monette's own) health. In Arthur W. Frank's formulation, then, *Borrowed Time* is ultimately a quest story (1995, 120). Monette tells of trips across the border to Mexico for ribavirin, one of the earliest anti-virals. The first of these trips for Monette is tinged with romance; he is an outlaw—"part of the nether world of the sick"—defying the U.S. government's Food and Drug Administration as well as its border patrols (1988b, 175). Partly through luck and partly through Monette's relentless charging ahead through the "AIDS underground," Roger is one of the first patients to get AZT. The drug has immediate positive effects, and Roger becomes, according to one of his nurses, "the miracle man" and the "AZT posterboy." In the poem "Black xmas," Monette reveals the boon AZT brings—nothing less than time itself:

> ... and '85 was yours Rog still
> still time home after 2 months in and the gift
> not anywhere near the tree but the newest drug
> rarer than myrrh drunk out of I.V. bottles
> 6 times a day because they hadn't got a
> pill yet the elixir that would give us 10
> months more ... (1988a, 18)

If AZT isn't, in fact, the magic bullet, it does, nonetheless, bring Roger back from the brink one final time.

Although Monette portrays his quest for the magic bullet as an active—heroic, even—response to AIDS, the heroism of such action, paradoxically, isn't about Monette's ability to take control of the situation in any real sense, to *choose* to do something that will save Roger and himself as well. Such action isn't about a real choice—heroic or otherwise—but is rather about acting in a moment where every action seems hopeless, where uncertainty is the only certainty. Because treatment options were so few and far between in the first years of the AIDS epidemic, and because many early options quickly panned out as worthless at best and deadly at worst, what I am describing here is similar to what Lawrence Langer has called a "choiceless choice." In an essay comparing the plague literature of Daniel Defoe, Albert Camus, Randy Shilts, Monette, and others, Laurel Brodsley notes that, "Shilts in *And the Band Played On* and Monette in *Borrowed Time* deal at length with the frustration, confusion, and impossibility of making prudent choices while the identity, attributes, transmission, and prognosis of HIV infection are not fully known" (1992, 21). According to Monette, throughout Roger's illness, the "profile of AIDS continued to be mostly a matter of shadows"; even that which garnered hope, in other words, was impossible to hold on to and see clearly. Hope itself is victim to the scourge of AIDS, nothing more than the "posture of last resort," and, for Monette, "as cruel as anything else [Pandora] released to the four winds" (1994, 254–55). Despite the "grammar of heroism and martyrdom" in Monette's writing, there is also, then, below the resilient surface, a grammar—or an un-grammar, as Blanchot might say—of chaos and disintegration as in the line from "Current Status 1/22/87": "is this how/ being a hero starts or just dying?" (1988a, 36).[7] In *Borrowed Time*, Monette tells us that he has learned that fear is "equal parts rage and despair," and that he is "up and down at the same time" (1988b, 48). The ambivalence between heroism and disintegration—being "up and down at the same time"—reveals again the temporality of AIDS and the impossible position of being between two deaths.

When Plagues End?

Arriving in 1995, protease inhibitors have changed the face of AIDS, in some cases quite literally: the faces of PWAs have themselves been transformed. AIDS is a disease that ravages the face as well as the body; the severe weight loss that is characteristic of AIDS creates a skeletal effect in which the face is reduced to bone and eyes. The skin becomes gray and waxy and loses its elasticity; PWAs age decades in a matter of months. For many PWAs, protease inhibitors have done nothing short of bringing them back from the dead in both appearance and actuality. In his essay "When Plagues End," Andrew Sullivan marvels at this phenomenon: "People I had seen hobbling along, their cheekbones poking out of their skin, were suddenly restored into some strange spectacle of health, gazing around as amazed as I was to see them alive" (1996, 60). Are protease inhibitors, then, the magic bullet that Monette and other PWAs and AIDS activists fought so hard for? All that is clear at this point is that it is still too soon to tell; even now, as Monette wrote regarding AIDS in 1988, "no one has solved the puzzle of its timing." Nonetheless, the signs of hopefulness are difficult to ignore; in many patients the HIV virus has dropped to undetectable levels in the blood. Yet, if the protease inhibitors are a magic bullet, they are an ambiguous sort of magic bullet. The phrase "drug cocktail," which has come into common currency to describe them, obscures the nature of a course of treatment that literally disciplines one's everyday life (see Sontag and Richardson 1997, 18).[8] There is also concern that if patients do not follow the course precisely, a more virulent strain of the virus will be unleashed; in other words, lurking within this magic bullet's gift of life after death is the potential that this gift of life is nothing more than a gift of death.[9]

I want to conclude, however, not only with the recent developments that have inspired many to speculate on the "end of AIDS," but also by considering briefly what the "end of AIDS" might mean for those who will survive. This brings us back, once again, to the encounter with death and the crisis of surviving the death of an other *and* one's own death. Can those who are HIV+ and who have witnessed the death of loved ones from AIDS ever say that they have seen the "end of AIDS"? Andrew Sullivan sums up the "difference between the end of AIDS and the end of many other plagues," explaining that, "for the first time in history, a large proportion of the survivors will not simply be those who escaped infection, or were immune to the virus, but those who contracted the illness, contemplated their own deaths *and still survived*" (1996, 58; emphasis in original). The promise of a future after AIDS transforms the present as well as the past, but to speak of a time after AIDS does not mean it is a time continuous with the time before AIDS; the gap between before and after cannot be filled by a future promise. Can a person return from the liminality of being between two deaths? The ontological rupture that is AIDS will not be bridged by a possible or even an actual cure. Like Monette, Sullivan knows that the "moment of mortality" he has experienced cannot be erased. "And not simply because I cannot dare hope that one day the virus might be wiped completely from my system," Sullivan asserts, "but because some experiences can never be erased" (1996, 76–77). The HIV virus may eventually be eradicated, one can certainly hope for that; but it will nevertheless leave a trace, a shadow of a rupture unassimilated not only within individual bodies but within the social body as well. We will all remain inside the time of AIDS as long as traces of this deadly virus remain in some of us.

Notes

1. For further discussion of what I call Monette's "practices of witnessing" to the AIDS crisis, please see Diedrich (2004).
2. In chapter 5 of *Treatments*, I discuss this figure in relation both to AIDS and to Alzheimer's disease (Diedrich forthcoming).
3. In a dialogue with Cathy Caruth and Thomas Keenan, AIDS activist and filmmaker Gregg Bordowitz remarks: "And when I see somebody getting sick, I don't say, 'That *could* be me,' I say, 'That *will* be me.' So it's very painful and sometimes intolerable" (1995, 267; emphasis in original).
4. The citations are from Maurice Blanchot's *The Writing of the Disaster*. In a fragment about the myth of Narcissus, Blanchot asserts that when Narcissus looks into the water and sees a face reflected there, he does not see a mirror image of himself, but rather the "Other within the Same, death in life," and "the invisible in the visible" (1995, 134).
5. The trope of the "half life" also returns in *Becoming a Man* (1992), which is subtitled "Half a Life Story," and which portrays the trauma of the closet as another death in life.
6. In *Globalizing AIDS*, Cindy Patton challenges the commonly held belief that AIDS activism began in 1987 with the formation of ACT UP. Patton contends that, "both leftist academics and the media made a fetish of ACT UP," and that "activism *began* when the first living person was acknowledged to have an unnamed but recognizable syndrome and had to cope with a hostile medical system" (2002, 4).
7. For more about chaos narratives, see Frank 1995, 171.
8. The cocktail trope implies that this regimen is as pleasurable as a martini before dinner, denying the fact that taking the combination of drugs has many side effects and entails a strictly delineated timetable that is difficult to follow over a short period of time, let alone for the rest of one's life.
9. Sontag and Richardson point out, moreover, that in some cases doctors are refusing the new drugs to patients who have proven to be undisciplined in the past. Intravenous drug users are most frequently presumed to be unreliable patients and, therefore, undeserving of this rigorous regime of treatment. Withholding drugs from patients is an ethical issue that has a long and rather sordid history (1997, 1 and 18).

BARBARA HAVERCROFT

Paper Thin
Agency and Anorexia in Geneviève Brisac's Petite

Feminist theoreticians of anorexia nervosa have observed that both the behaviour of women afflicted with this illness and the discourse used by anorectics to recount their experiences with the disease bespeak a number of paradoxes and binary oppositions endemic to Western culture. Perhaps the most basic of these oppositions is that between the body and the mind, where the body is considered as the animal element, the "prison" to be transcended in order for the subject to have full access to the life of the mind, to purity, to freedom. As Leslie Heywood (1996, 19–28) has demonstrated in her discussion of selected philosophical writings dealing with mind/body opposition, this division is a fundamentally gendered one, whereby woman is associated with the body, and the latter is conceived as a corpulent negativity hindering her access to spiritual and intellectual fulfilment. In cases of anorexia, this mind/body opposition engenders several related dichotomies, many of which bear heavy moral connotations: slimness versus obesity, good versus evil, reduction versus expansion, self-control versus lack of self-discipline, and so on. Indeed, as Susan Bordo claims, "the slender, fit body [is itself] a symbol of the 'virile' mastery over bodily desires that are continually experienced [in anorexia] as threatening to the self" (1993, 15). The constant tension between the terms of these various warring oppositions takes the form of a quotidian battle in the life of the anorectic woman, inscribing itself both on her body and in the rhetoric of her autobiographical narrative, when such a testimony to the illness exists.

The writing of anorexia, the discursive construction of its rhetoric, and the representation of its paradoxical oppositional logic are poignantly illustrated in a moving autofictional text by the contemporary French writer Geneviève Brisac, aptly entitled *Petite* (*Small*).[1] In this text the author recounts, some thirty years after the fact, the painful details of her battle with anorexia during several years of her youth.[2] Disturbed by a distant relationship with both of her parents and consumed by a voracious hunger to be loved, the young Geneviève decides to control her destiny by assuming control of her own body, through simply refusing food. However, the disease gradually gains the upper hand and the young girl, dangerously thin, is sent to a psychiatric clinic and, subsequently, to several foster homes, before returning to her parents' home and discovering love and happiness in her relationship with her grandfather. Skillfully constructed, the text oscillates between the uses of the pronoun *I*, the referent of which is both the adolescent and the adult narrator, depending on the context, and the pronoun *she*, which refers to the young protagonist.[3] A similar oscillation characterizes the use of proper names in the text, as the nickname "Nouk" denotes the young girl of the past, whereas the first name "Geneviève" refers both to the anorectic adolescent and to the author herself, sealing the text's autobiographical pact.[4]

The effects of her battle with anorexia, already inscribed on the body at the time of the narrated past events, find their textual expression in the narrator's retrospective autobiographical account, which features a lean syntax and a "non-fat," sometimes childlike, vocabulary, as well as a good number of rhetorical figures. At times, the reader has the impression that the style of the text and the narrator's young body are aiming for a similar emaciation. Despite this double movement towards physical and textual reduction, the writing of the disease assumes ample proportions in terms of its importance for the narrator's subjectivity. Life writing here is not only a matter of writing *about* one's life, testifying to the importance of past events, but also of writing *for* one's life. The narration of her former physical and emotional suffering allows Brisac to understand and examine it, while at the same time providing her with the means of retracing her steps along the difficult road travelled to attain agency in her life and become a subject of language. In addition, Brisac's narrative becomes a testimony, exposing the hidden and shameful aspects of this illness from which thousands of young girls and young women suffer in contemporary Western society.[5] Its symptoms, its effects, and its underlying logic are revealed by the many figures of speech that compose the carefully constructed rhetoric of Brisac's text. In *Petite*, the rhetoric of anorexia becomes a rhetoric of agency, as the aesthetic, ethical, and political dimensions of the text are closely entwined. Re-enacting the anorectic body through the recounting of its becoming, and by transcribing and inscribing the rhetoric and logic of the disease, Brisac combines the text's political dimension with a performative, therapeutic force, where writing itself participates in the emotional and psychological healing of the narrator, years after the physiological recovery has occurred.

The deployment of discursive agency in Brisac's text is, however, anything but simple and straightforward. The very act of starving oneself could well be considered a form of agency, for the anorectic allows us to read, on her lean body, a protest against patriarchal values that weigh heavily upon her: "In anorexia women transform the social meanings and practices through which the feminine body is constructed" (Macsween 1993, 8). The refusal of food, from this perspective, can be seen as an attempt at self-affirmation through the body become text, an unremitting effort to take control of one's life, or at least to voice one's discontent. In a paradoxical logic of reduction and expansion, reducing one's weight can itself express the attempt to lend weight to one's convictions, to inscribe, by subtraction, revolt on the body. As Gillian Brown (1991, 191) explains, this paradoxical agency of anorexia highlights the difficult relationship between the subject and her own subjection. In *Petite*, this form of agency, this protest uttered by the thin body through acts of physical deprivation, is expressed by the representation and description of past events that took place at the time of the illness. Although these actions succeed in writing resistance on Nouk's anorectic body, they should not be judged in a positive light alone. To deprive oneself of food is also to literally doom oneself to erasure; it is, as many studies of anorexia have indicated, a negative path that can at times prove fatal. The complex agency represented by the actions of the anorectic girl is ultimately destructive and, for that reason, Leslie Heywood labels it "the agency of negation" (1996, 147). The paradox is that actions demonstrating the subject's control over the body eventually lead to its destruction: "[the agency of negation] is a position where, deprived of all alternatives, a woman says: 'I negate what you make me (a powerless woman). I will show you I have power and agency by taking control of my body, the existence you say I don't own, by destroying it'" (Heywood 1996, 147). In the same vein, Gillian Brown insists on the self-destructive nature of anorexia, on its negative "accounting" practices. If a form of agency emerges from or is depicted through anorectic behaviour, it is an agency quite distanced "from conventional notions of consciousness and freedom" (Brown 1991, 191).

In her explicit portrayal of her own anorectic behaviour, including self-induced vomiting behind closed doors, Brisac thoroughly investigates the functioning of this agency of negation; the young heroine appropriates a self-destructive power that, far from freeing her as she imagines, puts her very life in danger. This type of agency dominates the representation of past events until the book's final chapter, which marks the beginning of the girl's recovery, made possible by the love of her grandfather. In *Petite*, the agency of negation is situated at the narrative level of what is recounted, of events long past, and not at the moment of telling the story.

Brisac's text also inscribes what I shall term a positive agency, which consists of her autobiographical act: the narrating, in the present, of the painful events of the past. This is continually emphasized by the use of comments temporally situated at the moment of narration, referring to the text that the narrator is in the process of writing, as well as to her fears regarding this undertaking, as the following passage illustrates: "This is a narrative, a quarter of a century has gone by. That seems immense to me ... This is a narrative, the interrupted narrative of what I call the time when I was crazy ... I would have wanted it to be amusing. That it would at least entertain people. I am not at all certain that people will find this amusing" (Brisac 1994, 63).[6] This passage precedes the darkest section of the text, where the author charts her descent into the illness, the period during which the disease governs her body, even her life. Seen retrospectively from this temporal distance, the unspeakable horror of the suffering can finally be told, at times indirectly, as in the ironic utterance cited above ("I am not certain that people will find this amusing"), when the narrator clearly wishes to express the contrary. *Petite* thus contains a temporal and enunciative division corresponding to the two different types of agency it inscribes, whereby the positive agency of the retrospective autobiographical act depends upon and is constructed from the agency of negation; that is, the self-destructive actions of the young anorectic girl. Consequently, it is by the act of recounting the dysfunctional story of anorexia, paradoxically, that recovery and witnessing can come about.

A number of textual features convey the shift from the rhetoric of anorexia to a rhetoric of agency. What catches the reader's initial attention is the brief but appropriate title, *Petite*, which provides few precise details concerning the text but captures its essential message. In this sense, the title functions as a euphemism, a figure which presents something in a more favourable light. Is it not more agreeable, more pleasing, easier to "digest," to simply say "petite" (which is often a term of endearment), rather than "the starving girl," or "the autobiography of an anorectic"? This title, accompanied by the drawing of a slim and sweet young girl on the cover, conceals the horrific aspects of the disease while clearly revealing the subject's gender, an important factor in this predominantly female disease. In addition, this concise title aptly depicts the state of the extremely skinny body described in the text, evoking the relationship between the body and writing, the inscription of anorexia on the body, and the body itself, which has been converted into text through the narrative. One could also read the condensed title as a synecdoche (a part for the whole), as it summarizes a long struggle that leaves the young Nouk "petite" in size, just like the brief text in which the story of the illness is told. The title already prefigures the text's pared down, "non-fat" style, as a minimum of words communicates a maximum of misery.

The skeletal style of the narrative is characterized by the frequent use of simple sentences, constructions well suited to convey the state of mind of a twelve-year-old girl. Or perhaps they also communicate a hesitation on her part to tell all, a fear of facing the horrors of the past or of failing to find the appropriate words to translate the body into discourse, as the following passage would lead one to believe: "I am groping my way along the path of those years; they are my little dark years ... While writing these lines, almost thirty years later, I am afraid, I am writing *parsimoniously*, with excessive prudence. I am doing this because it seems necessary for me" (Brisac 1994, 29–30; my emphasis). Brisac resorts to the use of many short sentences, in which the basic "subject/verb/complement" structure dominates, sentences that are deprived of wordy padding and reduced to the bare bones. This "slim" style is reinforced by the use of certain rhetorical figures, such as ellipsis and synecdoche, of which one example merits particular attention.

A single body part comes, significantly, to represent the (non) devouring self: the mouth, that part of the body through which ingestion occurs. It is through the mouth that one nourishes oneself, that bodily expansion or contraction occurs as a result of the food consumed; the mouth is also a borderline figure, an organ dividing the inside from the outside of the body.[7] This synecdoche of the mouth appears at several points in Brisac's text: "Nouk vomits everything, rivers [of vomit] flow together. Fasting is becoming slavery ... She is a spirit that walks, she is an immense mouth, she is nothing more than a mouth" (1994, 70). The mouth, a substitute in this passage for her entire body, for her entire being, acts as a double signifier, indicating both the thinness of the anorectic subject—there is nothing left of her but her mouth, since her body is so reduced—and, because of its enormous size, its importance as a literal and symbolic orifice, as well as the extent of Nouk's obsession with eating. Symbolically, she is nothing more than a mouth, since all of the other aspects of her life have been abandoned. A paradoxical image that unites the incompatible opposition of excessive size ("the immense mouth") and extreme slenderness (Nouk's entire person reduced to her mouth alone), the gaping mouth/hole also has eminently feminine connotations. As Leslie Heywood has shown in her study of anorectic logic in the works of Jean Rhys, femininity represents a radical openness in relation to the dominant cultural logic: "It is this radical openness, femininity, nothingness, that the anorexic tries to close down when she seals her mouth, refusing to let anything in" (1996, 161). In the same vein, Morag Macsween claims that "in the experience of anorexia, feminine bodily openness is centered on the mouth" (1993, 249).

Not surprisingly, as the illness progresses, Nouk closes her mouth ever more tightly, allowing increasingly small amounts of food to cross this threshold. In an effort to control and punish any infractions of her strict non-eating rule, Nouk seals her mouth: "Every day, my mouth is smaller, and my teeth more tightly clenched together. They try to force things into my mouth ... and I spit them out" (Brisac 1994, 51). The image of the sealed mouth heralds not simply a physiologically advanced stage of the illness—the concrete refusal to eat—but also Nouk's complete separation from others, a total lack of meaningful contact and relationships with other people.

Rarely engaged in eating or meaningful verbal exchange, Nouk does, however, consume words. The substitution of intellectual nourishment for ordinary food is demonstrated by Nouk's constant preference for reading over eating. This preference highlights the separation between mind and body which underlies both anorectic logic and rhetoric, operating in a manner akin to the logic of supplementarity as outlined by Jacques Derrida (1976, 144–52).[8] If, in Nouk's case, reading as a form of nourishment is initially a supplement to eating, an addition or a surplus, it increasingly comes to replace the latter: "it intervenes or insinuates itself *in-the-place-of*; if it fills, it is as if one fills a void" (Derrida 1976, 145). Necessary in the sense that it fills an emotional void and fulfills the desire to expand the life of the mind at the expense of the body, this intellectual food participates in the constant tension between the warring oppositions (mind/body, masculine/feminine, expansion/reduction, inside/outside) that define the disease and its discourse. Indeed, aiming for purity, perfection, and purification, Nouk can only swallow and digest books: "I know the essential parts of the history book by heart, I gorge on things learned by heart. This is part of [my quest for] perfection, like pedalling my bike until I am utterly exhausted" (Brisac 1994, 28). Numerous intertextual references are mentioned in the context of this intellectual nourishment, where words take the place of foodstuffs: "more reading meant less feeding; more words, less flesh. Since reading and writing mime the processes of eating and excreting they provide a kind of methadone for the obsession" (Ellmann 1993, 24). In this manner, reading acts as a kind of intellectual equivalent of the acting of feeding oneself, creating a relationship between mind, cognition, and digestion that transcribes itself on the lexical level. According to Maud Ellmann (1993, 29), one has only to think of expressions such as "to devour a book," "to ruminate an idea," or "a voracious reader" to observe the close link between thought, knowledge, and food. Moreover, it is books and words that provide Nouk with the comfort sought in her solitude, with a much-needed emotional sustenance. Perpetually rereading the final page of Solzhenitsyn's *One Day in the Life of Ivan Denisovich*, a poignant story of despair, Nouk is inspired and consoled by the dénouement, where the hero succeeds in "chasing pain away" (Brisac 1994, 98): "Sometimes books help you more than anything else" (98). It is, then, no accident that Nouk constructs her own means of rescue out of the words uttered by a former anorectic whom she meets: "ten years later, I would remember that sentence: 'I recovered.' I would make my lifebuoy from these very words" (61). Written and spoken words, ingested in the place of food, thus form the substance of another sort of nourishment, that of an intellectual and emotional nature.[9]

Two legendary, heroic figures form a prominent part of Nouk's intellectual nourishment: Geneviève, patron saint of Paris, and Roland, hero of the medieval literary masterpiece, the *Chanson de Roland*. Both names are used as examples (*exempla*) to denote models worthy of imitation, connoting courage, heroism, and a "terrible combat" (Brisac 1994, 11). In Nouk's mind, Roland and Geneviève recall her own battle with anorexia, for it is their thinness that constitutes the element to be emulated, as her description of the two renowned heroes reveals: "Roland doesn't have a gram of fat around his thighs ... She [Saint Geneviève] doesn't have a gram of fat around her hips" (11–12). It is by means of courageous, corporeal combat, indeed a truly heroic battle, that one eliminates surplus fat: this is the lesson Nouk learns from their exploits[10] and is the major factor motivating the adult narrator to include them in her retrospectively constructed account of anorexia. Significantly, Nouk's identification with the famous female saint occurs at a decisive moment in the autobiographical narrative, for it is precisely at this juncture in the text that the narrator reveals her real first name (Geneviève), consequently allowing the reader to make the extratextual link with the author Geneviève Brisac, and sealing the autobiographical pact. The author is able to play with the two identical names, of which one referent—the young anorexic girl—aspires to the noble destiny and the slender body of the other, the saint: "I stand up, all alone on a desert island, flushed with emotion, overwhelmed by this call of destiny. My name is Geneviève, it is my true first name" (12). Even the simple acts of naming and identifying the self, which are also instrumental in establishing the text's status as an autobiographical act, are closely connected to both anorexia itself and to the rhetoric chosen to narrate its role in the heroine's life.

At the time of the illness, during the narrator's adolescence, the body was already a highly signifying text; as Maud Ellmann states, "the starving body is itself a text, the living dossier of its discontents" (Ellmann 1993, 16–17). Brisac's transcription of her own former bodily codes and gestures into words results in the creation of a rhetoric of anorexia that eloquently expresses its underlying logic of irreconcilable oppositions. Brisac fashions her autobiographical text in the image of the anorectic body through a double movement that testifies to a twofold claim to agency. Recounting this painful, personal story by means of a public, autobiographical act is to offer it to others. In this sense, the entire text of *Petite* functions as an *exemplum*,[11] a story that sensitively discloses the paradoxes and pitfalls of anorexia. The claim to agency made in *Petite* does not proceed solely from its testimonial character, however. Narrating her battle with anorexia also gives Brisac the opportunity of re-examining it, and of commenting on her narration; in short, it allows her to transform the meaning of her adolescent experience through writing, an act which may well constitute the final phase of her recovery. As her scriptural strategies give textual body to the disincarnation of anorexia, and as the rhetoric of the disease becomes, through her autobiographical act, a rhetoric of agency, Brisac can finally "close the book" on this difficult chapter of her life.

NOTES

1 Geneviève Brisac is the author of several novels and autofictions (see note 4), including *Les Filles* (1987), *Madame Placard* (1989), *Petite* (1994), *Week-end de chasse à la mère* (1996; winner of the Femina literary prize and translated into English as *Losing Eugenio: A Novel*, 2000), *Voir les jardins de Babylone* (1999), and *Pour qui vous prenez-vous?* (2001). A journalist for the newspaper *Le Monde*, Brisac has also authored numerous books for children.

2 The anorectic subject in *Petite* represents a typical victim of the disease, as she exhibits the three principal characteristics associated with those who suffer from anorexia: she is an adolescent, she inhabits Western society, and she is a member of the middle class (see Macsween 1993, 1).

3 Antoine Jurga and Jean-Christophe Planche note that the first instance of the third-person pronoun occurs at a pivotal moment in the text, immediately following Geneviève's decision to cease eating. According to them, this passage from *I* to *she* marks an effort on the narrator's part to distance herself from the past events she is recounting, as she seems to "hide behind the use of the third person." (1997, 38; my translation).

4 In terms of literary genre, *Petite* corresponds to the major criteria of autofiction, as proposed by French theorists Serge Doubrovsky, Jacques Lecarme, and Philippe Lejeune (1993). On the back cover, Brisac's text bears the generic marker "novel," yet the author, the narrator, and the main protagonist all share the same name(s), a formal feature typical of autobiographical texts, according to Lejeune (1975).

5 The literature on anorexia has itself assumed great proportions. Among the many publications on this subject, see Marlene Boskind-White (2000), Hilde Bruch (1973, 1978), Kim Chernin (1985), Marilyn Lawrence (1984), and Susie Orbach (1986).

6 All translations from the original French text are mine. There is as yet no published English translation.

7 According to Maud Ellmann (1993, 105), the very notion of the subject is based on the regulation of orifices: "it is at these thresholds that the other, in the form of food, is assumed into the body ..." The self is established simultaneously by exclusion and by ingestion: "the ego is established by excluding what is not itself, by devouring whatever it is striving to become" (40).

8 The substitution of books and words for food is not the only one that discursively reflects the unremitting course of Nouk's struggle with anorexia. Whenever possible, Nouk secretly force-feeds her infant sister instead of herself, and with the very foods she desires and denies herself (Brisac 1994, 73).

9 Certain books do not belong to this beneficial category. During Nouk's sojourn at the clinic, intellectual books are forbidden. Instead, Nouk must devour "fattening books" (87), "which do nothing, which question nothing, which anaesthetize you a little" (97). They form part of the controlled and forced weight gain program, curing Nouk temporarily, until her release from the clinic.

10 Geneviève's identity as a saint and as a Christian virgin is most appropriate to this narrative of renunciation. In the Middle Ages, numerous women saints deprived themselves of food in order to control their sexual appetites and to attain a state of purity and piety. For a discussion of *anorexia mirabilis* in female saints of the Middle Ages, see Rudolph Bell (1985), Carolyn Walker Bynum (1987), and Joan Brumberg (1988).

11 If, as Lanham claims (1968, 139, 70), the *exemplum* is an example, a story which teaches a lesson, *Petite* provides an example of behaviour which is *not* to be imitated; it is a warning of the dangers of anorexia. The exposition of this negative counter-example, however, may well have positive effects on the lives of others.

ULRICH TEUCHER

THE INCOMPREHENSIBLE DENSITY OF BEING
Aestheticizing Cancer

In recent years, researchers in literature, health, and the social sciences have turned their attention to narrative and its potentially therapeutic effects. Many scholars propose that writing may help reconstruct meaning and psychological, even physical, health (Sacks 1985; White and Epston 1989; Metzger 1992; Shay 1994; Parry and Doan 1994; Schiwy 1996; Zimmermann and Dickerson 1996; Mattingly 1998; Schmidt 1998). Illness, in particular, is said to be "a call for stories," and the writing of those stories a moral act in educating others (Frank 1995). Cancer patients, too, are being encouraged to write and their narratives now constitute the largest share of the rapidly growing genre of illness narratives. Cancer narratives line the full literary spectrum, from brief testimonials on web sites to self-help books such as Anne Frähm's *Cancer Battle Plan* (1992) and highly crafted works like Audre Lorde's *Cancer Journals* (1980; see also Teucher 2001, 2006). However, the increasing number of such narratives should not obscure the fact that there are millions of cancer patients for whom talking or writing about their experience is very difficult, threatening, and even dangerous. Those who attempt to write such narratives struggle with the difficulties of finding adequate language to give voice to the density of an often overwhelming experience, and, in fact, there may all kinds of limits to narrativity (Chandler, Lalonde, and Teucher 2003); therefore, this essay cautions against indiscriminately encouraging cancer patients to write. Conversely, an examination of Maja Beutler's autobiographical novel *Fuss Fassen* ([Gaining a Foothold] 1980), suggests that the frightening density of life with cancer can be thinned better by writing with the artful instruments of literature and fictionalization. Understanding the art of literary representation as a guide to limiting experiences such as cancer may be of interest to literary scholars and health professionals alike.

There are more than two hundred different kinds of cancer. Each requires a particular course of treatment, and each cancer and treatment will be tolerated differently by individual patients. Some treatments are easily tolerated by the body; others are so toxic that they would be fatal by themselves if not offset, for example, by massive infusions of liquids. Consequently, cancer narratives reveal a wide variety of attitudes, ranging from those of writers who find few difficulties in describing their experience, to those who struggle to give voice to their suffering because they cannot find any adequate language. Additionally, there are periods of life with cancer and its therapy—sometimes extended periods—when patients can be overwhelmed with signs and symptoms, never felt before, that cannot be compared, categorized, and understood, eliciting visceral terrors. The sustained uncertainty of such sensations, the possibility of metastases and/or a relapse, and the threat of an early death can strip away the last vestiges of control over one's life. All of these sensations and emotions may occur at the same time, competing at various levels, overwhelming, threatening, and fragmenting familiar notions of the body and self. It is this density of experience that seems incomprehensible and therefore difficult to relate, and has been identified as traumatic by some (e.g., Stacey 1997).

Because of the current inflationary use of the term "trauma" for any fearful experience, a cautious use of this term seems justified. According to the Holocaust researcher Dominick LaCapra, "trauma brings about a dissociation of affect and representation: one disorientingly feels what one cannot represent; one numbingly represents what one cannot feel" (2001, 42); Cathy Caruth notes that trauma "is not experienced as a mere repression or defense, but as a temporal delay that carries the individual beyond the shock of the first moment" (1995, 9; see also Kirsch, 2001; Bronfen, Erdie, and Weigel 1999). Drawing on Caruth's work, the writer and cancer patient Jackie Stacey notes that recovery from genocide is "of a different proportion and different order" than that from "more private and *everyday traumas*" [my emphasis] such as cancer and its treatment; nevertheless, "some of the patterns may be familiar, if much less severe" (16). Whether life with cancer, or parts of it, qualify as traumatic or not, it is clear that many patients are terrified by their illness and that certain triggers, such as hospital smells, can trigger fearful memories even many years after recovery. During the course of my own work and research in Canadian and German cancer wards and with support groups, I have met many patients at various stages of their life with cancer. Some lay in their beds for weeks, literally shaking with fear, closed to the most gentle efforts by all those around them to draw them out. Others firmly made it clear to me that the time for reflection or writing was not now but, perhaps, after passing the five-year survival mark. Still others, who had left the five-year mark long behind them, explained with great anxiety that they did not want to reopen old wounds by reflecting on or remembering a traumatic experience that they had not been able to deal with then, and continued to feel threatened by. Often consumed by their terrors, many patients fear speaking or writing about their experience. In this, they are not unlike genocide survivors who wait for many years, sometimes decades, after their liberation before they feel safe enough to dare to give voice to their experience (e.g., Wiesel 1960, v; Semprún 1997, 194). For Elie Wiesel and Jorge Semprún, surviving trauma meant *not* to write; accordingly, one of Semprún's books is entitled *Literature or Life* (1997). To be sure, I have also met many patients who agreed to talk and write about their experience, hoping to contribute more information about living with cancer.

For reasons of space, I cannot discuss in this paper whether or not writing about illness is therapeutic, as a kind of "working through" (to use a term by LaCapra 2001, 22). Some cancer writers dispute such claims as too general; Maja Beutler, for example, points out that writing may worsen a crisis if a writer works him- or herself into a state of anxiety (Michel 1984, 50–51). The point that I wish to make here is that the ready availability of cancer narratives, whether published or unpublished, should not be allowed to obscure the fact that many patients choose, for good reasons, not to talk or write about their experiences. In fact, it should not come as a surprise that many cancer patients do not want to write, but that some succeed in doing so, leading us to appreciate the difficulties of such efforts even more.

Cancer is, obviously, an experience that is enormously difficult to put into language: how should the lived experience of suffering, uncertainty, and the fear of dying be expressed? Most autobiographical accounts of cancer adopt the medical chronology of cancer and its treatment for their narrative structure. This predominance of the medical trajectory as plot integrates the patient's narrative into a structural sequence and a larger whole of medical research. As a metaphor, it suggests that states of uncertainty are temporary and changes, hopefully for the better, are to be expected. However, in their portrayal of life with cancer, many of these narratives remain on a linear, descriptive level. For example, Gilda Radner's *It's*

Always Something (1989) contains many episodes where experience cannot be externalized and is left unexpressed. When Radner has a recurrence of her cancer and realizes that she may not "win," a short two-liner tells us that she was so frightened that "during the first four weeks after the recurrence, I spent a lot of time lying on the floor and staring at the ceiling" (231). Understandably, many writers do not want to explore the density of such profound terrors, but instead seek to demonstrate that one can make it "through the tunnel" and that life will continue "on the other side." However, the desire in illness for a conclusive ending, for closure, while quite common in contemporary culture, is rarely realized in cancer narratives. Radner's own book is a tragic testimony to these difficulties.

In contrast, the autobiographical novel *Fuss Fassen* (1980, written in German and unfortunately not translated), by the Swiss writer, dramatist, and cancer patient Maja Beutler, remains open-ended. In it, she manages to sort out for the reader prolonged periods of overwhelming density in her life with cancer, making it one of the very rare cancer narratives that is not only descriptive but uses a variety of artful literary tools to approximate the otherwise incomprehensible cancer experience. By doing so, Beutler contradicts Susan Sontag, to whom it had seemed "unimaginable to aestheticize the disease" (1977, 18).

Many of Beutler's literary writing techniques are consistent with those used in Holocaust accounts. Writers such as Boris Pahor (1995, 10–12) and Jorge Semprún (1997, 200–201) have noted that mere factual representation will not suffice in rendering their experience. This is not because language is not equal to the task; on the contrary, texts such as those by Aharon Appelfeld (*Story of a Life* 2005), Imre Kertész (*Fateless* 1992), Boris Pahor (*Pilgrim among the Shadows* 1995), and Jorge Semprún (e.g., 1982, 1997, 2001a, b) display their writers' confidence through the subversive strength of artfully crafted language. The difficulties, as Semprún notes, lie not with the articulation but with the density of such experience in the camps. In his account, "the only ones who will manage to reach this substance, this transparent density, will be those able to shape their evidence into an artistic object, a space of creation. Or of re-creation. Only the artifice of a masterly narrative will prove capable of conveying some of the truth of such testimony" (1997, 13). Such representation, Semprún adds, requires fictionalization in the service of a historical truth that, otherwise, would be too hard to believe: "How do you tell such an unlikely truth, how do you foster the imagination of the unimaginable, if not by elaborating, by reworking reality, by putting it in perspective? With a bit of artifice, then?" (123–24; see also 32, 45, 262,

284). Here, Semprún points out, from practice, what Dominick LaCapra theorizes in *Writing History, Writing Trauma* (2001): namely, that fictionalization in narratives may involve truth claims "by giving at least a 'plausible feel' for experience and emotion which may be difficult to arrive at through restricted documentary methods" (13–14).

In her discussion of Boris Pahor's *Pilgrim among the Shadows*, Ursula Maerz (2002) identifies a useful poetics of literary devices that might well be applied to other aestheticizations of the Holocaust, or to the cancer novel *Fuss Fassen*. Maerz lists four literary instruments: tremendous attention to detail, extension of narrative time, inclusion of the narrator's reflections, and abundance of lyrical metaphors. As the critic explains, attention to detail subverts the systemic reduction of the individual; extension of time works against the efforts to destroy life and individual time; narrative reflection asserts freedom of movement in a space where movement is confined; and the use of metaphor asserts creative choice, in the face of annihilation (35). These literary instruments are consistent with many of those used in *Fuss Fassen*. There, they are interwoven into a poetic hyperrealism that allows readers to be drawn into the midst of an almost indescribable experience so that they may glimpse at what is otherwise incomprehensible. These tools, artfully used, provide for a literary testimony that can disentangle and approximate the personal experience of illness and trauma much more closely than factual autobiography, and provide deeper insights into the incomprehensible density of being with cancer.

Fuss Fassen tells the story of Beutler's own illness. It is both autobiographical and very literary, transforming her experience into art. The book's cover presents the form of the account as a novel (in German, a *Roman*). As Beutler emphatically insists, the book's first-person narrator is not the author, and while some of the book's characters are real, others are literary constructions. It was important to Beutler for several reasons to put her account into the form of a novel. She has noted in various interviews that she sought to represent the crazed fragmentation of her life with cancer; a "schizophrenia-like state," as she called it (e.g., Michel 49, 51; Beutler personal communication with author, 7 June 2000). To this end, she put fictionalization into the service of experiential truth, seeking creative ways to involve the reader in her experience (52, 56). In addition, Beutler meant to subvert what she saw as common expectations among readers who may take a subconscious pleasure in the victimhood of the writer, especially if substantiated by his or her death—verified on the book cover by the publisher (personal communication, 7 June 2000). In contrast to such reader expectations, Beutler wanted to demonstrate that she had asserted and given creative shape to what had affected her, indicating her professional "intactness."

It is no accident when, early on in *Fuss Fassen,* a young woman (the narrator's alter ego) admonishes the narrator and, by extension, the reader, to "Watch for the details" ("Pass auf die Details auf," 50). In her book, Beutler attempts to put the pieces together anew, in a "play of combinations" that covers a vast area of literary and philosophical allusions. This is a difficult task because life with cancer is broken up into a myriad pieces, and the many details, spread throughout the book, are overwhelming. That, however, is both Beutler's experience and her point: the details are overwhelming, and the reality composed of these details becomes overwhelming, too. It becomes difficult to find one's footing in such a world. *Fuss Fassen* begins with a short excerpt from a lab manual that provides instructions, in chillingly distanced language, about how to conduct an empirical animal experiment. Beutler immediately contrasts this "objective" excerpt with the narrator's detailed, subjective experience of anxiety as her husband drives her on her first day of work after her initial recovery from surgery. Sentences, clauses, and words slow down and break against each other without connecting conjunctions. A disjointed subjective reality unfolds; the narrator's every perception, thought, word, body movement, and observation are externalized and described with acuity, evoking a sense of experiences that seem to click one after another like beads on a string but without context, where time has slowed down, proceeding from discrete moment to discrete moment. Here, abundance of detail and extension of narrative time work hand in hand in crafting space and time in the presence of cancer.

Many of the details identified with particular images or figures are spaced widely throughout the novel and interwoven with each other in different and changing ways. Frequently, capitalized or italicized sentence fragments and individual words from the lab manual, company notes, and suggestions by doctors, colleagues, friends, or the narrator's husband, interrupt the narrator's streams of thoughts, indicating the frantic workings of her mind as it races along on different levels. Thus, each word, with its possible meanings, appears as if under a magnifying glass, revealing "greatly enlarged details" (19). For example, when the narrator enters the cafeteria to look for her boss, Benz, on her first day of returning to her work place after months of recovery, she is overwhelmed by the crowded room: "Benz, my eyes should look for Benz only, LOOKING PAST EVERYTHING, who else counts but Benz ...?" (23). Overwhelmed by details, the narrator's life begins from these details, contrasted with, and written against, the superficiality of work relations and colleagues who awkwardly avoid her, and deny her experience and her voice. In an act of resistance, the narrator sets her reality, detail by detail, moment by moment, against the reality of her colleagues who have no time, and no time for her.

Within this fragmentation, the narrator is only one voice that competes with others: for example, there is a young woman who appears to function as a younger, more rebellious version of herself. Initially challenged by the young woman, the narrator and the alter ego interact with each other and, over the course of the narrative, begin to merge. Beutler notes that the young woman was originally a dream vision (personal communication with Beutler, 2000). Similarly, Pedroni, another cancer patient (and in fact, a real figure, though not with the same name), challenges the narrator. Both struggle initially with a high degree of self-involvement, common among cancer patients, and enforced by their constant need for vigilance regarding the continuous changes and possible signs of illness in the body. These voices, too, appear to merge over the course of the novel, as do others, adding to the sense of *Fuss Fassen* as a developmental novel. Beutler's point is to emphasize the process of fragmentation, struggle, and interlinkage in an interplay of combinations between all these voices. The first-person narrator begins to define herself by identifying herself with or against the positions represented by other voices. This play confronts the reader with ambiguity. On the one hand, the narrator invites the reader into proximity with her first-person perspective. However, the refraction of her voice into other characters conveys turmoil and fragmentation and suggests distance. As Beutler develops different characters, the reader becomes involved in the narrator's turmoil, torn between proximity and distance. By investing the narrator and other characters with these reflections, Beutler provides a close-up view into the terrified and frenzied mind of a cancer patient, struggling desperately to put the pieces of her life back together again.

For reasons of space, I shall restrict my analysis of metaphors in *Fuss Fassen* to some general comments. I have already referred to "play of combinations" as only one among an abundance of lyrical metaphors that saturate *Fuss Fassen*. Another central metaphor, that of "change as continuity," is used by Beutler as a means of writing regeneration into destruction, and she turns to many Romantic allusions (from, e.g., Goethe, Novalis, and Manzoni) for the literary and philosophical adaptations of this Heraclitean concept. Thus, Beutler invokes the support of, and writes herself into, a philosophical and literary tradition that spans more than two thousand years. Many other images and metaphors of death (e.g., "the black bird"), seasonal change ("falling of leaves," "evergreen trees"), and regeneration ("giving birth to language") also pervade *Fuss Fassen*. Turning to traditional Romantic language and imagery, Beutler refigures the act of writing as the practice of traditional handicrafts. The difficulties of finding words are likened to a birth ("Worte gebären," 79), with extending "umbilical cords" ("Nabelschnur," 31) of words, some of which may be taut, tentative, and provisional, or can be cut to provide freedom and survival. Beutler's use of this literary trope signals her creative rewriting of her present, asserting choice in an overwhelming situation where unhelpful doctors, colleagues, and well-meaning but misguided friends threaten the narrator's choice.

One of the main differences between most cancer narratives and *Fuss Fassen* is that patient-writers commonly attempt an identification of self that invites the audience, in turn, to identify with the writer, preparing the basis for a catharsis of pity and fear. Beutler, however, consciously subverts stable subject positions and the identification of writer, narrator, and character. This difference also plays out in the conscious fictionalization that occurs in this text. While autobiography is to some extent fictitious, most cancer autobiographers do not put out a sustained effort to fictionalize their narratives or to reflect on the inevitably somewhat fictional character of their accounts. Beutler, however, is very conscious of writing as a strategy for confronting cancer. Drawing on an abundance of details, slowing down time, refracting experience through the many narrative voices of the novel, and interweaving it all with an abundance of metaphors, *Fuss Fassen* shares the artful tools of literature with texts of trauma to unravel and represent the density of an otherwise incomprehensible experience. Presented as a novel, this text involves truth claims as Beutler accesses, better than any descriptive narration could, the subjective experience of living with cancer. By aestheticizing her experience, and revealing the importance and regenerative potential of language, Beutler articulates the difficult process of writing a present. While writing about one's own cancer experience can be dangerous—so dangerous that one should not indiscriminately recommend it to everyone—by using literary tools consciously, artful writing can involve readers more deeply, and generate more knowledge about the otherwise incomprehensible density of living with cancer.

HEIDI JANZ AND JULIE RAK

Challenging Subjects
Ruth Sienkiewicz-Mercer, Christopher Nolan, and Autobiography

On the back cover of Ruth Sienkiewicz-Mercer's 1989 book *I Raise My Eyes to Say Yes*, there is an excerpt from a review in the *Washington Post*, which, presumably, is supposed to help sell the book. This short blurb speaks volumes when it states, "What Sienkiewicz-Mercer has made of her fate is nothing short of triumph," succinctly summarizing much of what we feel is the problem with the public reception of autobiographies by people who have so-called "severe" disabilities. The implication in the reviewer's choice of words is that Sienkiewicz-Mercer must "make" something of her fate, which means that she is a victim of circumstances; she must triumph over what must be a tragic fate, rather than a difficult situation. That is the only way in which she can have a voice in the TAB (temporarily able-bodied) world. For this triumph and this only, she is to be revered and celebrated. This happens to Sienkiewicz-Mercer as it happens to other people with disabilities who, in the recent words of Thomas Couser, have been "hyperrepresented in mainstream culture; they have not been disregarded so much as they have been subjected to objectifying notice in the form of mediated staring" (2005, 603).

In this paper, we will consider two autobiographical narratives, the one by Ruth Sienkiewicz-Mercer and Christopher Nolan's *Under the Eye of the Clock* (1987), in order to identify the discursive barriers which work to construct an infantilized, disabled subject, a subject who is "challenged." Both of these writers have been characterized in what we call the "TAB celebratory process" as "special," but also have been made somehow universal, in ways which disable their own narratives. We refer to the nondisabled readers and reviewers of Sienkiewicz-Mercer's and Nolan's autobiographies as TABS in order to draw attention to the fact that, in many interesting and important ways, the distinction between able-bodiedness and disability is a tenuous and contestable social construction. Carol A. Breckenridge and Candace Vogler observe that "no one is ever more than temporarily able-bodied. This fact frightens those of us who half-imagine ourselves as minds in a material context, who have learned to resent the publicness of race- or sex- or otherwise-marked bodies, and to think theories of embodiment as theories about the subjectivity of able-bodied comportment and practice under conditions of systematic injustice" (2001, 35). In opposition to TABS, we call Sienkiewicz-Mercer and Nolan "crips." The term "crip" is a politicized reclaiming of the older term "cripple." Crips, unlike cripples, resist the tendency, in medicine and culture, for TABS to disempower them as subjects. We wish, therefore, within the domain of what we call "crip theory," and with the assistance of critical work on testimonials from autobiography studies, to "rehabilitate" these narratives ourselves so that we can expose the discourses of legitimacy that have been used against these autobiographies, both to celebrate them and to invalidate what these authors want to do, politically, with their stories. We want to shift the emphasis from subjects who are challenged, to subjects who challenge.

Since the 1980s, critics of autobiography have looked for ways to describe autobiographical writing done by people who have written in the genre under what are termed "extraordinary constraints." Autobiographical discourse, since the publication of Jean-Jacques Rousseau's *The Confessions* in the eighteenth century, has been understood to be a discourse of what Sidonie Smith (1993) has termed the universal male subject. This subject has been formed by a conglomeration of ideologies which includes enlightenment beliefs in liberalism, Darwin's progressive view of history, and the consolidation of Protestant ideology under the term individualism. Added to this mix are Victorian beliefs about psychology and Freud's ideas about the relationship of early experiences to the formation of the personality (Smith 1993, 5–10). Therefore, the person who is able to write autobiographically has to be able to conceive of themselves as someone who can be self-reflexive, or someone who has a self to "flex." The writer must have leisure time in which to write, possess print literacy, have a sense that (mostly) he or (less often) she has a private "self" which can be narrated, and, perhaps, a public life to which readers can relate. As Smith has shown, this has meant that traditional autobiographical discourse is most often produced by white, middle-class men who have access to the trappings of identity which can allow narration and publication (1993, 18–20).

What critics have noticed, too, is that there are many writers or producers of autobiography, or of autobiographical discourse which surfaces in non-autobiographical texts, who do not have access to the markers of identity privilege which are supposed to produce the desire to narrate a life story. Poor women, working class women and men, women of colour, members of fringe religious sects, lesbians, men of colour, print-illiterate people, and people with disabilities are just a few of the groups who have made use of autobiographical discourse in order to gain access to the privileges which the discourse affords. Critics have come up with many terms for this use of autobiography, particularly when people write or dictate in order to draw attention to injustice and to call for political change. These include generic terms such as "slave narrative" (Andrews 1986) or Latin American *testimonio* (Beverly 1991), which are specific to oppressed groups, Sidonie Smith's concept of the "autobiographical manifesto" for those works which contest the traditional subjectivity and ideology of autobiography for political purposes (1993, 154–82), and Caren Kaplan's term "out-law genres" for all those types of autobiographical works which contest generic boundaries as part of their protest against the other kinds of boundaries that keep inappropriate subjects out of autobiography, and out of social life (1998, 208–16).

Out-law genres, autobiographical manifestos: these are powerful terms. They hint at autobiographies which can be testimonials, and at what Mae Gwendolyn Henderson says are stories about a group experience of oppression as told in one life (Henderson 1998, 346). Autobiographical testimony refers to types of experience and types of subjects that are not usually admitted to public discourse. Both Ruth Sienkewicz-Mercer and Christopher Nolan take up autobiographical discourse in this way, for political reasons, because their use of it can draw attention to their own difference. Before we discuss how *I Raise My Eyes to Say Yes* and *Under the Eye of the Clock* could be narratives of resistance to able-bodied ways to tell a life story, however, we caution that both Smith and Kaplan do not talk about resistance as potentially unsuccessful, or as a negotiation in the public realm which depends on the understanding of those who have more cultural privileges than the authors themselves. In their negotiations with the TAB world, Sienkewicz-Mercer and Nolan have had to use a TAB-centered trope of normalcy as their primary point of contact in their narratives. In this sense, we agree with David T. Mitchell (2000) that the tendency in the genre of autobiography itself to stress the singularity of its subjects can work against the political messages which these authors may wish to convey. According to Mitchell, "Instead of serving as a corrective to impersonal symbolic literary representations, disability life writing tends toward the gratification of a personal story bereft of community with other disabled people. Even the most renowned disability autobiographers often fall prey to an ethos of rugged individualism that can further reify the longstanding association of disability with social isolation" (312). The discourse of singularity can help to make the stories of people with disabilities seem "exceptional" in ways which disable the political work of these narratives in ways similar to this romance of the normal. Autobiographies by people with disabilities may not be able to completely withstand the TAB romanticization of the borders of what is normal; a romanticization, we point out, which can look like the romanticization of resistance in autobiographical testimonial texts. The next section will examine what tropes occur in TAB romanticization. Then, we will re-read both texts in order to disable both types of readings so that we can clarify what resistance might be in these texts and how successful it is. Our reading seeks to rehabilitate, not cure, and it seeks to respect what these authors are trying to say, even when the discursive means of saying it is fraught with difficulty.

A common way in which TAB readers seek to apprehend the necessary otherness of autobiography by people with disabilities is to resort to common stereotypes which seem to be confirmed in those narratives. In this way, the TAB reader can gain at least a certain level of access to a realm of experience which seems, to him or her, to be otherwise impenetrable. As the blurb on the back of Ruth Sienkiewicz-Mercer's *I Raise My Eyes to Say Yes* indicates, her currency as a "severely disabled" writer of autobiography is based on the TAB construction and celebration of her as an exemplar of the "supercrip" stereotype. The supercrip, by virtue of her own determination and strength of character, has broken through physical and attitudinal barriers in order to gain some level of understanding and acceptance by the TAB world. Thomas Couser has observed that "confounding stereotypes by living and writing a life beyond presumed limitations is a time-honored phenomenon in narratives of disability" (1997, 203). However, Couser also notes that this carries with it the danger of simply replacing the stereotype of a passive disabled person with the stereotype of the supercrip: "A high-achieving individual with an obvious impairment is always in danger of becoming a Supercrip, an Inspirational Disabled Person who overcomes impairment through pluck and willpower" (203).

Sienkiewicz-Mercer and Nolan both risk this danger in their narratives, and it proves to be a high stakes gamble. In the quote above, Couser points to the very "challenge" facing both Ruth Sienkiewicz-Mercer and Christopher Nolan as they seek to make consciously political statements about disability, identity, and power inequities in a TAB-dominated world through the act of composing autobiography. Sienkiewicz-Mercer is most direct about the political ends she wishes to achieve in writing her autobiography: she "wants very much to address, and educate, professionals in all disciplines that deal with the physically handicapped" (1989, 224). Significantly however, this statement does not come in the form of a first-person utterance by Sienkiewicz-Mercer herself, but rather as a second-person observation made by her collaborator, Steven B. Kaplan. Although the narrative recounts, in the first person, the physical and emotional atrocities that she endured as a resident of Belchertown State School, Sienkiewicz-Mercer's account was not literally written by her. Her inability to speak orally, combined with her limited literacy skills, made it necessary for her to rely on Kaplan to construct a coherent narrative from her single-word cues. In the TAB world, the act of finding a way to communicate by someone who is "mute," and to speak, even through a surrogate, is sufficient to make Sienkiewicz-Mercer a supercrip. Ironically, however, the fact that TAB readers tend to view Sienkiewicz-Mercer as an overcoming supercrip threatens to undermine the stated political purpose of her autobiography, for, in admiring her plucky determination as a supercrip, readers can literally "read over" the stated political aims of the narrative itself. This reading of Sienkewicz-Mercer and her method of text production is, potentially, quite damaging to the intent of her narrative. However, there are other, more subtle, ways to misread this text and its intentions without making reference to the supercrip stereotype. In his article "Conflicting Paradigms: The Rhetorics of Disability Memoir," Thomas Couser suggests that *I Raise My Eyes to Say Yes* is not a narrative of triumph because Sienkiewicz-Mercer "never manages to walk or talk" (2001, 19). In essence, Couser raises the possibility that the core value of Sienkiewicz-Mercer's autobiography lies in her manipulation of the discourse of triumph in order to "speak" for a group of people who have traditionally been disabled by the rhetoric of rehabilitation. He collapses the rhetoric of rehabilitation, with its accompanying assumption from the medical model that the writer's desire is to be cured or to regain physical abilities, into the rhetoric of the triumph narrative (19). Sienkiewicz-Mercer may in fact be refusing to write about triumph not because her rehab has failed, but because she wants to facilitate political change.

Christopher Nolan's choice to write a fictionalized autobiography would seem to indicate that his objectives for writing autobiography are literary rather than political. Nevertheless, like Sienkiewicz-Mercer, Nolan too must stake out his own position in relation to the supercrip stereotype.

Nolan makes it clear throughout his narrative that not only is he aware of the probability that the TAB public will label him as a supercrip, he both invites and recoils from this public reaction:

> Newspapers bombarded constantly, each one eager to be the first with the story of how a cripple came to vie with able-bodied man, especially in the area of wanton frankness as applied to literature and its brash experts ... What am I garnering from all this jousting attention, pondered the alert boy. Casting glances of concern towards his family he noted the affront to their privacy, the yes associated with their handling of his hassle-filled, nodding-headed, creative though silent communication. He fought sadly to make his heartfelt plea—don't let the media create a monster out of me. (1987, 2)

Significantly, as Nolan's alter-ego, Joseph Meehan, comes to discover, even a supercrip can be turned into the converse stereotype—what Leonard Kriegel would call the Charity Cripple (Kriegel 1987)—simply by highlighting his/her neediness and dependence. This happens when Joseph discusses how the London *Sunday Times* spearheaded a charity drive for him. His initial response is gratitude for the readers who "responded so magnificently" (Nolan 1987, 84), but Joseph also recognizes that the charity he receives is based on the premise that his potential can never outweigh his abnormality. "Can I, he pondered, crippled as I am, spearhead a new drive to highlight the communicative needs of tongue-tied but normal-notioned man?" (84).

However, Nolan must be dependent on other people so that he can present himself as the mediator between "normal-notioned man" and his position as a "cripple." This creates a gap between the self-reliance Nolan wishes to project and the sympathy that he garners. There are a number of instances in his autobiography where Nolan seems to construct himself deliberately as a kind of hybrid supercrip/charity cripple, whose ability to attain any degree of success in the TAB world ultimately remains contingent on the physical and emotional support that he receives from the TABS in his life. For example, one of the biggest obstacles that Joseph faces is his inability to communicate with others. He is able to overcome this obstacle when Eva, his occupational therapist, devises a system which allows him to type with a head-stick. His mother, Nora, however, must act as his chin-steadier.

> Nora waited, her son's chin cupped in her hands. Then he stretched and brought his pointer down and typed the letter "e." Swinging his pointer to the right he then typed another letter, and another one and another. Eva finished speaking on the telephone and Nora, while still cupping Joseph's chin turned and said, "Eva, I know what you're talking about—Joseph is going for

the keys himself—I could actually feel him stretching for them." Eva brought [her fist] down with a bang on the table. "So I was right, I was afraid to say anything, I had to be sure," she said as she broadly smiled. Joseph sat looking at his women saviors. They chatted about their discovery while he nodded in happy unbelievable bewilderment. He felt himself float reliably on gossamer wings. Life hungered no more. (56)

Just as Sienkiewicz-Mercer must work with a collaborator in order to make narrative, Nolan's communication with the outside world can only occur through a collaborative effort between him and the TABs in his life. This appears to disable Nolan's agency as a supercrip. However, Nolan himself, somewhat problematically, seems to sanction and even to invite such a reading when he rhapsodizes about the virtues of his "two women saviors." Nolan's insistence on calling them saviours rather than helpers invites a sentimental TAB reading whereby Nolan's agency is dependent on the generosity of people from the TAB world.

Both Nolan and Sienkiewicz-Mercer attempt to prove their legitimacy as autobiographical subjects by presenting themselves and their narratives as being extraordinary in their normalcy. This is accompanied by rhetoric which also highlights their difference. In *I Raise My Eyes to Say Yes*, Sienkiewicz-Mercer makes no attempt to disguise her method of composition. She does work extensively with her collaborator, Steven Kaplan, so that the words from her word board can be made into complete sentences, but both Sienkiewicz-Mercer and Kaplan do all that they can to ensure that the narrative is in her own voice. In his introduction, Kaplan says that "if [he] found out the written version of her viewpoint accurately, if it felt right to her, she accepted it. Otherwise, it was corrected or deleted" (1989, xvii). In the narrative, sections are headed with Sienkiewicz-Mercer's words from her word board, such as "BOX" for the story of her imprisonment in what was meant to be a device to encourage socialization (1989, 96), ".C.A.R.L." which is her spelling of and introduction to her discussion of her friend Carol (81), or "FOOD.LIKE.SHIT," which should be self-explanatory for anyone who has ever experienced institutional food (40). In this way, the narrative disjunctures between her voice and Kaplan's serve to call into question a common TAB assumption that voice and consciousness must be connected. On the other hand, Sienkiewicz-Mercer does want to show that she is normal. She concludes her narrative with a conventional happy ending, in which she marries Norman Mercer, an event which bestows upon her the full status of a "normal" adult woman. This is prefigured by the section ".DREAM.TOWN.RED," where she says about her casual friend Bob, that "My relationship with Bob had a dramatic impact on my fantasy life. In my dreams Bob whisked me off to some exotic place like Hawaii or Paris, where we got married, raised a family, and lived happily ever after" (89).

Later on, Sienkiewicz-Mercer discusses erotic dreams that she has about her friend Hans, which would be "normal" dreams for a teenager to have. Even so, the abnormality of the situation in which she finds herself often invades even her normal dreamworld, when she imagines that Hans picks her up at the Belchertown State School and takes her away when she is disabled, and picks her up at home when she imagines that she is able-bodied (189).

Christopher Nolan deals with the idea of normalcy in a rhetorically different way. His chief method of representation is to consciously construct himself as a writer by telling his story in Joycean language. Since he himself is Irish, his style marks him as a direct stylistic descendant of Ireland's most famous writer, and this makes him appear as "normal" as any other contemporary imitator. At the same time, Nolan's style makes perception seem strange, even other, and this serves to highlight his position as disabled subject:

> In anchoring ship in Mount Temple, Joseph calmed foolish seas of vacant scanning, and cloyed bannered musings vacated his scolded, messaged notation. Austere casing wrapped him tightly, but fun, frolics and flutters marked out his future years' canvassed beat. (1987, 26)

The passage is about his schooling at Mount Temple and how learning activated his mind, but the richness of the prose with its alliteration and unusual use of nouns serves to show how he can imitate Joyce while resisting the stereotype of the disabled subject as simple, cheerful, yet alone. This is the literary equivalent of another type of resistance which Nolan practices: in a March 13, 2000 interview that appeared in *Publishers Weekly*, Nolan "has fun challenging visitors to understand his gestures" in a reversal of circumstances, where it is the interviewer who is "tongue-tied" and must work at meanings, and not himself.

Nolan and Sienkiewicz-Mercer contest what is expected of them even in the physical composition of their narratives. The structure of both their narratives serves notice to people who would see them as charity cripples, whose stories are to be revered because the writers are objects of pity. However, the critical reception of Sienkiewicz-Mercer's autobiography focuses invariably on the severity of her disability instead of the issues that she raised about the mistreatment of people in institutions such as Belchertown. While Nolan is introduced as a "literary genius" by Denise

Noe, in the same breath the author says that Sienkiewicz-Mercer "may be the most tragic figure under discussion" because her disabilities seem to be more severe (Noe 1996, 13). Although Sienkiewicz-Mercer intended this autobiography to be a catalyst for change, her narrative has been disabled by critics who insist on reading it only as an inspirational tale. P. Kaganoff in *Publisher's Weekly*, for example, calls Sienkiewicz-Mercer "a paralyzed cerebral palsy victim," a description which presents her disability both as her defining characteristic, and as an illness. The reviewer also depoliticizes her text by valorizing her as someone who has heroically overcome obstacles: " the imagery [in the book] of escape from a useless body ... pervades this inspiring account of victory over handicap" (1997, 60). In Nolan's case, he is acknowledged to be a talented writer in the tradition of James Joyce or William Butler Yeats because he is Irish, but even these discussions quickly move to troping him as a supercrip who overcomes adversity (Pearl 2000, 224), or to focusing on the fact that he "can neither talk nor control most of his physical movements" (Geracimos, 2000, 57). A *US News and World Report* article focused on Nolan's body as "his worst enemy," and quoted an Oxford University literature professor who said that "part of Nolan's value as a writer is that he comes from another planet— the planet of the paralyzed and speechless" (Sherrid 1988, 60). Thus disability turns a would-be James Joyce into Mork from Ork! Our reading of these autobiographies, therefore, is designed to begin a process of rehabilitation so that it is possible to read them as the authors intended. The extent to which these texts, ultimately, can be rehabilitated from the restrictions of celebratory TAB discourse will depend on the willingness of readers and critics to recognize and respect the challenge of otherness, and not to domesticate it as "challenged."

GAIL FINNEY

The Tectonics of Trauma
Father–Daughter Incest in Film

A woman butchers her husband in cold blood and is in turn killed by her son. A man murders his father and has sex with his mother. Another woman slaughters her small children.

Do these announcements sound like recent news headlines? Unfortunately, yes—but I have also just summarized the plots of several well-known tragedies by Aeschylus, Sophocles, and Euripides: *The Oresteia*, *Oedipus the King*, and *Medea*. One begins to understand why Plato wanted to ban theatre from his ideal republic. For the Greeks, who established the genre of tragic drama in the West, all that was necessary for a tragedy was a family—a family undergoing crisis, or even trauma. "Trauma" was originally the term for a surgical wound and was based on the notion that the body is surrounded by a protective envelope, so that when a rupture occurs in the skin, the entire organism experiences a negative reaction (Leys 2000, 19). The term came to embrace emotional or psychic, as well as physical, shock to the system, and the belief that trauma has global effects on the organism has persisted. Because the family is the first social unit with which we interact, family trauma can be characterized as primal trauma. Bennett Simon identifies this element as a distinguishing feature of the tragic genre: "war against the outside world in epic becomes war within the family in tragedy" (1988, 21).

Although the major narratives recounted in Greek drama were handed down as received legends, those involving family violence appear to have been particularly popular and to have survived through a process of natural selection. This preference is reflected by Aristotle's prescription in the *Poetics*, informed by the works of the great tragedians active in the preceding century, that tragic incidents should occur "between those who are near or dear to one another" (Aristotle 1961, 79).

The tragedies of Aeschylus, Sophocles, and Euripides, like the comedies of Aristophanes, were performed in vast, open-air theatres such as the Theatre of Dionysus in Athens. Audiences were heterogeneous and massive, with as many as 17,000 viewers at time (Walton 1987, 18). In fifth-century BC Athens, in other words, theatre belonged to popular culture. The same cannot be said about our own times. Today, the only live events that command audiences of the proportions of ancient Greek theatre audiences are athletic events and rock concerts, and plays are no longer performed in stadiums as a rule. Although family trauma has continued to fascinate playwrights and other writers and artists throughout the millennia, many of whom experienced it themselves, we should turn to the cinema if we are looking for the medium that, today, most closely approximates the theatre and its function for the ancient Greeks. Films can be viewed by hundreds of spectators in a single theatre, and by hundreds of thousands when shown simultaneously in multiple theatres. Box-office receipts of popular movies, which can climb as high as $115 million in one weekend (as for the opening weekend of *Spider-Man* in 2002) and $200 million during the first week (*Spider-Man 2*, in 2004), reflect the mammoth appeal of this medium, in which private and domestic concerns are rendered as mass public spectacle. The publicizing of films in contemporary culture, though reviews and advertisements on television, the Internet, and in print journalism, as well as by simple word of mouth, promotes a mass familiarity and sense of cinematic community that other media rarely command. While television of course also reaches a mass audience, its reception is private and intimate, typically occurring not in a public space but in the home, while more stringent mechanisms of censorship governing network television tend to inhibit the realistic portrayal of family trauma.

This, then, is my focus: the staging of family trauma in contemporary film, the medium whose mass dissemination most closely resembles the scope of classical Greek tragedy, and the first Western genre to bring family trauma before the eyes of large popular audiences. I will deal primarily, though not exclusively, with films made in the United States, since the "dysfunctional family"—a phrase I will henceforth avoid because of its catch-all imprecision—has become so prevalent in this culture.[1] In fact, insofar as my subject is the cinematic representation of families in severely traumatic situations, I am examining what could, more accurately, be called the "hyper-dysfunctional family." Whereas, in Greek tragedy, family trauma, presented as the result of fate, possesses mythic significance and is dehistoricized, contemporary films depicting severe family trauma do not arise in a vacuum but often reflect actual social pathology.

It is telling, therefore, that there appears to have been an increase in the number of American films dealing with family trauma during the 1990s and especially around 2000, such as *My Own Private Idaho* (1991), *What's Eating Gilbert Grape* (1993), *Bastard Out of Carolina* (1996), *A Thousand Acres* (1997), *Affliction* (1998), *Happiness* (1998), *The Ice Storm* (1998), *Buffalo 66* (1998), *American Beauty* (1999), *Magnolia* (1999), *The Virgin Suicides* (1999), *The Cider House Rules* (1999), *Panic* (2000), *In the Bedroom* (2001), *Monster's Ball* (2001), *Frailty* (2001), *The Safety of Objects* (2001), *White Oleander* (2002), *Antwone Fisher* (2002), *Mystic River* (2003) *21 Grams* (2003), *Monster* (2003), *The Door in the Floor* (2004), *Winter Solstice* (2004), and *Mysterious Skin* (2004). Yet my interest is not so much sociological (why has this increase occurred?) as psychological and aesthetic: I want to explore the tectonics of family trauma—how these films are structured and how they stage family trauma, with an eye to discovering how these films, through the evocation and resolution of primal fears and fantasies, can function as productive cathartic mechanisms for our times.

The indirect means through which mythic incidents of family violence are conveyed, or told rather than shown, can begin to shed light on a typology of modes for staging family trauma in contemporary cinema. The treatment of family trauma in film can be said to range along a spectrum of formal modes extending from the performative, to the narrative, the dramatic, and the scenic, a progression that manifests a decreasing degree of self-consciousness or distance from the traumatic event(s) portrayed. I would like to illustrate the last two of these modes through two turn-of-the-millennium films, *A Thousand Acres* and *The War Zone*, that deal to varying degrees with the same form of trauma: father–daughter incest.

Incest is one of the most universal taboos, common to cultures around the globe, recurring throughout millennia of human history. In *Totem and Taboo* (1950), Freud's interpretation concurs with the findings of anthropologist James G. Frazer that the reason for the prevalence and vehemence of the taboo is not the horror of incest, but the opposite: "The law only forbids men to do what their instincts incline them to do; what nature itself prohibits and punishes, it would be superfluous for the law to prohibit and punish" (Freud 1950, 153). Yet the incest taboo is so long-standing and so internalized in civilized societies that to break it, particularly by sexually molesting one's own child, can cause the child substantial psychic damage. It is this kind of damage that the two films in question explore.

Although a cinematic rendering of Jane Smiley's Pulitzer Prize–winning novel of the same title, itself a modern recasting of *King Lear*, *A Thousand Acres* (1997; directed by Jocelyn Moorhouse) can stand on its own, worthy of autonomous appreciation, by virtue of its visual beauty and psychological power. Its surface calm and order belie the amorality that lies hidden at the film's center. The first shot, with its symbolic use of landscape that is typical of the entire film, intimates the ambivalence of its vision: a pan over well-appointed farmhouses, large farm equipment, windmills, opulent crops, with storm clouds on the horizon. The father–daughter relationships at the heart of Shakespeare's play are echoed in the decision of Smiley's wealthy Iowa farmer Larry (echoing Lear) Cook, played by Jason Robards, to divide his large farm between his two elder daughters, Ginny and Rose (echoing Goneril and Regan), after it appears that the youngest, Caroline (echoing Cordelia), has become disloyal to him. In an inversion of the *Lear* story, however, it is gradually revealed that the authoritarian patriarch who commands so much respect in the community secretly had sex with Ginny and Rose as teenagers for years and that this experience, which the girls kept hidden for decades, continues to wreak psychological, emotional, and sexual damage on them as adults.

The narrative mode through which this secret comes to light can in many ways be read as a cinematic recreation of Freud's trauma theory and of the classic therapeutic situation, in which the therapist encourages the patient to recall repressed traumatic experience in order to free her/him of neurosis (Freud 1939, 90–101; 1961, 6–29). Although *A Thousand Acres* does not accord with all details of Freud's theories on trauma, enough of a parallel exists that the analogy is hermeneutically illuminating. Both Rose (Michelle Pfeiffer) and her older sister Ginny (Jessica Lange) are unhappy in their marriages, Rose as full of anger and bitterness as Ginny is conciliatory and self-deprecating. Rose has told her husband about the molestation she experienced, whereas Ginny claims to remember nothing. Viewing the film through the lens of the Freudian therapeutic situation casts Rose as therapist or analyst and Ginny in the role of patient or analysand. The "therapy," which occurs in stages, is previewed by the unwitting question Caroline (Jennifer Jason Leigh) exasperatedly puts to Ginny because of what Caroline regards as Ginny's unfeeling treatment of their father: "What *happened* to you?" The first explicit step in Rose's attempts to bring Ginny to recollection, however, occurs during a scene in which Rose, angry because of Larry's erratic and brutish behavior since giving away his farm, claims that she sometimes hates him and prods Ginny to "Tell me what you really *think* about Daddy."

Rose's confession, designed to elicit a similar one from Ginny, occurs in the precise middle of the film, during the storm: "You don't remember how he used to come after us, do you?" She then tells Ginny that their father came to her room regularly and had sex with her at night when she was between thirteen and sixteen years old, and that he seduced her by telling her he loved her and that she was special. Although Rose is certain that he had done the same thing with Ginny first, Ginny still claims to remember nothing. Not until Ginny overhears Larry talking in a soft, seductive voice to Caroline, with whom he has reconciled, does the "recovered memory" of her incestuous experience suddenly come back.

The connection made in both Moorhouse's film and Smiley's novel between incest and patriarchal power suggests a link to Judith Herman's influential book *Father–Daughter Incest* (1981), a feminist reading of the incest story which endeavors to explode many of the underlying myths of incest, and recounts several so-called "recovered memories" from the 1970s.[2] *A Thousand Acres* should not be viewed as support for the recovered-memory movement, however, for while Ginny's breakthrough is transformative, it is not redemptive (see Doane and Hodges 2001, 76).

In examining how the trauma is staged at the center of the film *A Thousand Acres*, a close look at the scenic apparatus shows that, rather than exploiting the sensationalist potential of cinema, the film visualizes the incestuous acts largely symbolically through striking images of purity and filth: on the one hand, the family's pristinely white farmhouses and glistening green fields are repeatedly shot against the horizon beneath a tranquil blue sky, along with abundant white bed linens that are forever being hung up, taken down, or shown drying in the breeze; on the other hand, there are repeated depictions of the family using its water supply, which is ultimately revealed to be poisoned by fertilizers—fertilizers Larry had used to enhance his production. Jess, the neighbor (and lover) of Ginny and Rose, tells them that while the well-water is polluted and could cause health problems, it "affects different people in different ways"—a highly ironic observation in view of Ginny's miscarriages and of the cancer that afflicts Rose and killed their mother. Larry's considerable wealth, in other words, is based on his poisoning—literal and psychological—of his wife and daughters. These images provide a contrast with the film's numerous references to the girls' fascination with the drainage grate and other allusions to the way in which their father, grandfather, and great-grandfather had worked to drain the land and turn it into arable farmland. Foregrounding these images through visual repetition, the film conveys the ironic contrast between surface order and tranquility and underlying corruption and greed in a manner unavailable to verbal narrative.

If the visual focus of *A Thousand Acres* is on cultivated nature, which belies the uncivilized drives of the patriarch who farms it so successfully, these same drives are visually paralleled by a setting of wild, untamed nature—a rocky seacoast in Devon, in southwestern England—in *The War Zone* (1999). In an ironic inversion of the conventional dichotomy between corrupt urban space and unspoiled rural realm, the film treats a lower-middle-class family—a father, a highly pregnant mother (Tilda Swinton), their eighteen-year-old daughter Jessie, and their fifteen-year-old son Tom—who have recently moved from London to Devon, and are destroyed over the course of the film by the father's sexual relationship with his daughter. This British film, which represents the directorial debut of actor Tim Roth, relies so heavily on the visual or scenic mode and so little on dialogue and narration that one could almost imagine it being done in mime. The film signifies not through speech but through image. The camera lingers on several recurring settings whose starkness underlines the power of primal sexual instincts that seem to predate or transcend human civilization. Foremost among these settings are the family's house, which stands like a monolith in a vast windswept landscape with nothing around it and is repeatedly shot in the middle of the frame, as if in a painting; the narrow road, overgrown with vegetation, that leads to the house; the steep, craggy coast near the house, with wind blowing and surf crashing loudly; and an abandoned bunker, situated high on a bluff overlooking the ocean. The disturbing power of Roth's film, with its alternately understated and graphic portrayal, far transcends that of Hollywood treatments of father–daughter incest.

The initial scene inside the family's house, in which the children sit in the living room staring at each other and saying nothing while their mother washes their father at the kitchen sink, is emblematic; it is appropriate that our first view of the father is of his back, which he will, in so many ways, turn on his family. The typical family scene depicts mother and children silent and inactive in the living room while their father talks on the telephone, separated from them in an alcove off to the side. Although the telephone appears to be the family's main link to the outside world, the father's telephone conversations, like most of his dialogue, are nearly incomprehensible to the viewer, reflecting his utter self-involvement. The road leading to the house, which emphasizes the isolation of house and family, figures most prominently during the night when the family takes the mother to the hospital to have her baby and the father, distracted by his children, wrecks the car. The camera lingers so long on the overturned car that the viewer is invited to regard the accident as a metaphor for the life of this family. Ironically, this is one of the most positive scenes in the film, since no one is seriously hurt and the baby arrives on-site—though it is significant that the baby is born, literally, into a wreck. The bandages the family wears after the accident can be read as symbolic of the bruised nature of all of them.

The untamed sea coast near where the family lives, to which the camera returns often, assumes the function of mythic backdrop and visually dehistoricizes the secrets the film reveals. The rocky coast is also the location of the abandoned bunker that helps to give the film its name. In *Beyond the Pleasure Principle*, Freud begins his discussion of traumatic neurosis by referring to the many cases of this illness brought about by World War I (1961, 6). The metaphor of the psychic battleground, or war zone, for traumatic neurosis follows logically, and it is fitting that the scene that reveals this family's war zone occurs in a bunker. The film approaches the bunker in stages: our first view of it, like so much else in the film, is through the eyes of Tom (the voice and vision of morality in this family, from whose perspective we see much of the film), when he sees Jessie and their father enter the bunker from down below, at a distance, so that it looks very small. We next see the bunker from the outside but close up, when Tom buries an old videocamera next to it, as he became aware, earlier in the film, that something is going on between his sister and father. Finally, as he films through an opening in the wall, we witness a horrifying perversion of the primal scene inside the bunker through Tom's eyes, as the boy sees his father having sex not with his mother, but with his sister. For a film to portray the scene of father–daughter incest directly is very rare. This scene—in the middle of the desolate bunker, empty except for a few articles of clothing, Jessie on all fours and weeping as, behind, her father has anal intercourse with her—is intensely stark and disturbing, doubly so because the camera cuts repeatedly to Tom's watching eyes: our shock is magnified by our awareness of his. The scene reads as a perversion of the voyeuristic constellation so popular in pornography, in which the viewer's pleasure in watching sexual acts in a film is heightened by the presence of a spectator within the film, typically a male spectator, who is watching the same sexual acts. One of Tom's most telling gestures in the entire film is his hurling of the videocamera—recorder and preserver of the traumatic moment—down the steep cliffs into the sea, as though he can eradicate the reality by destroying the image. Appropriately, the film's final scene is set in the bunker, where Tom has retreated after stabbing his father.

As these illustrations should have demonstrated, the progression from the narrative to the scenic mode is a move away from self-consciousness and mediation toward directness and immediacy. When dealing with a subject as emotionally laden as family trauma, however, both modes can be powerful and cathartic, each in its own way.

Notes

1. This awareness is so ubiquitous that it has even penetrated country music: in the song "The Little Girl" (2000), country singer John Michael Montgomery tells of a girl growing up in a home in which she is neglected, her mother is addicted to pills, and her father drinks heavily and physically abuses her mother. One night her father comes home and shoots his wife and then himself. The girl is adopted and acquires a home where she learns about Jesus and becomes religious. Several songs on Rodney Crowell's CD *The Houston Kid* (2001) treat similar themes.
2. My thanks to Janet Walker, who illuminated this connection in response to a version of this paper I presented at the University of California Interdisciplinary Psychoanalytic Consortium at Lake Arrowhead, CA, May 2002.

SALLY CHIVERS

THE SILVERING SCREEN
Age and Trauma in Akira Kurosawa's Rhapsody in August

Akira Kurosawa's penultimate film, *Rhapsody in August* (1991), commemorates victims and survivors of the August 9, 1945 atomic bombing of Nagasaki. Set during a summer in the early 1990s, the film depicts the adult children of the central character, Kane, leaving their children with their grandmother while they travel to Hawaii in order to investigate reports of a previously unknown dying uncle. Kane lost her husband to the atomic bomb and witnessed her brother going mad as a result of trauma caused by the explosion, and herself shows physical signs of the effects of radiation, which mingle indistinguishably with visual signs of aging on her body. Her grandchildren contemplate stone war memorials in the schoolyard where their grandfather died, and subsequently feel compelled to listen to their grandmother's stories. In the process, the children's new recognition of the experience in Nagasaki merges with Kane's continued struggles to reckon with the tragedy. The film concludes with what appears to be Kane's descent into mental confusion, so that—in her mind—she lives within the moment that has physically and emotionally marked her.

In order to grasp the film as a form of commemoration, and to abide its rather thin plot, viewers must develop an understanding of the narrative and visual signification of old age, and of the late life of a particular Japanese woman who survived the attack on Nagasaki. In the character of Kane (played by Sachiko Murase), the film embodies a memorial for Nagasaki as both cultural agony and cultural memory. The film situates age as a culturally specific identity marker and demonstrates the ways in which cohort affects age identity. Especially, the film argues that a cross-generational connection may contribute to a revaluation of age and the particular experiences of the aged—in this case, Kane's experience of an atomic bomb. Kane's body evokes her engagement with historical time in a double fashion: the traumatic effects of atomic radiation denote a past sudden physical change, visually represented through her nearly bald head. More typical, gradual change, visually represented by her stooped posture and wrinkled skin, provides evidence of her encounters with time.

The narrative structure of *Rhapsody in August* is based on the notion that old age is a time of memory and a time to pass on memories, especially in the form of stories, to a subsequent generation. As Mitsuhiro Yoshimoto explains, "*RIA* is about the possibility of talking about and remembering as much as the fact of the Americans' atomic destruction of Nagasaki on August 9, 1945" (2000, 369). This fairly typical connection between age and memory is fraught with certain assumptions. The link comes from a negative interpretation of the physiology of old age, expressed quite pessimistically in "Trauma and Aging: A Thirty-Year Follow-up," by Henry Krystal:

> Particularly severe losses are accrued to the things one *does*, in all spheres of activity, from sexual through occupational, avocational to recreational. These losses force a shift from doing to thinking, from planning to reminiscing, from preoccupation with everyday events and long-range planning to reviewing and rethinking one's life. (1995, 82)

Stephen Prince articulates a similar transition to retrospection as he sees it manifest in Kurosawa's later cinema: "At its end, Kurosawa's became a cinema of recollection, not action, one suited to an advanced age in which activity has given way to memory" (1999, 324). However devastating Prince's wording, which contributes to the troubling acceptance of decline as inevitable, younger generations do tend to turn to elders for stories of the past and treat older people as the embodiment of cultural heritage, rather than thinking of them as active participants in a social sphere. In *Rhapsody in August*, as Kane's grandchildren witness prominent public memorials to the bombing, they begin to think of their grandmother as a private memorial and seek to draw from her stories of the bombing and see its effect on her as exemplary of a larger cultural effect. Further, though her family turns to her as the arbiter of family and cultural history, Kane faces the impending death of a brother she does not remember. The family's association of their grandmother with a past that she only partially and periodically remembers (or chooses to remember) demonstrates a tension that arises with the assumption that an elder literally embodies the past. The connection between age and memory is fraught not just because the automatic association may be inappropriate, but because, at a time associated with memory, memory itself falters for many and becomes even more unreliable and inaccessible than previously. Kane does not remember her brother and, later in the film, she can no longer determine whether she lives in the past or the present.

In her contribution to Kathleen Woodward's *Figuring Age*, E. Ann Kaplan tries to elucidate a thorny connection between trauma and aging. She focuses her argument openly on Western white women, arguing that "aging need not *necessarily* be a trauma for women, but that western cultures may produce this result—particularly perhaps for white women—through prevailing gender constructs, and specifically the anxiety of (white) males about their own aging and their own death" (1999, 172). To explain what she means by trauma, Kaplan draws on the American Psychiatric Association's *DSM-III-R* definition: "The person has experienced an event that is outside the range of human experience" (1987, 250).[1] She goes on to support Laura S. Brown's assertion that because the "human" in that definition is gendered male, women's experience of abuse "at the hands of men" can be labelled trauma. For a number of reasons, this unconvincing argument cannot apply to Kane's situation in *Rhapsody in August*. She is outside of Kaplan's "Western, white" rubric, and her experience of unquestionable trauma makes the supposed trauma of growing old seem rather trivial.

In *Unclaimed Experience: Trauma, Narrative, History*, Cathy Caruth explains that "in its most general definition, trauma describes an overwhelming experience of sudden or catastrophic events in which the response to the event occurs in the often delayed, uncontrolled repetitive appearance of hallucinations and other intrusive phenomena" (1996, 11). Kurosawa and Murase's depiction of Kane's response to what seem to be impinging memories of the Nagasaki bombing enacts this definition of trauma, particularly at the climactic close of the film. In her chapter on Alan Resnais's *Hiroshima mon amour*, Caruth suggests "that the interest of *Hiroshima mon amour* lies in how it explores the possibility of a faithful history in the very indirectness of this telling" (27). *Rhapsody in August* also invests in indirect telling, particularly in Kurosawa's refusal to visually depict the bomb—offering instead only a twisted jungle gym as evidence—and in Kane's circuitous story-telling techniques. In part, the "rethinking of reference" that Caruth claims arises from the attempt to understand trauma occurs in a deflection through the topic of aging (11). The depiction of aging in this film is also a depiction of trauma: not because age is trauma, but because people of a particular cohort in a particular location all experienced catastrophe.

At the opening of the film, Kane does not appear to have spoken previously to her grandchildren of her experiences with the bombing. They resent her old-fashioned ways and complain about her cooking. On a trip to Nagasaki to buy their own culinary supplies, three of the grandchildren (one of whom becomes disconcertingly wise as she takes up the narration) pay their tribute to the bombing by visiting the statues sent by countries such as Cuba, Bulgaria, China, Czechoslovakia, Poland, and the USSR (the absence of a memorial from the United States does not go unremarked). At this point in the film, when Kane has not yet told her stories, perhaps because of gaps in her memory, the stone memorials take the place initially of her storytelling. In scenes criticized for their awkwardness and praised for their evocation of visual stasis, the grandchildren develop a new understanding of their grandmother's experiences (or think they do) and subsequently turn to her for stories, some that she tells willingly and others that she would rather not discuss. As the film progresses, Kane's stories take over the awkward narrations, although "the ambiguous point of view and Kurosawa's uncertain control over the perspectives and voices embodied in the narrative," as Stephen Prince puts it (1999, 320), remain a problem for the film.

In addition to commemorating Nagasaki in this filmic elegy for its victims, Kurosawa comments throughout *Rhapsody in August* on the disjunction among three generations: "those like Kane (and Kurosawa) who are pre-war, those born in the 1940s, and the youth of today" (Prince, 1999, 317). In doing so, Kurosawa reiterates a longstanding tradition of excluding the middle generation from cultural transmission, so that disparate generations relate across age and cultural differences. In *How Societies Remember*, Paul Connerton describes Marc Bloch's research into the transfer of cultural knowledge:

> When the ancient Greeks called stories "geroia," when Cicero called them "fabulae aniles," and when the picture illustrating the Contes of Perrault represented an old woman telling a story to a circle of children, they were registering the extent to which the grandmother took charge of the narrative activity of the group. In such a context we should not envisage communication between generations as being conducted, [in a linear fashion], the children having contact with their ancestors only through the mediation of their parents. Rather, with the moulding of each new mind there is at the same time a backward step, joining the most malleable to the most inflexible mentality, while skipping the generation that might be the sponsor of change. (1989, 39)

Though it resists the troubling connection between age and inflexibility, as opposed to youth and malleability (and, in fact, demonstrating the opposite), *Rhapsody in August* does represent the middle generation as the agent of change, embracing the Hawaiian relatives and, especially, their wealth. However, after going to the memorials and before hearing Kane's story, Shinjiro—the youngest grandchild—assumes that his grandmother does not want to travel to Hawaii because she hates America. She corrects him, explaining: "It was a long time ago that I felt bitter about America. It's been forty-five years since Grandpa died. Now I neither like nor dislike America. It was because of the war. The war was to blame. During the war many Japanese died ... and so did many Americans." Though she is not explicit about it, Kane's choice is not between Japan and America, stasis and change, or even unremembered family connection and remembered spouse. Rather, she must choose either to visit a forgotten relative simply because he is dying or to remain near her home to attend the commemoration of August 9, 1945, and, in particular, the death of her husband. She must choose between rituals for brother or husband and compete with the family's expectations of her in that regard.

As the grandchildren's awareness of the atomic attack increases, they realize the impossibility of understanding Kane's experience from a previously learned version of events, and a more generous reading of the film's ambiguous perspective becomes possible. Minako says, "Neither we nor our parents know about war. Sure we've heard about the destruction ... but it seemed only like a scary fairy tale. We could never understand the feelings of the victims. We never stopped to think." When Kane overhears this, she enters the room to take on the role of storyteller. However, as James Goodwin explains, "The memories of those who lived through the bomb are largely unspoken in Kurosawa's film ... This past remains tangibly present only in a few physical vestiges of the devastation, such as a half-standing playground apparatus that was melted into a twisted, misshapen figure by the bomb blast" (1994, 138). Rather than narrate the bombing, as the grandchildren seem to desire, Kane tells a fairy tale–like story of one brother's elopement and retreat into the forest. In resisting the perspective required of her, Kane follows through on the film's refusal to take an easy or direct perspective on the bombing. As reviewer Vincent Canby explains, "*Rhapsody in August* vividly recalls the atomic holocaust, but entirely by indirection" (1994, 223). The next night, Kane moves closer to speaking of the bombing, but is still vague in telling the story of another brother, Suzukichi, whom she describes as "slightly weak in the head"—"after he lost his hair from the radiation ... for some strange reason he kept drawing eyes." While the children go swimming and encounter a snake whose eyes bring to mind Suzukichi's illustrations, Kane attends a Buddhist service for the souls of the departed, after which she makes a decision and is able to explain the exact nature of the eye to the children—to explicate the "strange reason" which somehow eluded her before. "Snake eyes? The eyes of Suzukichi's drawings are not snake eyes. They are the eyes of the flash," she says. A perspective previously refused to the grandchildren, and more largely refused to the audience, floods the film and a lurid image of an eye over the hills near the house takes over—an image much criticized for its literalness. The image comes with Kane's explicit description of the effect on Suzukichi, but not of her own attempt to run to Nagasaki to save her husband.

When news of her forgotten brother's death reaches her, Kane breaks down with grief and appears to become demented. As Yoshimoto puts it, "Kane's recognition of her elder brother is traumatic because the missing memory returns to her only when it is too late for her to see him. The untimely recovery of the memory is so shocking that she becomes delusional and mistakes the death of Suzujiro for that of her husband" (1994, 370). Further, she confuses her son with her brother, which makes her subsequent attempt to protect her grandchildren from the bomb seem like insanity. However, it could also just be that she is reading an impending storm as an attack because it replicates the conditions that preceded her husband's death, conditions that were ignored because they seemed like a storm. Her reaction may be delusion, and it may not be. Her relatives and friends explain the strangeness in relation to her memory. One of the grandchildren, Tateo, says, "The clock in her head is running backwards. She is slipping back into the time of Grandpa." When a neighbour arrives to tell of her attempt to run to Nagasaki, she says, "Maybe she remembered what happened that day." Then she changes her mind. "No," says the neighbour, "she's reliving that day now."

The subsequent closing scene presents the most memorable and widely known image from the film. Beginning with the youngest, the grandchildren run into the rain followed by their parents. A series of shots of the family running from right to left across a still frame concludes with their arrival at a fork in the road. There is a cut to Kane running uphill into the background. Shots of the family running from right to left without camera motion again follow but, this time, there are cuts between shots of the male grandchildren, the female grandchildren, and their parents. Next, Kane attempts to move right to left but is stopped by the wind and rain. She resolutely steps forward and sideways in an attempt to continue her journey. Quick cuts follow with separate shots of the four grandchildren, and this time the camera moves with them, emphasizing their movement in comparison to Kane. Her daughter, Yoshie, falls and gets up again; cut to Kane making steadier progress, and the camera panning with her. Again, a succession of shots of the grandchildren follows, each of them shouting, "Obachan!" The pattern repeats without the middle generation. Finally, Kane's umbrella blows inside out and, at that point, the soundtrack of the storm is replaced by the Schubert chorus "And a boy saw a rose …," this time sung by a group of children. After another series of separate shots of the grandchildren, there is a slow motion shot of Kane struggling, nearly faltering, but steadily moving towards Nagasaki with an expression on her face that could be read as a grimace or a slight smile, either of which connotes pure determination. Slow motion shots of the grandchildren follow, with Shinjiro falling and standing back up, and Tateo stumbling. The film closes with a shot of Kane, almost still and then moving forward again, her bent umbrella brandished against torrential wind and rain.

Stephen Prince interprets Kane in this scene as "immobilized" in her "efforts to escape the history to which her latter life has been subject" and "her inability, pushed back by the headwind, to recover or re-enter the past" (1999, 328). A consideration of the integral intergenerational connection between Kane and her grandchildren, however, allows for an alternate reading. Following Prince's reading, the middle generation is cut from the scene as they fall back physically, and in their efforts to recover the past. The grandchildren fight hard to catch up and, in doing so, they too stumble. Yet because of their youth, perhaps, or because of how youth is typically understood, they nimbly regain balance and press on to reach their grandmother, who does not even try to accelerate her pace but still remains ahead. Kane has the *least* difficulty in the face of the storm. The children stumble and recover and the middle generation completely falls behind, but she continues steadfast. At the close of the film, in this scene and in the narrative, the grandchildren are closer to their grandmother than her own children are. It is always difficult to discern whether the middle generation chases their mother or their children, whereas Kane's motives are clear, even if her imagined time frame is not.

Rhapsody in August does not portray age as trauma, in the way that E. Ann Kaplan has attempted to describe the connection. However, the film investigates how trauma ages and how trauma affects the intergenerational relationships examined by Paul Connerton and Marc Bloch. There is a strong link forged between Kane and death: she quietly insists on remaining in Japan for her husband's memorial; her relatives want her to participate in the rituals surrounding her brother's death; and memories of another brother's death, along with news of her forgotten brother's passing, push her into memories of trauma and leave her no time, past or present, to "be in" comfortably. Kane's grandchildren need her to play the role of memory provider, but when memories intrude on her present she is sent into an episode that evokes what has been read as mental illness and as metaphor/allegory. When Tateo and Tami tell each other, as reassurance, "Grandma is pretty good at telling make-believe stories. We shouldn't take them so seriously. At her age, she's probably senile," they mean to comfort each other by leaning on a stereotype of old age. Whether Kane's later dislocation from the present is the result of trauma or old age or a combination of the two, the result, rather than tethering her to a negative conception of age as immobility, joins her to her grandchildren's recognition of the need and desire for the stories only she can tell, and leaves her physically quite strong. The film commemorates not only the victims of Nagasaki and its survivors, but also the cross-generational bonds that transmit trauma and define age identity.

Note

1 Anne Hunsaker Hawkins discusses the revisions to the *DSM* definitions in "Writing about Illness: Therapy? Or Testimony?" (this volume).

PART II

Representing the Subject

THE EDITORS

Introduction
Narrative in Qualitative Research and Therapeutics

The stories made public in writing or film discussed in Part I are consciously framed and presented in a "finished" format that lends itself to detailed textual analysis, and the narrative has an acknowledged author. In qualitative research in the health and social sciences, narrative methods often involve a different type of storytelling that is based on individual interviews or oral life history. The narrative exchange may have a strictly therapeutic and private function or it may be more oriented towards a social or political goal, but whatever the focus of the research, ethical guidelines usually insist that researchers relay their exchanges anonymously, to protect the identities of the participants. The researcher is not a reader or viewer invited to digest the story at leisure, but is involved in a face-to-face exchange that entails co-construction, interpretation, and representation of other people's stories. This additional level of mediation (as in ghost-written auto/biographies) raises a further set of difficult questions. What do narrative approaches in qualitative research or therapy have in common, and how relevant are literary methods of analysis to these contexts? What are the limitations of narrative methods, when something has to be "demonstrated" by "scientific" criteria? How do apparently "objective" researchers shape the narratives they receive through the subtle background noise or interference of their own stories? These issues were among those raised at the Wall project conference in a panel discussion entitled "Narrative Methods" that included sociologists Arthur Frank (author of *The Wounded Storyteller* [1995] and *At the Will of the Body* [1991]), Catherine Riessman (author of *Narrative Analysis* [1993]), and Anne Hunsaker Hawkins, a literary analyst specializing in pathographies.

Both Frank and Riessman chose to focus on the relationship of self to narrative, as Frank spoke of his experience as a sociologist writing his own memoir of illness, and Riessman explained how she has become increasingly aware of the need to be critically self-reflexive in mediating other people's stories. Riessman's work over the past twenty years has focused on the narrative analysis of individual qualitative research interviews. Moving away from an essentialist and static notion of the self to one that is performative and dynamic, Riessman's current work attempts to break down the distinction between "artistic" narratives and informal oral accounts, seeing both as interactive performances requiring engagement from both speaker and listener (as analyzed by Langellier, 2001). In the discussion, she noted a current trend to over-personalize the autobiographical narrative, neglecting its socio-historical context and the limits that institutional discourses place both on what stories can be told, and what forms they can take. Wary of the ubiquitous use of the term "narrative" to designate almost all forms of communication, she reminded us that narratives always convey a sequence, although it may not necessarily be a temporal one. Recalling Cheryl Mattingly's list of narrative components (1998, 2000), Riessman situated the essential elements of desire, trouble, risk, plot, and suspense as all depending on the co-construction of an exchange based on translating one person's idiom and experience into another's. Calling for greater self-awareness and responsibility on the part of those who solicit narratives from research subjects, Riessman urged us towards greater self-reflexivity, while also acknowledging the risk of our own confessional selves interrupting and displacing the fragile stories waiting to be heard.

Frank described his approach to narrative as both therapeutic (by reintegrating his own illness into a life-story) and emancipatory (in allowing illness to be spoken about, and others to hear such stories). While retaining a firm belief that each individual story is unique, he has also turned his attention to what he calls "narrative templates," the frames or culturally preferred narratives that shape individuals' stories. He suggested that the influence of the dominant stories disseminated in popular media can be minimized by the narrator's reflective awareness of them. Reflexivity is required on the part of the story teller as well as the receiver.

The third panelist, Anne Hunsaker Hawkins (author of *Reconstructing Illness: Studies in Pathology*, 1999), related the concept of "narrative templates" to her work on modern ideological myths, such as the myth of progress. She asked whether narrativity itself may be such a myth, colonizing various disciplines and running counter to postmodern destabilization of the self and of master narratives. Hawkins hypothesized that personal narratives are popular because of their apparent authenticity, although the narrative may in fact supersede actual memories and be far from factually "true." The anonymity required by ethical review boards in the interests of reducing potential harm to participants prevents the kind of verification supposedly possible in published memoirs, where the "autobiographical pact" (Lejeune 1975, 1989, 2005) depends on the signature of the author, who acknowledges responsibility for the authenticity of the account.

Part II of this volume brings together a variety of papers that illustrate and expand on the issues raised by the conference panelists. In the first paper in this section, Hunsaker Hawkins raises the question of the balance between therapy and testimony in the telling of personal narratives. While the therapeutic function may require no public audience (and, indeed, frequently precludes a public audience due to rules regarding confidentiality), the emancipatory goal associated with testimony demands that the story be heard as widely as possible. Drawing on trauma theory, Hunsaker Hawkins examines how the act of writing or telling a story can function to connect the narrator to others for effective healing and recovery. The success of the therapeutic function may, in fact, lead to the desire to inform and help others.

In the next paper, Barbara Schneider illustrates the value of the personal story as a tool for social and political action through personal narratives collected in research interviews with four people diagnosed as schizophrenic. Her analysis of the participants' accounts shows how they simultaneously contested medical definitions and expectations of who they are, and actively used medical discourse to redefine a distinctive "schizophrenic" self. Schneider attends to the issue of self-reflexivity by foregrounding her own theoretical understanding of identity formation, providing the reader with tools to analyze the relationship between identity and narrative when both are imposed from outside, and provoke a counter-narrative from the individual.

Lourdes Rodriguez Del Barrio looks more closely at one person's experience of psychosis to show how difficult it is for that person to be heard. Using a phenomenological approach, she pays close attention to the images this individual's discourse evokes. The metaphors central to his story reveal how the illness affects his subjectivity, as he vacillates between a temporally constructed narrative line and a spatially defined non-narrative perception of what is happening in his life. His life history exemplifies a socio-cultural frame determined by a diagnosis condemning him to an exclusion that, paradoxically, is intensified by his treatment. Del Barrio raises issues that will be taken up in Part III by Richard Ingram and by James Overboe regarding the status of non-stories or anti-stories as means of communication and co-construction (or refusal) of meaning.

Joy James, author of the next contribution, bases her discussion of a collective reaction to psychiatric treatment on a published text, Persimmon Blackbridge's *Sunnybrook: A True Story with Lies* (a title that recalls Lauren Slater's memoir, *Lying*). Blackbridge records and discusses a group art installation project in a closed psychiatric hospital, that enabled former inmates to take over the space and express their memories and reactions. In contrast to a typical qualitative research study or a personal memoir, Blackbridge provides what James terms a "highly imagistic autofictive form of hypertext." The format of the text explodes the space of the page (as the art installation opened up the hospital), providing a multiplicity of subject positions in an innovative challenge to a normative, linear storyline. This formal aesthetic experiment reflects the refusal of a straitjacket "normality" that denied the former patients the right or opportunity to tell their stories. James also relates this example to the concept of "amplification" (developed by Ross Chambers and Thomas Couser, and illustrated by Geneviève Brisac's autofiction as discussed by Barbara Havercroft in Part I), as a means to enable the stories of those who otherwise have no agency or access to being heard.

Another type of interactive narrative can occur when caregivers come together with patients to share their experience. L'Arche, an international, residential care operation, represents an alternative type of residential setting that brings together people with mental or physical disabilities and their caregivers on a model of mutual respect. Pamela Cushing has studied, as a participant observer, how the exchange of stories with and about the residents is central to the integration of new caregivers into the community. These stories are essential in articulating what eventually becomes self-evident, but is not clear initially to newcomers. They illustrate a dynamic that reflects the role of narrative in establishing socio-cultural norms and turning visitors into inhabitants in any setting.

Janet McArthur illustrates another type of participatory research. Using herself as a case study to represent the notion of disruption of self, she discusses her experience as an academic living with a chronic illness, lupus. This self-study enables the eye of the researcher to examine the specifics of the experience with a degree of detail that is not possible when discussing the experiences of others. McArthur echoes Susan Sontag's (1977) image of "entering" illness as comparable to becoming a citizen of another country. In the case of lupus, this alienation is intermittent since the illness "flares" and subsides, and the subject is constantly readjusting to becoming "other." As the condition is incurable, battle images are less useful than those that evoke a remapping of the self's territory. Since those with lupus bear no visible external signs of the illness, others are not aware when shifts in the terrain occur and suspicion reigns, along with a denial of accommodation for those with this type of disability.

While MacArthur tells her own story directly, Sharon Dale Stone does so less directly by including herself in her sample of six women who experienced hemorrhagic stroke at a relatively young age. All of the participants in this project mention positive as well as negative effects from the stroke, although they all, like MacArthur, feel left out in contexts where others have no understanding of their experience. As in many other qualitative research studies, quotations from the participants illustrate specific points. What is unusual about Stone's study is that one of the interviews from which she quotes is an interview with herself. This experiment illustrates concretely the fluid boundaries between researcher and researched, without becoming, as do some of the other papers in this collection, overtly autobiographical.

The juxtaposition of Stone's paper with a study of fourteen men with spinal cord injuries also leads into issues of gender difference that are raised more directly in Part III. The reactions of the women interviewed by Stone are very different from those of the men studied by Brett Smith and Andrew Sparkes. Using a traditional qualitative approach, Smith and Sparkes collected narrative data through open-ended interviews, which were then transcribed and analyzed. The analysis revealed that participants had a complete change of attitude to a previously taken-for-granted body. Even after twenty-two years, one man still does not recognize himself in the mirror. This major life change affected their professional and family life, as well as their recreational activities and friendships, and forced them to reassess the values associated with "masculinity." Rather than accepting the changed situation, many of them resisted it, continuing to dream of being restored to their former state while feeling emasculated because they could no longer attain a model of heroic virility. A few participants, however, used the opportunity to tell another story, reflecting different values that enabled them to (re)establish coherence in their life.

These last studies reflect the presence of ideological metanarratives that shape individual experiences, echoing the template stories categorized by Arthur Frank (1995) of recovery and restitution, destitution or loss, chaos and quest. The papers in Part II draw attention to the interaction between life and story and between teller and receiver, which may be ongoing and in flux. Disease, disability, and trauma disrupt the body, the self, and the life-as-story. They challenge the sense of being a self/subject, and both propel and impede the urge to project a self-representation or image that can re-establish coherence. Often mediation is required, entailing other issues of representation, as the subject speaks through the researcher or therapist, who ends up speaking for someone else. There is a possibility for what Hilde Lindemann Nelson (2001) calls "narrative repair," but what Howard Brody (1991) referred to as the "broken story" may require major surgery or reconstruction to be made comprehensible. As some of the papers in Part III suggest, the re-covering may be as painful and damaging as the injury itself, and not everyone has equal access to restorative storytelling.

ANNE HUNSAKER HAWKINS

Writing about Illness
Therapy? Or Testimony?

Some seven or eight years ago, a woman I'll call Yvette asked me if she could come and talk to medical students about her experience with breast cancer. She had had a mastectomy, followed immediately afterwards by reconstructive surgery. I invited her to my class, "Pathography and the Patient's Experience of Cancer," which was made up of second-year medical students. Yvette had written poems about her experience, as had her husband. Both of them came. The students read these poems beforehand, then Yvette and Emil came and talked with the students. It was a powerful and emotional event for both wife and husband, who seemed to me to be reliving aspects of the experience as they read their poems aloud and talked with the students. For the students it was a wonderful learning experience, one that strongly reinforced what I was trying to teach about the importance of understanding and empathizing with what it is like to be a patient. Yvette and Emil were enthusiastic about their encounter with the students, and indicated that they hoped they could come again next year. As it turned out, I was responsible the next year for a large core course for all first-year medical students. I talked with Yvette and her husband about this larger pedagogical setting, and they were still enthusiastic about presenting their writings and their story. I decided to begin the course with a plenary session in which they would talk to the students—the point being to emphasize the importance of patients and their experience of illness and treatment. Once again Yvette and Emil did a marvelous job; once again their presentation seemed to be emotionally powerful; once again it seemed as though they were reliving their experience.

I became concerned about the implications of their reliving the experience in this way. Most of all, I wondered if they were being helped by coming back again and again to talk about a very painful experience. It certainly seemed a powerful exercise in learning about patients for the students, though some of them asked questions that were a little disquieting. One student told me that she thought Yvette and Emil, in different ways, were "overreacting." It had by now been three or four years since her surgery. The student asked: "Why isn't Mrs. B. more concerned about a recurrence of the cancer?" I wondered, too, about Yvette and Emil themselves: what did their encounter with the medical students do for them? I talked with them about this, and they told me that they were gratified that the students were so appreciative of their presentation, and that they felt they were providing an important service in demonstrating how it felt to be a patient (or husband of a patient). When I asked about the emotional outpouring that was a part of their presentation, however, they seemed ambivalent to me. On the one hand, they felt exhausted—drained by their presentation. "It really takes a toll," Yvette confided, but she also claimed that it was helpful for them in coming to terms with their experience.

I wondered, though, whether Yvette and Emil were being helped to get beyond their experience by reliving it in this way, or whether, like the Ancient Mariner of Coleridge's poem, they were compelled to keep reliving their story every time they told it. Also, I wondered what my role should be in this. Was I exploiting them to create a good learning environment for my students? Or was this performance-like testimonial a part of their healing process? The uneasiness I felt about this issue caused me to reconsider the question as to why people want to tell their stories of illness. I had published *Reconstructing Illness*, my study of autobiographies of illness, several years previously, and thought I understood what motivated people to write about their illness, to "publish" an experience of illness: but, now, I wondered how much I really understood.

I turned to trauma theory, where I found a wealth of information. My question as to why people "publish" their illnesses—whether orally or in writing—seemed to find an answer (or perhaps two answers) in the models of "therapy" and "testimony." Does a personal narrative about illness, intended for an audience of listeners or readers, serve as a way to "treat" illness, with the intent of getting past or "over" it? Put differently, is the primary motive self-healing? Or do these narratives serve as a kind of witness, testifying to the reality of the experience and all the feelings that went with it? A related question is, do these performative narratives help people get past their experience and incorporate it into their sense of self so they can get on with their lives? Or do such narratives serve to embed them even further in the experience, in the way that trauma victims often seem compelled to enact an experience over and over?

In thinking over these questions, I found the metaphoric substrate of both models to be helpful in itself. The root metaphor for therapy, or treatment, is medical, whereas the basic metaphor for testimony, or witnessing, is legal. Thus, the therapeutic model is based on the assumption that trauma is a wound or disease, whereas witnessing assumes that a traumatic experience violates some basic sense of right. In one model the victim of trauma is hurt; in the other the victim of trauma has been wronged. Both models can help survivors come to terms with traumatic experience, but the sense of injury in both these models has its psychological perils. All of us are familiar—in our own selves if not in others—with the narcissism of sickness: pain has a wonderful way of focusing one's attention on oneself. The therapeutic impulse to tell one's story can become narcissistic in this way. Similarly, the feeling of injustice can become an obsession that narrowly defines the sense of self in terms of having been wronged. Both these ways of dealing with trauma focus on the self, and both perpetuate the trauma they try to confront. These are the potential dark sides of the processes I call therapy and testimony.

Trauma Theory: Its History

It may help our understanding of trauma theory today to glance back at its history. Since the mid-eighteenth century, there have always been two parallel explanations of trauma: the organic and the psychological. In 1886, the British physician John Erichsen studied the "trauma syndrome" in individuals suffering from the fright of railway accidents: he attributed the problem to whiplash injuries and "railroad spine." In 1889, German neurologist Paul Oppenheim called this syndrome "traumatic neurosis," and ascribed it to some undiscovered neurological damage. On the other hand, as early as 1859, French psychiatrist Pierre Briquet found that individuals demonstrating symptoms of hysteria often suffered trauma during childhood. Jean-Martin Charcot, in the 1880s, had linked trauma with hysteria and treated both with hypnosis; Pierre Janet developed this approach further in his examination of the idea of trauma as a dissociative state (van der Kolk, Weisaeth, et al. 1996, 48–49; Leys 2000, 3–4). For Sigmund Freud, in his early years, the etiology of neurosis lay in childhood trauma (usually of a sexual nature). Later on, he determined that neurosis was caused by repressed fantasies of trauma rather than actual traumatic experience—a view that survived an unconscionably long time, into the 1970s.

In the United States, an early, and also neurobiological, version of trauma theory developed in conjunction with the treatment of Civil War wounded. Neurologist Silas Weir Mitchell took an interest in the condition of Civil War soldiers who displayed symptoms of what he then called "acute exhaustion," and later identified as a "neurosis" (1904, 368). Mitchell himself traced the source of his idea of the "Rest Treatment"— a therapeutic modality later used almost exclusively for neurasthenic, upper-class women—to his work with Civil War soldiers with neurological complaints (368).

Shell shock, or combat fatigue, was a major problem on both sides of the Atlantic in World War I and World War II. Though there were organicists who associated it with neurological or cardiac problems, trauma began increasingly to be perceived primarily as a wounding of the mind, rather than a lesion of the brain or nervous system. The treatment of choice in the U.S. and England was hypnosis and catharsis: repressed traumatic memories were uncovered, or brought to the surface, where they were "abreacted" and thus released. Treatment of soldiers suffering combat fatigue in World War II was based also on an approach drawn from early Freudian theory, though advances in pharmacology made a kind of drug-induced hypnosis and narcosynthesis possible, so that traumatic memories could be remembered and then abreacted (Leys 2000, 3–5; van der Kolk, Weisaeth, et al. 1996, 48–59).

Trauma theory developed and changed in the years after World War II. In the 1960s and 1970s (a surprisingly long time after the war ended), studies began to appear of the effects of the Holocaust on survivors and of the bombing of Hiroshima on Japanese civilians. In the 1980s, trauma theory began to reflect concern over sexual abuse and incest during childhood—which, increasingly, were coming to be seen as real experiences rather than as fantasies, as Freud had claimed—and with the concerns raised by the women's movement about the frequency of rape and spousal abuse. Indeed, there seems to have been a kind of "memory boom" in the 1980s, when remembering traumatic experience gained a certain level of cultural legitimacy. By 1990, trauma theory had been shaped and reshaped to include a variety of conditions and issues: these included the problems faced by returning veterans (this time from Vietnam) in rejoining mainstream society, the threat of biological warfare, the fact of genocide, the condition of people victimized by political torture and terrorism, and the problems of rape, spousal abuse, and violent and/or inappropriate sexual acts directed towards children.

When I began researching pathographies, it was the work of Robert J. Lifton, and his 1967 book about survivors of Hiroshima in particular, that I found most useful in helping me understand what goes on when people write books about their illnesses. I took two ideas, in particular, from Lifton. The first was his idea of "formulation"—the process by which trauma survivors recover (if they recover) from their experience. Lifton defines it as a kind of "psychic rebuilding," the construction of certain inner forms or configurations that function "as a bridge between self and world"—a psychological process whereby the individual suffering from trauma "returns" to the world of the living (1967, 367, 525). Formulation, for Lifton, involves the effort to re-establish three elements essential to psychic function: the sense of connection (between self and other), the sense of symbolic integrity (seeing one's life as meaningful), and the sense of movement (the capacity for change) (1967, 367).

Lifton's idea of formulation, I realized, was very close to the way many literary critics describe the autobiographical act. Autobiographical reconstruction, like formulation, is often described as a process of selective remembering, ordering those memories into a narrative form, and in so doing discovering—or imposing—meaning.

I am also indebted to Lifton for the way he emphasized the role of symbol, image, and metaphor in representing and coming to terms with traumatic experience. "The image," he writes, "is integral to human life. Its absence or breakdown threatens life" (1979, 38). The trauma survivor with impaired formulation retains an "indelible image" of the experience; "a tendency to cling to the death imprint." (1967, 482–83, 526; 1979, 170). The indelible image is extraordinarily compelling, and often felt to be qualitatively different than any other image or memory drawn from earlier or later life experience (1967, 482).

In researching pathographies, I had been struck by the extent to which authors use images and symbols, and even fully developed myths, to describe their experience. It occurred to me that, perhaps, the myth or image that served to enable people to recover from the trauma of their illness was the reverse of the "indelible image" that inhibited the recovery of Lifton's Hiroshima survivors. The myth of the journey, for example, enables some pathographers to perceive themselves, disoriented by the trauma of physical injury, as moving into a distant and strange country from which they would return to the ordinary world. So Oliver Sacks (1984), in his pathography about a leg injury, describes his recovery in spatial imagery consistent with the journey metaphor that dominates the pathography: each literal move to a new room or place is accompanied by an existential movement out of the contracted world of illness and into a new and wider dimension. Thus, early in the pathography, he characterizes his experience as a Dantean "journey of the soul ... to despair and back" (1984, 113). Later on, he sees his recovery as "a 'pilgrimage,' a journey, in which one moved ... stage by stage, or by stations" (1984, 160–61).

I believe that images and symbols, even in this present "age of narrative," are more important and more central than we may realize. For me, personally, media coverage of national and international events has emphasized the reality of Lifton's "indelible image." I find I am still haunted by the terrible photograph—one you all must have seen—of the Vietnamese child, a young girl, absolutely naked, running in terror from what was probably an explosion of napalm. I find a not dissimilar reaction to the terrible image of the World Trade Center as the plane flew right into it and the building exploded into flames, an image played and replayed hundreds and thousands of times on television. I should add that I was not traumatized by these images, and I realize that in no way did I "share" the trauma. However, I was deeply affected by them, and the way I was affected has shaped my sense of the purpose of my work.

Lifton's work was published in the 1960s and 1970s. Given the fact that what had been variously called war neurosis, shell shock, or combat fatigue was a recognizable condition affecting U.S. soldiers for more than a hundred years, it seems surprising that it was not until 1980 that the American Psychiatric Association officially acknowledged "Post-traumatic Stress Disorder" (PTSD) as a psychiatric condition in the *DSM-III* (*Diagnostic and Statistical Manual for Mental Disorders*, 3rd edition). The "historical moment" for this seems to have been our responsibility, as a nation, for the many disturbed and dysfunctional veterans who had returned from the Vietnam War. These young men seemed unharmed, psychologically, when they returned to their homes after the war; however, they began having trouble several years later. The initial psychiatric definition of PTSD reflects their condition, and includes a kind of latency period between the event and the appearance of symptoms.

Another aspect of the original, clinical description of PTSD, which has been discussed frequently in trauma scholarship, also deserves mention here. When first described in the *DSM-III* in 1980, PTSD was perceived as a response to an event that is "generally outside the range of usual human experience." Such experiences as "simple bereavement, chronic illness, business losses, or marital conflict" were excluded because they were considered "common experiences" (1980, 236). This definition of PTSD was repeated in the revised manual that came out in 1987, the *DSM-III-R* (1987, 247), but it continued to be the source of much controversy, especially with the discovery that child abuse, incest, and rape were not uncommon experiences. The phrase was dropped in 1994, with the publication of the *DSM-IV*, though the controversy as to what events are traumatogenic continues.

The omission of that important phrase, "generally outside the range of usual human experience," seems of great importance because it marks a cultural recognition of trauma as a part of normal human experience—as ordinary, not extraordinary. This decision both represents and legitimizes the present, widely inclusive, notion of what constitutes trauma. Ronnie Janoff-Bulman (1992) emphasizes that the key element in trauma is the loss of one's basic assumptions about the world, not the common symptoms of fear and anxiety. Jeffrey Kauffman, building on Janoff-Bulman's "assumptive world" thesis, points out that the difference between traumatic loss and non-traumatic loss "lies not in the nature of the event but in the nature of the experience," and the impact of that experience on the individual (2002, 205). Laura Brown (1995) offers a feminist perspective: alluding to the *DSM* definitions, she suggests that "all of those everyday, repetitive, interpersonal events that are so often the sources of psychic pain for women" be considered potential causes of trauma. (1995, 108). Suzette Henke extends the notion of trauma even further, observing that "trauma configures the parameters of modern life, as each of us is forced to endure a series of losses through the death of parents and loved ones, the disappearance of cherished friends, or the diminution of physical faculties through aging and illness" (2001, 40). Certainly, then, the category of trauma today includes conditions like sickness, loss, and grief that are, indeed, a part of ordinary human experience.

Contemporary Trauma Theory

The understanding of trauma and the treatment of trauma survivors has been remarkably consistent over the years in that it frequently consists of the same three stages—stabilization, processing, and integration—described by psychologist Pierre Janet in his work on hysteria early in the twentieth century (van der Kolk, van der Hart, et al. 1996, 319; Herman 1992, 155–56). According to Janet's dissociation theory, the traumatic experience is cut off from other parts of the self, resulting in a dissociative state, and the process of recovery requires an integration of traumatic memories. By this reasoning, people who develop problems after trauma are incapacitated not because of the traumatic experience itself, but because they are unable to integrate it into their consciousness of self, their ongoing lives, and their sense of reality. Trauma theorist Bessel van der Kolk is elaborating on Janet's theory of dissociation when he describes the way that traumatic memories are stored in the mind: "as sensory fragments that have no linguistic components ... [with] no verbal (explicit) component whatever ... as fragments of the sensory components of the event: as visual images; olfactory, auditory, or kinesthetic sensations." As people become more aware of those memories, he observes, "they construct a narrative that 'explains' what happened to them" (1996, 287–89).

Judith Herman, in *Trauma and Recovery*, a book based on her work with victims of sexual and domestic violence, indicates that her own, three-stage approach is indebted to Janet's work. She describes each of these stages, which she calls "safety," "remembrance and mourning," and "reconnection," at length (1992, 155–213). The first stage involves the identification of the problem; the second involves the work of reconstruction, delving into and confronting whatever remains in the psyche of the traumatic experience; and the third is that of integration, whereby the traumatic memory is integrated into the mind and life of the survivor. Herman's second stage, in which the individual "tells the story of the trauma," lends itself very well to pathography, as she describes in some detail the importance of reconstructing experience and of organizing an historical account of what happened (175–95). Herman's third stage emphasizes the restoration of human connections. There is a difference, though, between Herman's idea of the third stage and those of earlier trauma theorists, like Lifton. For Lifton, establishing connection is a psychological dynamic—it occurs between people. For Herman, establishing connection also has a political dimension whereby the larger community must take some action to recognize the trauma and repair the injury. This third stage for Herman is transformative, and often involves "discovering a meaning" in one's experience "that transcends the limits of personal tragedy" (73).

I have found that a number of contemporary trauma theorists working within Janet's three-stage formula sometimes emphasize narrative, and sometimes image. Lifton does both. His idea of formulation involves the creation of a narrative representation, but he is also very interested in "the indelible image" left by the traumatic experience. Herman sees traumatic memories as either non-verbal, involving "iconic" images or "frozen imagery and sensation"; or, if they involve a chronology of facts, as "prenarrative," leaving out the survivors' feelings and interpretations of what happened (1967, 175–77). Images are important, particularly during "unbearable moments" in constructing the narrative account, and at these times patients often turn to non-verbal forms of communication, such as drawing. Ultimately, however, the goal is "to put the story, including the imagery, into words"; into a narrative that includes facts as well as feelings (1967, 177). Herman's explanation privileges a narrative construct— and, ultimately, a narrative solution. She acknowledges non-verbal components—image and isolated sensations—but these are treated as "pre-narrative," to be identified in the first stage, woven into a coherent narrative in the second stage, and the resulting whole integrated into the ongoing sense of self and life in the third stage.

Since the mid-1990s, trauma theory has tended to de-emphasize stage models of recovery, focusing instead on individual (rather than universal) coping styles and on the ways human beings construct meaning out of experience (Neimeyer 1998; 2001); looking at cultural differences in the way individuals respond to trauma (Nader et al. 1999); and sometimes perceiving the very idea of recovery as problematic (Tal 1996). The latter is of particular importance for understanding pathography and illuminating the experience of Yvette and Emil in my classroom. Kalí Tal, in *Worlds of Hurt* (1996), attests to the impossibility of recovery from certain kinds of traumatic experience and to the value, both for the individual and for society, of providing testimony about it.

Tal treats the Nazi Holocaust as a "paradigm case … [a] precedent and yardstick to measure trauma in contemporary U.S. culture" (1996, 7, 8). It is from this position that she examines other kinds of traumatic events in the U.S., particularly the Vietnam War and sexualized violence against women and children. Tal is interested in the way a given culture interprets individual trauma and how these interpretations become tools for the construction of national and cultural myths. Her writings are helpful in understanding pathography in several ways.

First, she adopts the myth of recovery as a process only to explode it: for Tal, once one has been traumatized there is no return to "ordinary" life. "Trauma," she writes, "is a transformative experience, and those who are transformed can never entirely return to a state of previous innocence" (1996, 119). Second, though Tal's understanding of trauma is different in a number of ways from other writers, she similarly emphasizes the strong urge "to bear witness, to carry the tale of horror back to the halls of 'normalcy' and to testify to the people the truth of their experience" (120). Finally, Tal emphasizes the importance of images, metaphors, even mythologies in conveying traumatic experience, but she takes a decidedly pessimistic view of the possibility of recovery or even representation of the traumatic event. Trauma for her is essentially incommunicable, inexpressible—and thus to find language for it is a huge task, and here is where metaphor and image play an important role. "As it is spoken by survivors, the traumatic experience is reinscribed as a metaphor"(16). It seems to me that there is an interesting correlation between Tal's pessimism, her emphasis on image and symbol, and the way she downplays narrative, since the reconstruction of a trauma through creating a story is almost always seen as a part of the process of recovery.

Importantly, Tal, like Herman, sees the creation of a story to be told to others as not just something that benefits the trauma survivor, but something of benefit for the larger society, and observes that these authors believe that each of them is a storyteller with a mission; that their responsibility as survivors is to bear the tale. "Each one also affirms the process of storytelling as a personally reconstitutive act, and expresses the hope that it will also be a socially reconstitutive act. The whole point of testimony, she writes, is to "change the order of things as they are, and working to prevent the enactment of similar horrors in the future" (121).

Similar in some ways to Tal's thinking is the Yale school of psychoanalytic practitioners and scholars, perhaps best represented by Shoshana Felman and Dori Laub. Felman and Laub (1992) also base their ideas about trauma on the Nazi-generated Holocaust. Paradoxically, though asserting that the actual experience is incommunicable, they also emphasize the testimonial value of its representation. It is possible that the emphasis by writers like Felman and Laub on the idea of testimony, in a legal sense, derives from the concern with the need for widespread public recognition of the Holocaust. Narratives of trauma are thus "testimonials," never "confessions," so that the emphasis is on the truth-value of the narrative and the wrong done to the teller. Felman suggests, citing Elie Wiesel, that "testimony is the literary—or discursive—mode par excellence of our times, and that our era can precisely be defined as the age of testimony" (Wiesel, quoted in Felman and Laub, 1992, 5). The growing popularity of the term "testimony" for trauma narratives clearly reflects the legal world of courts and accusations, victims and judgments. Shoshana Felman acknowledges this, and both Tal and Herman imply this in their idea that resolution of traumatic injury involves some reparative act on the part of society.

Also, there are the trauma therapists who fall outside the medical and psychoanalytic paradigm, particularly those who would facilitate healing through writing. James Pennebaker is a psychologist who has conducted controlled clinical research on the therapeutic value of writing about traumatic experience. Pennebaker's claims are based on research demonstrating that "when people put their emotional upheavals into words, their physical and mental health improved markedly" (2000, 3). For Pennebaker, there is an inherent link between "building a narrative" and insight and understanding. He is somewhat vague about just what goes on in this connection between writing and recovery, but he has been able to document that in order for such writing to be felt as valuable for the author, it must involve both cognitive processing and the expression of emotion. An emotionless chronicle of events will not bring about a positive reaction for the author, nor will the venting of emotions without an attempt at understanding.

The research model of Pennebaker and others like him is problematic in its emphasis on measurement at the expense of other, important considerations. For example, these studies do not distinguish as much as they should between the act of writing and the act of writing for an audience. I certainly do not mean to discredit writing therapy: each year I supervise medical students who are involved in creative writing projects with patients, which are then published in our medical center's literary journal. Our patients seem to find both the act of writing and the fact of publication a positive, even healing, experience. I have come to believe, however, that the presence of the student and the possibility of an audience of readers are as much a factor in the patient's feeling that this was a helpful experience as the act of writing itself. Similarly, people who write pathographies about their experience of illness are not just writing for themselves, they are addressing an audience—even if only an imagined, future audience. Trauma theory tends to support this assumption, as it emphasizes witnessing *to* someone or giving testimony *for* an audience.

Trauma Theory and Pathography

There is a striking parallel between the gradual broadening of trauma theory to incorporate more and more conditions as traumatic, and the rapid growth and development of pathography as a genre, both trends which took place between 1980 and 2000. When I began researching my book about pathography in 1980, there were few published narratives about illness to be found at all. Moreover, the pathographies that were available then were mostly about cancer, heart attack, and stroke, with a few about disabilities. In general, people either died from their disease (in the case of biopathographies) or they recovered (in most autopathographies).

Not only did the number of pathographies multiply during this twenty-year interval, but the kinds of conditions that people were writing about changed. I examined this phenomenon closely when I prepared the second edition of my book in 1999, comparing the numbers of books published for particular disease categories between 1988 and 1992 to those published between 1993 and thereafter. I found that in recent years, though cancer remained a popular topic to write about, books about heart attack and stroke were much less prevalent. It seemed as though pathography had undergone a kind of paradigm shift, with acute illness displaced by chronic illnesses. I also found that people were writing much more about disabilities, both major and minor—conditions that one tends neither to recover from or die from. Increasingly, moreover, pathographies appeared about conditions that might not, earlier on, have been thought "serious" enough to justify an autobiography: stuttering, for example, or asthma (Jezer 1997, Brookes 1994, DeSalvo 1997). The revision in the *DSM-IV* (1994) of the parameters of PTSD to include ordinary experience as traumatogenic points to a cultural legitimization of a whole variety of experiences as potential causes.

Trauma theory and psychiatric definitions of PTSD are helpful in a number of ways in better understanding pathography. First, both the therapeutic and the testimonial models of trauma encourage the act of writing about one's illness. On the one hand, the orthodox treatment of PTSD, with its three stages, makes the narrative reconstruction of experience a therapeutic act that integrates dissociated memories of trauma into a sense of the ongoing self. The role that various kinds of iconic expressions such as image, metaphor, and symbol play in "storing" and encoding traumatic experience explains why these should be so prominent features of pathographical writing. On the other hand, the motive to testify to one's experience—often taking place as a ritual action—emphasizes the truth value and the factual nature of autobiographies about illness. Though allowing that they are constructed and not remembered narratives, trauma theorists would stress the factual over the fictive dimension. This emphasis on the factual nature of testimony reflects our cultural preoccupation with the authority of personal experience. Perhaps, then, autobiographies about illness or trauma have achieved a validity and an authenticity that is in part a reflection of the way we in our culture privilege personal narrative.

Second, the general agreement among theorists on the need for human connection in recovering from trauma encourages writing about one's illness experience. Lifton discusses "the sense of connection" as an essential element of psychic function, but he sees this as only one of several essential elements, which include "connection with non-human elements" as well as "connection to other human beings." (1967, 367). Subsequent scholars have placed more emphasis than Lifton did on the primacy of the need for human connectedness in recovering from trauma. Tal observes that "the survivor's perception of community is a crucial element in the shaping of her new myth" (1996, 125), and Herman concurs: "Sharing the traumatic experience with others is a precondition for the restitution of a sense of a meaningful world" (1992, 70).

Pathography supports the primacy of human connection in coming to terms with illness. People write about their experience of illness because they expect to find readers. It does not matter that they do not know who the reader is and will not (in most cases) find out what his or her response was to their book—they write so that others will read what they wrote. In the simplest terms, this is a way of establishing connection with the larger human community. As author Kenneth Shapiro observes, "I exist in the world as most people see it, but I live in the world of the person with terminal cancer" (1985, 130). Other pathographies are written as testimonies with the ultimate aim of bringing about institutional and cultural change. Many authors are critical of the medical establishment: Jory Graham deplores "the inhospitability of hospitals" (1982, 18); Esther Goshen-Gottstein observes, "We are all reared to believe in the efficacy of the medical profession, so the realization that the doctors could contribute absolutely nothing to Moshe's recovery came as a total shock" (1990, 12). Others see their illness as a product of environmental toxicity, so Fran Peavey writes about AIDS as the result of "a world of chemistry and radiation and pollution that our bodies are telling us we can no longer tolerate" (1990, 43). What happens in many pathographies is that the intent to "tell" others becomes the wish to "help" others. As Bernice Kavinoky remarks about her illness narrative, "I wrote it originally for myself, because it clarified my thinking and emotions. Then I began to ponder over it and felt perhaps it was for everybody—not only those who had my operation but everyone who had been through an experience of shock and loss, and who had eventually—after the flying of flags and lifting of the chin—to face it, in his own waiting room, alone" (1966, 71–72).

Third, recent trauma theory emphasizes the way in which personal recovery is frequently linked with political or social action. Indeed, this seems an extension of the emphasis on human connectedness in the way people deal with traumatic experience, and the activist dimension of recovery may be a function of the broadening of what constitutes trauma. If we all have experienced trauma to a greater or a lesser degree, we can all take part in a sense of community based on the mutual need to give and to receive. Herman writes about the way the phase of reconnection can extend for some into finding a survivor mission. "A significant minority [of trauma survivors]" she observes, "recognize a political or religious dimension in their misfortune and discover that they can transform the meaning of their personal tragedy by making it the basis for social action" (1992, 207). Tal writes about how survivors of trauma can believe "that he or she is a storyteller with a mission ... [affirming] the process of storytelling as a personally reconstitutive act, and [expressing] the hope that it will also be a socially reconstitutive act" (1996, 121).

Pathography demonstrates the frequency with which authors go on beyond their illness story to become engaged in social action of one kind or another. Augusta Hicks Gale, an African-American woman with breast cancer, not only wrote a book about her experience but also became involved in a movement called Advocacy-for-Empowerment for breast cancer patients, and then went on to get a degree in health care administration in order to educate others about medical issues. Dennis Kaye wrote a pathography about living with ALS (amyotrophic lateral sclerosis); he also instituted an advocacy organization to bring together persons with this disease. Of course, not all survivors survive their illnesses, like poet Audre Lorde. In her essay "A Burst of Light," she described how she confronted the recurrence of her cancer by using alternative therapy (it didn't work) and also by continuing the political work in the United States and South Africa that was so important to her. Lorde employed visualization exercises to bring these two causes—the political and the medical—together, visualizing the disease process in political images. For her, cancer, racism, and apartheid were similar in that they are all destructive processes that must be combated by any and all means (1988, 133).

Conclusion

In closing, I'd like to return to Yvette and Emil, the couple I mentioned at the beginning of my talk who wanted to tell their story to medical students. I have kept in touch with Yvette over the years. She is a woman with lots of energy and lots of ideas, and has been able to continue to teach our students in various ways. Her recent and latest venture is an extension of the set of poems she wrote for medical students, which certainly is appropriate to "the need to find a mission" that Herman and Tal have found in many of the trauma survivors they write about. Yvette has undertaken a collective project along with other women in our hospital's breast cancer support group, with a book called *Show Me* (Breast Cancer Support Group, 2001) that is beginning to receive national recognition. The book consists of photographs of the women in the breast cancer group after mastectomy and, in some cases, after breast reconstruction. *Show Me* is intended for women diagnosed with breast cancer whose physicians recommend mastectomy: these are women who must make a sudden decision as to what to do, and who would benefit from being able to see what it would look like to have various kinds of breast reconstruction, or no reconstruction at all. *Show Me* is a picture book of whole body views—these views include faces, and on all the faces there are smiles. In this case, what might be an "indelible image" has been transformed into a liberating one.

In very different ways, I've learned a great deal from Yvette and from trauma theorists about the motives and function of pathography. They've taught me that the medical and legal models for trauma and recovery that I call "therapy" and "testimony" are not without their psychological risk. Either can so fixate and imprison the survivor in the trauma that it is so much survived as it is perpetuated. Perhaps this is a difference between victims and survivors: victims are not just those who repress or deny traumatic experience but also those who seem to become it, rather than assimilating it into an ongoing sense of self. I've also learned that neither treatment nor testimony ever can fully achieve its goal—healing, in the case of therapy, or witnessing, in the case of testimony. With neither model is there a total and final cure or reparation: survivors of trauma are never able totally to put the experience behind them and move on in life as though it didn't happen. Finally, I've learned to value the importance of human connectedness in recovering from traumatic experience even more. It is this exchange—and I do believe that it goes both ways, the act of telling and the act of listening—that creates the sense of human community needed to turn trauma victims into trauma survivors.

BARBARA SCHNEIDER

Constructing a "Schizophrenic" Identity

Schizophrenia is one of the more incomprehensible conditions to afflict mankind. It is hard to express just how cruel and tragic schizophrenia is for both individuals and their families. It is estimated to affect approximately 1 per cent of the population (Torrey 2001) and occurs in normal, intelligent people from all walks of life. It occurs in every society and culture, and some observers believe it has been part of the human condition since ancient times (e.g., Shorter 1997).

There have been a number of ways of talking about schizophrenia over the centuries: individuals were thought to be possessed by the devil or be in the grip of mysterious powers. Now, of course, we no longer think of the devil when we think of madness, but over the course of the twentieth century, there have been a number of ways of viewing schizophrenia: as a result of unconscious conflicts; as a creative response to an untenable family situation; as a sane response to an insane world; as a result of poor parenting or schizophrenogenic mothers; as a response to being labelled; and so on (e.g., Laing 1969; Szasz 1972; Scheff 1975). Now, in the early part of the twenty-first century, the medical version of schizophrenia as a brain illness, "a broken brain" (Andreason 1984), has become the dominant, perhaps the only available, discourse for understanding schizophrenia. Certainly the medical discourse is hegemonic. Edward Shorter (1997), in his history of psychiatry, describes the biological approach—"treating mental illness as a genetically influenced disorder of brain chemistry"—as a "smashing success" (vii).

In this essay, I examine the personal narratives of people with schizophrenia to show how people who have been diagnosed with schizophrenia use this medical discourse as a resource in the construction of identity. Although the medical discourse for understanding schizophrenia is, for all practical purposes, the only one available, and it would seem that individuals have very little choice in taking it up as a way to understand themselves and their behaviour, this is, nevertheless, something that people actively do, rather than something that just happens to them. It is this active process of taking up medical discourse to describe experience that I examine here. I begin by outlining my theoretical approach to understanding how identity is constructed in personal narratives, and then examine extracts from interviews I conducted with people with schizophrenia to illustrate how medical discourse is both taken up and resisted in the narrative construction of a "schizophrenic" identity.

Narrative Practice and Identity

Identity is an extremely complex construct that has been defined in a number of different ways in a variety of literatures (see Holstein and Gubrium [2000], and Widdicombe [1998], for detailed discussions). Here, I shall draw on a view of identity as something that is narratively constructed and communicated (Chase 2005; Daiute and Lightfoot 2004; Holstein and Gubrium 2000). As George Rosenwald and Richard Ochberg observe, "Personal stories are not merely a way of telling someone (or oneself) about one's life; they are the means by which identities may be fashioned" (1992, 1). Jaber Gubrium and James Holstein's (1998) notion of narrative practice elaborates this active process of identity construction and its relation to the social circumstances in which particular stories are told. They use the term "narrative practice" to "characterize simultaneously the activities of storytelling, the resources used to tell the stories, and the auspices under which stories are told" (164). In this view, narratives are not simply reports of "the facts" of past or present experience. Rather, they are artful, situated constructions assembled to describe and constitute, or ascribe meaning to, experience in particular ways. In an "interplay of discursive actions and the circumstances of storytelling" (Gubrium and Holstein 1998, 164), storytellers select those aspects of experience that are relevant to a particular circumstance of storytelling and to the construction of a particular identity from a vast memory storehouse of life events.

Personal narratives, however, are not simply individual productions; rather, they are, as Catherine Kohler Riessman puts it, "both an individual and a social product" (1992, 232). Stories are mediated and constrained by the local and institutional circumstances of the storytelling and by available social and cultural resources, which people draw on to shape their stories, and their identities, in particular ways. Andrew Giddens (1991) uses the term "institutional reflexivity" to refer to the way in which what he calls abstract, or expert, systems provide people with material from which to construct identities. Individuals appropriate expert discourses to describe their own experience, a process he calls "reskilling" (7). For Giddens, to live in the context of institutional reflexivity is to actively engage in this filtering of expert knowledge into daily life. A diagnosis of schizophrenia provides an expert discourse that allows, and in fact requires, people to "redefine their past, present, and future in illness terms" (Karp 1996, 63), using expert knowledge as a framework for the narrative construction of a "schizophrenic" identity. Giddens (1991) also points out that the way in which people take up medical discourse works back into the abstract system of expert knowledge, in turn reshaping it, although an examination of this process is beyond the scope of this essay.

Although the expert discourse provides a resource for interpreting experience, as both Giddens (1991) and Gubrium and Holstein (1998) point out, neither medical discourse nor local and institutional circumstances determine how individuals will construct identity. Rather, all of these provide narrative resources, and possibilities for who the self can be, that are actively taken up by individuals in diverse ways through interpretive practice. There is no doubt that the medical version of schizophrenia is a powerful discourse that limits the possibilities for self construction by exerting a strong degree of narrative control over those to whom it is applied. In framing their own experiences in the language and understanding of medical discourse, individuals reproduce and reinforce that discourse as an appropriate resource for understanding themselves. Nevertheless, within the limitations imposed by the discourse, individuals engage in interpretive activity and make choices about how and to what degree they will take up or resist the discourse.

In the next section, I will examine this interpretive activity in the construction of "schizophrenic" selves in the narratives of four people with schizophrenia. The narratives presented here were collected during a research project in which I conducted unstructured interviews with people with schizophrenia. The interviews were taped and later transcribed. Participants ranged in age from eighteen to about fifty-five. All had been diagnosed with schizophrenia and were taking medication to control their psychotic symptoms. With the exception of the eighteen-year-old, who still lived with her parents, all the participants lived independently, with some working part-time or attending school.

I will look at three ways in which the speakers in these narratives draw on the resources provided by the medical discourse of schizophrenia to construct identity. The first two of these have to do with how the interviewees adopt medical language to describe their experiences, or what Giddens (1991) would call "reskilling": the acquisition of medical knowledge about schizophrenia, and the reconstruction of past experience in terms of this medical knowledge. These actions are closely related, although not exactly the same, and because they are difficult to separate in the narratives, I have combined them in the analysis. I then look at how interviewees resist the application of the medical discourse of schizophrenia to themselves. In my analysis, I show the narrative construction of identity in action.

Adopting Medical Language to Describe Experience

In the following excerpts, we can see medical language being used and medical knowledge being displayed as the speakers talk about their illness. In addition, we can see the way in which past experience or behaviour is actively reconstructed in light of knowledge provided by the medical version of schizophrenia. What once was a certain kind of experience and identity is now understood as another kind of experience and identity. Donald (in response to a question about what he tells people schizophrenia is) says:

> Yes, it's a mental illness, a biochemical brain disorder with too much dopamine, and serotonin inhibitors are out of control. And then I would tell them that I have delusions, I have delusions and paranoia, but I never hear the voices or those things ... I thought I did awful things, which I know I didn't do now, but definitely at the time I thought I did awful things ... Those delusions have been absent for about two years now.

Donald uses a medical vocabulary of dopamine and serotonin to describe schizophrenia as a biochemical brain disorder. He also talks of delusions, paranoia, and hearing voices. This is a vocabulary that many people will recognize in relation to schizophrenia and readers in an action attesting to the power and hegemony of the medical view of the disease, might well ask if there is any other way to describe the symptoms of schizophrenia. From the point of view of people who are in the grip of schizophrenia, however, their experiences, perceptions, and understandings of the world are real. Donald thought he did "awful things." He did not in fact do these things, but at the time he believed that he really had done them. Having been told, presumably by his medical practitioners, that they were not real, he has now learned to use medical vocabulary to describe these apparently real experiences as delusions and himself as a person who once had delusions. In a later excerpt, Donald again redefines past experience:

> When I was young, in college, I thought people thought I was really stupid because I couldn't—chemistry experiments, physics experiments—I couldn't do them because I was so slow and weighing things on scales and stuff like that. I couldn't think it over because I got so nervous with people watching me, you know. I think people thought I was stupid, which I wasn't. It was the illness.

In the previous excerpt, Donald described experiences that he now knows were not real. Here, he describes what he regards as real experiences, in which others, and perhaps he himself, thought he was slow and stupid. He had trouble doing lab experiments in university science classes and got nervous if people were watching him. Now he sees these experiences in a different light: it wasn't that he was stupid, it was that he had schizophrenia. His narrative presents a person who once had certain kinds of thoughts about himself and told a certain kind of story about himself, but now has incorporated medical knowledge of schizophrenia into his personal biography to tell a quite different story. He now presents an identity as a person with schizophrenia rather than as a stupid person, and, clearly, he prefers to be a person with schizophrenia. He uses medical discourse to legitimate his incompetence in the chemistry lab by describing it as a result of an illness, something that is clearly not his fault. He also seeks to establish his current competence as a person by demonstrating his understanding and acceptance of the medical version of his experiences, using medical discourse to assign "reality" to some but not other experiences and perceptions.

In this excerpt, Marie presents a veritable lecture about the involvement of the thalamus in schizophrenia:

> My perceptions are all different because the thalamus—do you know the brain is constructed to create this, the symptoms?... Well the thalamus generally is smaller. The thalamus is the relay center for all the perceptual experiences. So our thalamus, people with schizophrenia, the thalamus gets overwhelmed at times by the influx of perceptual experiences, which gets translated, because it can't take all the information in, it obscures it and it gets translated into these symptoms.

We can see that Marie has incorporated medical knowledge into her resources for understanding herself. She is a person who has symptoms of schizophrenia because her thalamus gets overwhelmed by perceptual experiences. In the next excerpt, we see her actively using this knowledge to understand and redefine her perceptual experiences:

> I also know that when these things called delusions are occurring in my mind, I can kind of separate myself from it. And if I can voice at some point, "This is too bizarre. Even though it seems very real, it's probably a delusion," you know, it's more manageable.

She has experiences that seem quite real to her, but she now knows that some of her experiences are "delusions," caused by an abnormality of brain function. When she has certain kinds of bizarre thoughts or experiences, she now actively defines them as delusions and "separates" herself from them, allowing her to manage these experiences and not let them interfere with her life. She is no longer a person who can rely on her thoughts to be "real" (at least some of the time); she is someone who can identify thoughts as delusions, and thereby manage them.

In the next excerpt, Luanne describes the moment in which she redefined herself. Describing some pamphlets on schizophrenia she read, she says:

> I remember feeling that way or thinking that way [referring to what she read], so that must have been part of it. Because I never realized how many symptoms I had, you know. I thought it was just that I heard this voice. But reading over the negative and positive symptoms, whoa, I had this and I had this, and those.

Before reading the pamphlets about schizophrenia, Luanne thought of herself as a person who heard a voice. Then she read the pamphlets, and suddenly aspects of herself that she had previously thought of as personal characteristics became symptoms of schizophrenia. In the time it took to read the pamphlets, she went from being a person who heard a voice to being someone whose personality and life experience were in large part symptoms of schizophrenia. She constructs her present schizophrenic self from what the pamphlet directs her to notice in her biographical history.

Taking on an identity as a person who has an illness is very useful for people with schizophrenia. Many have strange and frightening perceptual experiences and often engage in quite bizarre and anti-social behaviour. At the very least, their behaviour is different than it was before and this is usually very troubling for them and those around them. Using medical discourse to describe this behaviour helps both people with schizophrenia and those around them to make some kind of sense of these experiences and behaviour. As well, socially unacceptable behaviour for which individuals would normally be held morally accountable is now redefined in terms of an illness over which they have no control. From the point of view of the medical community, getting people to take up the medical discourse and agree that they have schizophrenia is seen as an important step in helping them to get better. One of the hallmarks of schizophrenia is that people insist, in the face of their increasingly bizarre behaviour, that there is nothing wrong with them. It is only if people agree that they have an illness that they will participate in (or, in medical terms, comply with) treatment, which in the case of schizophrenia mainly consists of massive doses of extremely heavy sedatives, which sometimes have very troubling side effects. The construction of schizophrenic selves may be seen to serve the interests of individuals themselves, the medical community, and society at large, but that does not mean that it happens automatically. In all of the excerpts presented so far, the speakers are people who actively participated in learning to present various aspects of their biographical history in the medical language of schizophrenia. In the next excerpts, the speakers actively resist medical discourse as a resource for identity construction.

CONTESTING THE MEDICAL DISCOURSE OF SCHIZOPHRENIA

Throughout our interview, the next speaker, Jane, had demonstrated her ability to use medical language to describe herself. At one point she also said: "Yeah, I had a breakdown. I was diagnosed as a schizophrenic. I don't feel very schizophrenic even though I know what schizophrenia is." Jane knows what schizophrenia "is," according to the medical discourse, and she knows that the medical profession applies this label to her, but she confides that she still does not "feel very schizophrenic." A psychiatrist listening to this statement would probably regard this as evidence that she does indeed have schizophrenia, because, as noted above, one of the signs of the illness is denial that there is any problem. However, Jane's assertion can also be understood as a statement that she is not willing to give herself over to the medical version of herself, and reserves the right and ability to define herself in terms other than those offered by medical discourse. Here, Jane is resisting the totalizing power of the medical version of schizophrenia; perhaps she is doing so only in her mind, and privately to me, but she resists none the less.

In the next excerpt, we see Marie actively and explicitly resisting what she understands as the medical discourse of schizophrenia, drawing instead on what she regards as a more productive discourse in the construction of her identity:

> When I first went into the mental health system, when I was nineteen, I was told by a psychiatrist that I would never go to school, I would never work a job. Basically I would never live in the real world ... Hearing that kind of information, it dispelled a lot of my hopes for a normal future. It was debilitating, actually ... The focus on the sick model as opposed to the able model is creating a lot of self-perceptions that the person is sick. That's what I learned in community rehabilitation [a course she took at university] ... That a disability is uniqueness, and you're not broken, you do not need to be fixed ... They have a philosophy of self-actualization, how can a person become all they can be. Now that's not the focus with mental illness. The focus is on the problem. When you focus on the problem, then the person internalizes that they are a problem. They are ill. They are sick...
>
> So now I find it's very fundamental to think of schizophrenia not as a problem ... I don't want to see myself as a problem. I want to see myself as somebody who is not unusual or bizarre, [but] as somebody who is unique ... By removing myself from that identification, I know I have schizophrenia but I'm not going to consider myself as sick in the mind, I'm not going to make it a fundamental aspect of who I am. By doing that I think I'm going to develop and grow and integrate into this society more competitively than I would if I would be dependent on the system. That's a fact.

In this stretch of talk, we can see Marie doing very explicit identity work. She does not deny that she has schizophrenia, which, as noted above, is a dangerous move for someone who has been identified as having it. Rather, she delicately negotiates her relationship to the medical version of schizophrenia. She identifies it as a way of talking about the self and contrasts it with other ways of talking about the self. She rejects the "sick" model for understanding schizophrenia and herself, selecting instead aspects of what she regards as an alternate model and discourse, the "able" model of disability discourse, as a resource for the construction of her identity. She regards herself as unique rather than sick or a problem, and believes that this will help her to be successful in integrating into society. In her narrative we can see how much autonomy individuals can have in calling on various resources for self construction, and just how active this process is.

Conclusion

While larger cultural discourses—in this case medical discourse—are very powerful resources for identity construction, my research and analysis has shown that neither biographical particulars nor available discourses determine the self. People engage in what Holstein and Gubrium call "biographical work," in which they "assemble aspects of personal history that can be used to bolster present claims of and about" themselves (2000, 169). Details of lives are "mobilized to become part of local-selves in-the-making" (169). This is quite an ordinary process, something most people all do all the time, and even though it seems that people with schizophrenia may have little choice in taking up a "schizophrenic" identity, it nevertheless is something they actively do, not just something that happens to them. Receiving a diagnosis of schizophrenia does not mean that an individual must adopt a particular "schizophrenic" identity. Rather, both available discourses and past and present experience provide a set of resources that individuals actively take up in various ways in the narrative construction of distinctive "schizophrenic" selves.

While schizophrenia is a biological illness, it is also very much a social phenomenon. I believe that understanding identity in the way that I have illustrated has implications for how schizophrenia is understood generally in society. In closing, I want to refer to the other half of Giddens' (1991) ideas about reskilling, which were beyond the scope of this chapter to examine in detail: that changed social environments work back into expert systems, in turn, changing them. As Giddens shows us, it matters how we take up the expert discourse, how we talk about schizophrenia generally, and what kinds of stories we tell when we talk to and about people with schizophrenia, because personal narratives feed back into that expert discourse, influencing and shaping it. Change in the expert discourse then affects how schizophrenia will be understood in future talk about it. This means that we have the potential to change how schizophrenia is understood generally in society, and thereby to change the resources that are available to people with schizophrenia in constructing identity. As Marie so eloquently shows us, this opens a powerful possibility to "provide those with schizophrenia better opportunities to participate more meaningfully and inclusively in the social world" (Doubt 1996, xi).

LOURDES RODRIGUEZ DEL BARRIO

Space, Temporality, and Subjectivity in a Narrative of Psychotic Experience

The life histories of people who find themselves in need of psychiatric care are often marked not only by difficult living conditions and violence but also by limitations that stem from an inner world troubled by psychotic experience. This experience of psychosis has a direct effect on their experience of self: their personal sense of emotional and cognitive integration, their relationships with others, their connection to their bodies, and their perception of reality. It destabilizes the everyday signposts of body, identity, society, and culture, and thereby compromises the fundamental parameters of the subject.

The terms developed to describe this experience, and the practices designed to help psychosis sufferers face it, have many pitfalls. Whether one uses terms such as "madness," "mental illness," or "mental health problem" or diagnoses such as "psychosis" or "schizophrenia," these words all belong to and reflect the theories and practices of the historical and socio-cultural context upon which they are based. Such terms—and the practices that go along with them—come from attempts to understand, make sense of, cope with, and master experiences that come up against suffering, the unknown, and the strange. However, these terms are also a source of pain, exclusion, reclusion, incomprehension, and various forms of violence, and shut out the voices of the people most directly concerned (Rodriguez 2000).

This paper will delve deeply into the process of listening to psychosis with a phenomenological ear (Binswager 1971; Blankenburg 1991; Corin 1990; 1998), a process that takes into consideration the complex web of links between people, society, and culture through the mediation of language. By analyzing the life history of a psychosis sufferer, whom I will call "Francis," I will study the modes of speech used to create a personal discourse and recreate the psychotic experience within the social and cultural context that forms, provokes, reinforces, or allows that experience to be reconfigured after the fact, always from Francis's point of view.

The Life History and the Socio-cultural World

In this context, the life history becomes the fundamental mediator for understanding and accounting for the processes of "subjectivation" (Rodriguez 2000). The notion of subjectivity refers to a person who is able to think of himself as an effective being whose actions have an impact on the rest of the world. In contemporary hermeneutic, phenomenological, and critical circles, the personal narrative is considered an indispensable form of mediation among the dynamics that allow for self-constitution (Ricoeur 1985, 1990; Foucault 1994; Habermas 1995). It allows the subject to emerge, imagine potential avenues, and choose from among the weave of various elements that make up his experience (desires, events, circles, etc.).

The text of Francis's history illustrates a clash between two types of discourse that differ in the emphasis they place on temporality and on the flow of action. The first type is narrative discourse, in the sense that the events and actions in his account are articulated according to when they occurred. Despite a multiplicity of densely interwoven scenes, a single linear account can be established by reorganizing the events chronologically and identifying the evolution of one or several initial events toward a final situation. This timeline—or *fabula*—is an essential part of any narrative (Eco 1996). The text of Francis's account, which organizes events and actions according to their temporal positions, would seem to be in conflict with another form of discourse in which the articulate element is "space." In general, the description of places within an account moves the action ahead or specifies its context. However, in Francis's account, these descriptions shape the discourse itself, as though the important thing was both to describe the spaces he associates with "impressions," states, and moods and to establish the borders of these spaces (or between different spaces), rather than simply relating a personal history through a chronological series of events and experiences. Using broad strokes, I will use the "conflict" between these two forms of discourse to reveal the content of Francis's account. In the first section, I will try to reconstruct the *fabula* and the narrative's temporal "rhythm." Next, I will deal with the impressions that emerge from a semantic analysis of the text's articulated meanings but that defy narrative logic. Finally, I will show how these two readings of the text help us to understand the roles played in his life history by the various institutions and socio-cultural practices to which Francis had access or consulted.

Temporality and the Life History: The *Fabula*

Francis builds his narrative by recounting anecdotes and scenes that overlap in time. He often comes back to an episode to provide further details, trying to explain his difficulties and experiences. His account contains many attempts to situate events and actions in time and to find the initial appearance of the fear and troubling experiences that he has come to name "psychosis" and "illness."

Reference Points

This is the story of a thirty-year-old man who, since the age of seventeen, has spent long periods of time in psychiatric care. For him, his problems began with a "street fight" he had when he was thirteen years old. A "gang of bikers" attacked him in an alley, and, ever since then, he has had "fears" that confine him to his home. While discussing the origins of his strange behaviours with his brother, Francis learned at the age of seventeen that he was schizophrenic. While the word "schizophrenia" gave a name to Francis's state of fear and isolation, the diagnosis transformed the meaning of this state, assigning him an identity that made it impossible for him to imagine a "normal life" (i.e., having a job, a family, etc.) or "getting better." Francis viewed the diagnosis of schizophrenia as something coming from the outside—as a transferral to him of a strange identity that he kept at a distance. Even today, after twenty years in the psychiatric system, he doubts the validity of this diagnosis. The battles, the fears, the schizophrenia, and the "psychiatry" make Francis feel abandoned, all alone, "on the street"—lost in the threatening world he has become part of.

"The accident"

At the beginning of his narrative, Francis speaks mysteriously of a particular event, to which he returns several times to add details. However, he does not refer to this experience as an episode but, rather, as "the accident." It is only much later in the account that Francis reveals the true nature of this "accident."

After a long period of isolation, when he once again found himself "all alone," Francis lost all contact with reality, stopped paying his bills, stopped eating, and stayed indoors all day. At this point, Francis was twenty years old. In a moment of great despair and panic, and after several failed attempts to get help, he seriously mutilated himself. After the "accident," the fears that Francis had experienced since the age of thirteen increased significantly: "I was in the hospital every three months; they increased my pills."

Over a period of more than ten years, there seems to have been a succession of episodes and hospitalizations. During this long period, Francis accessed resources in the mental-health services network such as a psychologist, a centre for agoraphobics, community crisis centres, and alternative mental-health resources with a critical view of psychiatry.

The World of Impressions

Highlighting the various scenes that make up the *fabula* of Francis's account has familiarized us with him enough to approach other possible readings of his story. The account is studded with descriptions and impressions that lead to a different logic than that of the narrative—a logic in which time becomes so heavy and dense that it seems to stop entirely. Thus the text becomes a description of places and people, descriptions that seem to break down the story rather than advance it.

Francis's account is constantly interrupted by attempts to explain his problems by means other than telling a story or referring to past events, and his discourse prioritizes metaphors: *street*, *holes*, and *gardens*. The doorway into this world is one of "impressions." Both the events and actions of Francis's life and socio-cultural resources such as institutions, families, and help networks take on a new light depending on the relationship he has with these powerful symbols. Thus, his *psychotic episodes* seem like attempts to break through the boundaries of the "street" world, dominated by emptiness, a lack of vitality and contact with other people, and violence. Certain institutions and practices would appear to strengthen this world, while others help Francis find support and build a new space of calm and relative well-being.

Metaphors of Strangeness: The Street and Gardens

The "street" is a central metaphor in Francis's text, one in which several paradoxical meanings overlap. It is a place of violence, abandonment, solitude, and survival, where a lack of stimuli means he cannot fully experience life. He uses "the street" as a metaphor for evil, and as an experience of excess and extreme loss. "I believe that evil exists in society and in life," Francis says clearly, toward the end of the account. On the "street," however, evil has several faces. It is a violent place, one of "wars" and "battles."

Francis describes more of his experiences with violence as his account continues. In addition to the physical violence that has scarred his body, he also underwent another, more subtle, form of violence that consisted of people "blocking" his way. This feeling of being blocked, in his narrative, leads to a loss of control and panic. Eventually, the threat of being blocked becomes increasingly anonymous, more blurred, until it reappears toward the end of the account. There it is associated with his self-mutilation, as Francis says he cut himself to release something. When the "accident" happened, the threatening characters predominant in previous scenes were not present; rather, there was a feeling of isolation, loss of identity, emptiness, and abandonment.

At several points in the narrative, the street appears as a place of abandonment, and represents the feeling of not knowing where to go, of not having one's own place: "At first, there weren't any mental health resources for me, so I was like put on the street, and when I was scared, I was on the street." The street is also associated with a sort of solitude other than that produced by "abandonment": the solitude created by a lack of stimuli. Being alone also means no longer having feelings or desires (especially sexual desire). For Francis, the worst thing is not the violence that harms both his body and his ego integrity. He uses the word "hell" rarely, but when he does, it is associated with a lack of stimuli—with the form of solitude he relates to a feeling of isolation and loss of vitality, libido, and connection with the world. This experience of "non-life" seems more terrifying to him than physical injury: "You need your feelings to live too; it's important to have feelings and sensations, to not be completely alone [...] at one point, you no longer have sex. It's hell; you're on the street."

Several times, Francis refers to an image of a garden, a symbol which contrasts with the world of the street described above. The garden is a bright image, "where there are fountains" and people stroll about. However, the brightness of the garden is ambiguous; it is a metaphor for happiness but it also represents the danger of the psychotic episode and of excessive vitality. Gardens are linked with his most significant episode—Francis's self-mutilation occurred after moving into a place with gardens nearby, and the hope for well-being seen in gardens is associated with the impressions and fear of "being psychotic": "When I'm excited, it seems as though, in the spring ... I get all excited ... I end up in the hospital." In its most positive expression, the garden symbol is associated with nature and a habitable space that exists far from the "street." For some time now, Francis has avoided the places where he has had trouble and is slowly establishing a less threatening and dangerous space, symbolized by the garden.

The garden image can be understood as a signifier running through the text that stands in opposition to the signifier of the street, the emblem of a threatening "outside world." This outside world—with its impressions that threaten the "bright" and ambiguous opening that the garden image seems to represent—is "always there."

Spaces and Practices of Exclusion and Support

Francis's life history makes reference to a supra-narrative world—to a social context historically created by institutions and social practices. Indeed, the relationship between Francis's account and this context goes beyond that of the referential. Uncovering the subjective meaning of the practices, resources, and socio-cultural discourse with which Francis was confronted will transform our understanding of what happens to him, his relationship with himself, and what the future holds for him.

We can identify certain social spaces in the narrative (institutions, practices, discourses) and the specific panorama of experiences, expectations, and projects that each space makes possible: his family, bad places or company, psychiatric institutions, alternative mental-health resources, an agoraphobia group, psychologists, etc. Francis also identifies a "space" he feels excluded from, which includes work, friends, love, and being a "normal" part of society: what he calls "real life." In particular, we can ask what signifiers he associates with the resources, institutions, and practices that are specifically targeted to psychosis sufferers. I will now illustrate the signifiers associated with each of the potential "spaces of assistance" that appear in Francis's account.

Francis's hospital experience has much in common with that of the "street," and he refers to being hospitalized in several anecdotes where he highlights acts of aggression and violence he suffered while in hospital. He often associates the space opened by his diagnosis of psychosis and hospitalization with feelings of abandonment—of being "dumped in the street." To him, the experience of hospitalization is almost like the threat of death: it is a place where time seems to stand still. As a result, Francis fears being forced to go back to the hospital "for the rest of his days" and takes action to avoid this fate because "I knew some people who were miserable in 'psychiatry.' I'm scared of ending my days in a psychiatric institution."

This feeling of not living life fully is associated particularly with psychiatric medication. Medication "flattens" life because, among other things, it reduces sexual desire, and sensations, moods, and desires are all "regulated" by the schedule of the medication. Psychotropic drugs artificially provoke stimulation, which is why Francis associates medication with a lack of spontaneous sensation, which is itself associated with a feeling of extreme solitude—a lack of contact with other people. "It's important to not be stimulated only by medication," he says. "We also need our own sensations to live; to not be completely alone." This sensation echoes the psychotic feeling of "being blocked" that he describes in his account, which strengthens the sense of lack of freedom and control that he feels over his own life: "'Psychiatry' is like a prison, it's like a chemical prison inside of me; you can't work, it's always 'you can't' when you're on medication. If you take more medication to one day get out of 'psychiatry,' you can't. So you don't have any freedom. I feel like I always need chemical help with me … Many times, I would have liked to have my freedom to stop feeling like a prisoner."

For Francis, alternative mental-health resources represent the hope of a place where he can find refuge from the world of the "street." "Often, you have to deal with a lack of understanding, from the psychiatrist, from your family, no one understands you. At first, I didn't have any mental-health resources, so I was like out on the street. When I was scared, I was on the street." Further along in the account, however, his descriptions of these resources become permeated with a mood that recalls his descriptions of "the street." First, Francis associates these resources with the same impressions of a lack of sensation and stopped time that he feels when hospitalized: "I had the feeling that I would spend my life in there [going from one resource to another]. At some point, you want to get out of that world, you want to feel more stimulation." Then he recounts conflicts with individuals within these alternative resources, and that he felt judged. Finally, he tried to reduce his use of these resources or avoid them because he began again to experience the world of "fights" and "wars" that characterize "the street": "And at one point I went to some places … that were against any kind of psychiatry, and when I came out of there I was really screwed up, I didn't know where I was going, I was against everything." Alternative mental-health resources thus risked becoming a part of this negative ambiance at the very point when they seemed to be the only spaces in which Francis could move and establish relationships with others.

A Habitable Space

At some point, Francis seems to have built spaces that are isolated and that protect him from the "fights" and "abandonment" of "the street." These "survival" spaces are based on a new medication, certain relationships, and habits that help him avoid psychosis and, thus, the worst kind of "abandonment," the worst kind of solitude: psychiatric hospitalization. He has also built a world in which he has developed habits that keep the evil "outside world" at bay; the emblematic image of this world is, perhaps, a walk in a park. He associates happiness above all with the frequenting of certain places and the avoidance of others: "Last week there were times when I felt good. It's encouraging."

He also has to create this positive space within himself. Thus, when he refers to spirituality, he talks in terms of space: "Spirituality is the positive that goes inside you." One can imagine the importance of this sentence for someone who has always felt threatened by the outside. Francis feels that spirituality has a very positive influence on his life. Through prayer, he can face his fears and avoid certain thoughts; when he feels a psychotic episode coming on, he recites the Lord's Prayer. He also writes poetry, composing poems that, primarily, play with paradoxes. He was able to read his poems during a "poetry conference" organized by Les Frères et Soeurs d'Émile Nelligan, an organization for people who have experienced "severe breakdowns" and whose members identify with the definition of this illness. This group organizes a number of recreational, contemplative, and creative activities around the experience of "madness."

Thus, an important dimension of Francis's process of "subjectivation" is the creating of borders between various spaces: the space of evil, isolation, and abandonment (the street), and the space of good, calm, and communication (the garden).

Understanding Practices from the Perspective of the Inner Experience and Its Paradoxes

This analysis has tried to grasp how the mental changes caused by psychosis conflict with efforts to use the temporal logic implicit in narrative to articulate this experience. Right from the start, the limits of the narrative process became obvious. Taking its limits into consideration, however, allowed the tensions and constituent paradoxes of Francis's discourse to be emphasized, which led to a better understanding of his effort to maintain or reconstruct meaning both in psychosis and in the face of its effects; it also helped to identify the socio-cultural resources his effort was based on. These resources were approached from Francis's subjective perception of them, and from their place in the world of signifiers set out in his account.

It is clear, however, that the temporal logic of narrative is incapable of collecting or expressing all of the experiences Francis wishes to convey. Much of his account uses "space"-related metaphors to describe a world of threatening, "outside-of-time" impressions that cannot be integrated into or expressed by the narrative. The symbol of the "street," for example, can be interpreted as a metaphorical expression of Francis's overwhelming feelings detachment and exclusion created by psychosis, feelings that are experienced as profound abandonment and the sense that one can never be part of the "normal" world.

This analysis shows that certain socio-cultural resources, such as a diagnosis of schizophrenia or a psychiatric hospitalization, can be "absorbed" by the dynamic of the "street"; one might even say that they strengthen the isolation and the atmosphere of suspicion and violence that dominate this dynamic. The roles of other resources are more ambiguous for Francis: his family, with whom he had difficult relations for many years but who also helped him considerably; medication, which for Francis represents both a "prison" and a tool that allows him to be calm and feel well; and alternative resources, where Francis thought he had found a place for himself but where, at the same time, he feared being trapped, either in isolation or in a world of conflict and struggles (against medication, psychiatry, and the family).

Unlike other studies that give priority to the simple criteria of effectiveness or impact assessment, a phenomenological and narrative approach highlights the paradoxical effects of intervention. The meanings that support services take on in relation to the inner worlds of the people they serve are multi-faceted and contradictory. By highlighting these meanings, we can improve interventions and better synchronize them with the mechanisms that the person with these experiences has put into place to deal with psychosis. One can certainly hope that by listening more attentively to the discourse of people suffering from psychosis, we can prevent support services from actually reinforcing their experiences of violence or exclusion.

JOY JAMES

Re-sounding Images
Outsiders in Persimmon Blackbridge's Sunnybrook

This essay constitutes a return in that it enacts a dialogue with concepts introduced by Ross Chambers in his keynote address to the 1999 symposium "Facing Life: The Body in Dis-ease."[1] The symposium, held at the University of British Columbia in February of that year, immediately preceded the start of the Narratives of Disease, Disability and Trauma project, that culminated in the conference at which the paper that forms the basis of this essay was first presented in 2002.

First, I will first introduce Persimmon Blackbridge's book *Sunnybrook: A True Story with Lies* (1996), and investigate its relation to the concept of "agencing" as formulated by Ross Chambers. Next, I will offer a Nietzschean reading of Blackbridge's text as a basis from which to perform a re-sounding of Chambers' ideas concerning the functions of audibility and amplification in processes of agencing. Reading *Sunnybrook* through Friedrich Nietzsche's understanding of the multifarious ways of experiencing that make up a life allows us to stand back from particular assumptions embedded in theories and practices of narrativity. Once these assumptions are suspended, it becomes possible to hear the singularities of the refrain that runs through *Sunnybrook,* and to understand how the text works to activate spaces from which there is the potential for multiple subjectivities to emerge.

My involvement with Chambers' use of the concept of agencing, and its attendant notions of audibility and amplification, has revolved around questions about how new ways of existing are imagined by those who are designated/diagnosed as outlaws and outcasts. By necessity, this research has taken me into the realm of those who perform acts of designation and diagnosis, as well as those who suffer their imposition. This aspect of my study has resulted in my recognizing that moral considerations are ultimately unproductive in attempts to understand the "becomings" entailed in the generation of subjective modalities.

Persimmon Blackbridge's book *Sunnybrook: A True Story with Lies* entertains these questions from the outset. The ambiguity of Blackbridge's title in relation to definitions of "truth" sets the tone for the duration of the readers' engagement with the text. It is not without significance that the book's title calls to mind Friedrich Nietzsche's essay "On Truth and Lying in a Non-Moral Sense" (Nietzsche 1999, 139–53). Like Nietzsche, Blackbridge shows that notions of "truth" and "lying" are not moral propositions, but rather consist of determinations that are thoroughly context based. In so doing, she takes on the weight of Western logocentric thought. This is a particularly apt move, in that Blackbridge's book counters the moral imperative towards rationality and coherence with a celebration of the productive possibilities present in processes of fragmentation. Blackbridge's revaluation of what constitutes "normal," "mental illness," and "the realm of the rational" complicates any easy understanding of these terms and their histories in Western discourse. Moreover, Nietzsche's admonition to approach serious and weighty issues as play can be seen to have been illustrated to good effect in *Sunnybrook*. The playfulness of the text is in keeping with its content in that it provides modes of access that are not dependent on—that, indeed, eschew—dominant narrative forms that privilege linear ways of thinking. Instead, Blackbridge uses the entire field of the page to blast open spatial and temporal continuums, incorporating textual strategies that allow her to animate a multiplicity of subject positions while steadfastly refusing to construct unifying concepts within which to contain, codify, and overwhelm the specificity of experience.

The "Sunnybrook" from which the book takes its name was an Ontario psychiatric institution that was closed down by the province during a period in which systems of care for those designated as "mentally ill" were reorganized in compliance with changing perceptions of treatment protocols. Blackbridge's highly imagistic, autofictive form of mock hypertext is the most recent emanation of a transdisciplinary project that began as a testimony to the struggles of those who have been psychiatrized. The book incorporates and then goes beyond its earlier life as a fine art installation—a large scale exhibition of painting and sculpture that was shown in venues across North America—to engage in a form of witnessing that chronicles a litany of complex difficult topics: adult illiteracy, learning disabilities, mind problems, and outlawed sexual identities. The many scenarios described in the text stand as testimony to the dangerous terrain that those who are locked up in the asylum must negotiate. Moreover, Blackbridge shows that these dangers do not stop at the locked doors of the institution, and the similarities of the outlaw/outcaste territories of the lesbian, the learning-disabled, and the economically disadvantaged are thrown into sharp relief as they are held beside the misguided and malevolent practices cloistered inside Sunnybrook's walls.

The problem with which Ross Chambers was grappling in his 1999 lecture, and that I want to revisit in relation to Blackbridge's *Sunnybrook*, was this: how is it possible for that which cannot be spoken, or more properly, that which cannot be heard, to reach a level of audibility? Chambers, who was working on narratives of witnessing at the time, juxtaposed François Lyotard's sentence-based theories of narrative—an extremely simplistic reduction of which can be reiterated as "sentences speak us"; that is, subjects are produced by and in language or, in Heideggerian terms, "sentences sentence"—with Gayatri Spivak's famous question, "Can the subaltern speak?" (Spivak 1988) . Chambers' counterpoising of Lyotard's and Spivak's ideas facilitated a focus on the problematic of audibility and agency that I want to pick up again in this essay.

In his lecture, Chambers invoked a theatrical device, prosopopoeia, used in ancient Greece. In Greek theatre, actors spoke through elaborate masks, or prosopone, that rendered the sound of their voices uncanny. This altered speech was important because the action of donning the mask, in effect, displaced the actor, who then became an orator through whom others spoke. This magical auditory transformation made it possible to give voice to those that were thought to be present—ancestors, animals, Gods—but could not speak.

Chambers brings this model to his understanding of texts involved in the process of giving voice to the unvoiced, or audibility to those who cannot be heard. The Latin word for prosopone is persona. In prosopopoeia, the mask that the actor wears substitutes as the persona of the unvoiced subject of speech. As Chambers explains, prosopopoeia entails:

> a kind of switch and the switch goes like this: it starts with the actor, the actor wears the mask/the orator produces the sentences, which in turn produce the speaking subject: that which cannot speak. So you go from the actor producing the mask, the orator producing the sentences, via the sentences now having a subject that is *not* the actor, but, those who cannot speak—to the situation where those who are deprived of voice have acquired, not exactly a voice, but a voicing, which they borrow from the actor's voice, transformed—they also acquire authority ... audibility, amplification.[2]

He goes on to explain that "the actor has an agency here, but the actor's agency consists of an agencing..., an agencing through which what doesn't have a voice achieves audibility." So then, in Chambers' formulation, the unvoiced—that which is present but does not speak, or more properly, cannot be heard—becomes audible through a process in which an/other (literally) becomes its agencing.

In Chambers' interpretation of the potential present in the powerful device of prosopopoeia, it is possible to read Blackbridge's text as one that through the construction and animation of a number of personae—of masks—gives voice to those who otherwise could not be heard: in this case, those incarcerated in the psychiatric asylum, along with those locked into the exclusions involved in various forms of embodiment and identity deemed transgressive by, or that are invisible to and silenced by, mainstream society. I suggest, however, that Blackbridge's text performs more vital and dynamic functions.

What Chambers describes is a coming together, a cohesion of the unvoiced with one who functions as an agencing that becomes a voicing. However, in *Sunnybrook* it is precisely the act of breaking apart, undoing, fragmenting, and of narrative coherence—and Blackbridge does this in both metaphorical and material ways—that creates gaps and aporias with the potential to activate differently figured processes of coming-to-voice. The practical necessity that is required of *Sunnybrook*'s readers to acknowledge the gaps and vault the aporias results in a multiplicity of singular readings. Every reader puts the text together differently according to their associative processes, the emphasis they place on particular registers, their involvement with political/psychic necessities, and so on. Far from tracing a linear progression such as that evoked by Chambers in his prosopopoeia model of voicing—actor to orator to a voicing of the unvoiced subject of speech—Blackbridge's text suggests that any move toward cohesion, such as in the progression noted above, must always be held in productive tension with a simultaneous movement of fragmentation. Furthermore, her text shows that it is the tension resulting from an oscillation between cohesion (unity) and fragmentation (multiplicity) that makes it possible to avert the dangers that would result in simply "speaking for," in the place of, an/other. For while it is the case that in theory the model of prosopopoeia works well—and has a long history—it becomes difficult to maintain that, as a practice, it does *not* entail one person speaking for an/other, or multiple others.

In *Sunnybrook*, Blackbridge does not speak *for* anyone. Nor is she in a position of having to translate, amplify, or bring to audibility the voices of those who cannot be heard. Those whose stories are re-presented in the text—and whom Blackbridge acknowledges by name in the foreword—along with *Sunnybrook*'s readers, and Blackbridge herself, do this work together. In what follows, I will show how Blackbridge's book indicates that the emphasis in Ross Chambers' theory of the agencing capabilities of prosopopoeia-like interventions is perhaps mis-placed. Instead of dwelling on the processes of amplification of that which cannot be heard, Blackbridge's text demonstrates that it is equally necessary to underline processes of assemblage and processes of oscillation. That is, the condition of possibility in this scenario is not found primarily in the relation of the one who becomes an agencing to the unvoiced, but rather in the ongoing activation of spaces between the audience and the play, the reader and the text, and in the *affective* constitutive work that is done in these in-between spaces of trans- and intra-cultural encounter.

The shift in emphasis from agencing to agencing in correspondence with processes of assemblage and oscillation is significant for thinking about how conditions of possibility are activated by outlaw/outcaste constituencies, and the place of cultural production in these processes. Blackbridge's *Sunnybrook* both resonates with and extends Chambers' conceptualization of "agencing" in just these ways.

The French word from which "agencing" is derived is *agencement*, and *agencement* has a number of meanings. For the purposes of this discussion, the most relevant of those meanings, and one that has been popularized primarily by the work of theorists Gilles Deleuze and Félix Guattari, is "assemblage" (Deleuze and Guattari 1987). Chambers himself refers to this translation of Deleuze and Guattari's concept of *agencement*, but sets it aside in favour of "agencing." So, then, agencing/assemblage. Now, in Deleuze and Guattari's work, the term "assemblage" also incorporates notions of desire. The assemblage is characterized as a "desiring machine." Desire in this understanding is both potential and the affirmation of that potential. Desire is the attraction or force that brings and holds together any particular assemblage: the force of the form, as it were. Moreover, Deleuze and Guattari's term "desiring machine" is closely aligned with Nietzsche's "will to power," wherein power is potential, and will the affirmation of that potential.[3] It is precisely in this register of desire as affirmation that I find a productive resonance between Blackbridge's *Sunnybrook* and the work of Friedrich Nietzsche.

Reading *Sunnybrook* through Nietzsche is useful in that it reveals, by way of contrast, particular assumptions about what constitutes a subject that are embedded in the prosopopoeia theory of agencing. Privileging notions of becoming over being—"*becoming* with a radical rejection even of the concept of *being*" (Nietzsche 1992, 51)—Nietzsche tells us that the subject, far from being a static entity, is the expression of a kind of attention or attending to the becoming self: to its rhythms, desires, needs, pleasures, and aversions; to its health and continuance. This attention, or attending to, takes the self directly into the flow that is the constant of its "isness," and is why Nietzsche can admonish us to "become what you are!" So nothing stable or autonomous here, but rather an acute consciousness, or sensation of flux-movement-ephemerality that is nonetheless embodied in a singular physicality of greater or lesser duration. This is a distinctly different idea of "subject" than the one called up by the linear, coherent narrative of prosopopoeia with its presumption of a subject, a "one," who even though it can provisionally "become" an/other (i.e., the speaking subject who speaks through the subject who is its agencing), remains, nonetheless, the condition of possibility for that which cannot be heard to attain audibility.

I would like now to turn to Blackbridge's *Sunnybrook*, and show how her orchestration of a fragmented fluid subjectification, one that is in keeping with a Nietzschean idea of the subject—the subject as a series of events, eventful subjectivity—illuminates an alternate understanding of how this process of coming to audibility might unfold. Rather than being constrained and contained by the limitations involved in a cohesive tyranny of narrative—or, as in the case of prosopopoeia, a subject who has enough coherence to be able to become another's voicing—Blackbridge's text animates flows of images and imaginings that eddy into a multitude of possible realities, and possible "becomings." As I continue, I will be looking at *Sunnybrook* as a form of desiring production; a desiring machine.

How is desire set to work in Blackbridge's text? What forms of desiring production are activated? In Blackbridge's self-description, desire is figured as capacities and abilities. In her bio in *Sunnybrook*, she refers to herself as a "learning-disabled-lesbian-cleaning-lady-sculptor-performer-video-artist." This is reminiscent of the way that Nietzsche describes his own desiring production. In his autobiographical text, *Ecce Homo*, he talks about the challenges of negotiating his multiplicity:

> An order of rank among these capacities; distance; the art of separating without setting against one another; to mix nothing, to "reconcile" nothing; a tremendous variety that is nevertheless the opposite of chaos—this was the precondition, the long secret work and artistry of my instinct. (254)

Nietzsche's words provide a map to the embodied territories of experience opened up in Blackbridge's text. Seen in this light, Blackbridge's introduction is not just a trendy attention-catching nomenclature, but rather its multiplicity (the "subject" experienced as many rather than one) and its singularity (an assemblage that defies duplication) signal the abiding concerns of the text. Blackbridge sets in motion a number of technologies of desire, two of which I want to talk about here, as one imbricates the other. The first is her dynamic use of images and of text-as-image, and the second is Blackbridge's invocation and contestation of the ideal through reference to its shadow form.

Throughout the book, the all-over placement of images and text on the page, and the shape given to each textual unit, keeps our eyes (and our minds) glancing across surfaces. In addition to disrupting, and in fact, disallowing habitually linear patterns of reading, the close association of images and text shapes that incorporate a wide variety of font types coaxes us into seeing the text-as-image: that is, as seeing the blocks of text as imagistic components with the capacity to be constitutive of a number of different assemblages, rather than understanding the textual units as fixed moments in the unfolding of a particular narrative. The different types of fonts used in the physical text further encourage us to respond to the book as the inscription of a polyvocal telling that describes multiple voices tracing a multiplicity of subject positions. For instance, most of the pages contain sidebars of text that provide, in turn, running commentaries on events and conversations, moments of internal dialogue, factual and historical information about institutional practices, and anecdotal accounts of experiences. These textual elements are characterized by a number of different font types that are suited to the information they carry. Most of the personal and private internal dialogue asides, for example, are printed with an old-style typeface—the kind associated with early manual typewriters. With that association, the typeface itself conveys a sense of intimacy, and gives us the feeling that these are personal messages written directly to us. It is tempting to interpret these asides as adhering to a specific voice, that of a narrator. However, just as we come to believe in the voice of a single narrator who is overseeing the proceedings, we realize that, seemingly without our notice, a shift has occurred and that this voice is no longer located where we thought it was. Furthermore, even when the several typefaces used *can* be tentatively traced to particular positions, a variety of inflections produce a multiplicity of voices that together radiate geographies of experience even as they relinquish any sense of subjects as discrete and knowable entities. Because of this, any attempts by the reader to distinguish a single trajectory moving through all these linguistic and imagistic eruptions—that is, to narrativize—are thwarted. There are, at best, only partial correlations to be made between typeface and the voice of a particular subject. These discrepancies have the effect of orchestrating a reading that again privileges Nietzsche's idea of the "subject" as a fluidity that rests in other flows.

The restlessness entailed in the fleeting movements of the glance that this text demands does not, however, limit its power as a desiring machine that produces possible realities. Why should it? In making my point I call on Nietzsche again, who in his approach to difficult problems, brushes aside the usefulness of the depths in favour of the "quick look":

> I approach deep problems like cold baths: quickly into them and quickly out again. That one does not get to the depths that way, not deep enough down, is the superstition of those afraid of the water, the enemies of cold water; they speak without experience. The freezing cold makes one swift.—And to ask this incidentally: does a matter necessarily remain ununderstood and unfathomed merely because it has been touched only in flight, glanced at, in a flash? Is it absolutely imperative that one settles down on it? that one has brooded over it as over an egg … as Newton said of himself? At least there are truths that are singularly shy and ticklish and cannot be caught except suddenly—that must be *surprised* or left alone … (1974, 381).

Indeed, the power of *Sunnybrook* is in part its uncanny ability to provide lightning-strike revelations that surprise readers with potent "truths" that persist as afterimages to be taken up in other imaginings, other assemblages.

Blackbridge's all-over use of images (each page is awash with evocative collages of image, colour, and texture), including her use of text-as-image, is entwined with a second technology of desire. I am referring here to her method of summoning an ideal by reference to its shadow form. Blackbridge takes delight in uprooting ideality, and by association, "normality," in all its hideouts. The "ideal form," that which my colleague Jim Overboe calls the normative shadow, is figured as a shaded and silent aspect of any event, or that which haunts all becomings.[4]

For example, one of the scenarios encountered in *Sunnybrook* is the hiring of a young woman, Persimmon, who uses her "real" name, Diane, when applying for the position of a one-to-one counsellor in a psychiatric institution. Persimmon/Diane gets the job by putting on the application that she was employed at a clinic where she was in actuality a patient. Soon after beginning work at Sunnybrook, Persimmon/Diane comes across a novel, *Honeymoon for Nurse Holly*, which has been left in a downstairs staff washroom where Diane/Persimmon goes to escape the uncertainties entailed in her new professional undertaking. Nurse Holly quickly takes on the role of "the normative shadow" to Diane/Persimmon's becoming nurse. This normative shadow is further bifurcated by the ghostly presence, in Diane/Persimmon's imaginings, of Florence Nightingale. The crossings and connections between and among these three figures—the becoming-nurse Diane/Persimmon, the ideal Nurse Holly, and the beyond reproach but sacrificial Florence Nightingale—imbue the harrowing events relayed in the sound bites of text with a sense of hilarity that sharpens the drama of the real risks and dangers that are encountered by those embodying positions that remain constantly under threat. It is, therefore, in the fissures, gaps, and tensions among all these different tellings that the engendering of space I spoke of at the beginning of this essay is affected. In Blackbridge's re-soundings, the sheer excess of the many opens onto the clamour of voices that rise up from *Sunnybrook*'s pages and dissemble all notion of "the one." In the final analysis there is in *Sunnybrook* no "subject," nor unifying system of any description, of which to take hold. If there is any logic here, it is the logic of images, the logic of the prism, which is located by the light glancing off its surfaces.

In conclusion, I would like to suggest that Ross Chambers' theorization of "agencing" benefits from the active incorporation of the additional definition of *agencement* as assemblage. When *agencement* is understood as *both* agencing and assemblage, focus is shifted away from the figure that is said to make agencing possible, and placed instead on the *affective* relationality of the processes' constituent parts. It is a question of emphasis. In this formulation, agencing is refigured precisely as the activity of assemblage itself: the activation of the desire that brings into correspondence the author/artist, the multiple participants who provide accounts of the events and activities of their lives, the textual object and its readers, and the resonances of the multiple sites that provide the context for the assemblage. Social structures, institutional practices, and politics of identification have the ability to lock individuals and communities into untenable lives. The very definition of the "subject"—of what it means to be human—on which these structures, practices, and politics rest, also carries life-affirming/life-diminishing powers. This is an important consideration, because it is exactly this process that is problematic when attempting to understand where the points of leverage are for political actions that work towards a more broadly defined and inclusive social order.

Notes

1 My analysis draws on an audiotape of Ross Chambers' keynote lecture "Can the Body Speak?" and on the unpublished summary of that lecture prepared for the Narratives of Disease, Disability and Trauma Project by Richard Ingram, doctoral candidate, Individual Interdisciplinary Studies Graduate Program, University of British Columbia.
2 Transcribed from an audiotape of the lecture.
3 See Brian Massumi, *A User's Guide to Capitalism and Schizophrenia: Deviations from Deleuze and Guattari* (Cambridge, MA: MIT, 1992), 82, 174n. 56.
4 This is a concept formulated by James Overboe in his dissertation "Articulating a Sociology of Desire: Exceeding the Normative Shadow of Phenomenology" (University of British Columbia, 2004).

PAMELA CUSHING

(Story-)Telling It like It Is
How Narratives Teach at L'Arche

The research presented in this essay illustrates how informal, experience-based narratives shared among caregivers about *individuals*, not types or labels, can be deployed as a humanizing complement to formal training. In particular, it shows how storytelling about the particulars of individuals with developmental impairment/disabilities and their everyday desires is shown to be a fluid and effective mechanism of enculturation into the local, moral world of L'Arche, an international, residential care organization with a radically inclusive, relational approach to caregiving and disability. To operationalize the counter-cultural philosophy of L'Arche into quality care, the organization must assist new caregivers to overcome their initial, narrow perceptions of people with developmental disabilities, and does so by enhancing the moral imaginations of new caregivers through narratives. Limitations of the narrative teaching style will also be identified.

Research about the conditions of life and care for people with developmental and intellectual impairments/disabilities[1] often emphasizes *process* conditions and structural issues. This essay directs attention instead to the *attitudinal* conditions which influence quality of life and care: in other words, how people around people with developmental and intellectual impairments/disabilities feel for and care *about* them as individuals, not just care *for* them as a category of client. In doing so, a narrative-based teaching approach for the strategic (re)enculturation of caregivers in one organization is elaborated upon, to demonstrate how it shifts cultural attitudinal frames and results in improved quality and mutuality of care.

Hilde Lindemann Nelson has written of the need for a better understanding of how to put narratives to "moral use" to do "moral work"

(2002b). This essay illustrates how narratives are used as strategic, cultural tools to do the moral work of countering prevailing negative stereotypes of disability. Storytelling among caregivers about the people with developmental disabilities with whom they share daily life can have a radically humanizing effect on care relations if done within a progressive, ideological framework.[2] Particular kinds of narratives can change and shape how new caregivers experience people with developmental disabilities and how they imagine supporting them. The research results presented here also suggest that such (re)shaping of its caregivers' perceptions, away from mainstream standards, is a necessary prerequisite for the mutually respectful care relations that L'Arche advocates. These newly shaped perceptions create a strong foundation for quality of care, and encourage shifts in the conventional caregiver–client power imbalance, rather than reproducing it.

Project Background

The research presented here draws on over a year of anthropological fieldwork gained through living in L'Arche community homes across Canada. L'Arche was formed in the 1960s in France and Canada by Jean Vanier, as a social justice–oriented response to the ubiquitous sub-human conditions then found in large institutions (Vanier 1995). It has since grown into an international organization, with 130 alternative caregiving and life-sharing communities for people with developmental disabilities in many countries (Vanier 1998). Their *relational* ethic of care involves most community members[3] living together in the homes, sharing meals, common space, and social time.[4] L'Arche aims to work against processes of exclusion by promoting greater public awareness and acceptance of the intrinsic and social value of people with disabilities (L'Arche 2006). They believe that, for many people, genuine inclusion is often better facilitated through rich social relations, belonging, and opportunities for growth than through the material trappings of independent living (Cushing 2003b).

Critical histories of the cultural construction of developmental disability in the twentieth century have revealed how stigma and negative perceptions of disability have been built up, often intentionally, and often by professionals in the field (Trent 1994, Simmons 1982). Many scholars and activists have been calling for a reversal of these attitudes for decades, but changing deeply held public perceptions is difficult, and, as the prevailing existence of discrimination shows, that challenge has not yet been adequately addressed (Braddock and Mitchell 1992).

Active culture-shifting is needed, therefore, in order to alter the publicly perceived negatives of life with a developmental disability, and to encourage social inclusion of people *as they are*. Policy-makers, on the other hand, have appeared in the past to believe that merely pushing idealistic aphorisms and rules about "respecting and empowering" the client onto front-line caregivers is sufficient to create change. In fact, such rhetoric is generally unconvincing: it provides no compelling rationale for why the caregivers should adopt this culturally unsupported perception of disability. Some rationale is vital if people are, fundamentally, to reorganize their work where power, authority, and role definitions are at stake.

Caregivers need better tools to help them learn how to reframe and revalorize disability, and the difference it implies, in practice. What I observed in the L'Arche sub-culture is that narratives can be one such tool. Through everyday storytelling about their experiences, the caregivers there have inadvertently developed an effective tool for producing a new perspective on disability, difference, and caregiving in their organization.

Multiple Uses and Types of Narratives

L'Arche uses a variety of strategies to enculturate and socialize new caregivers into their ideology and practice, and narratives are one of them (Cushing 2003a; 187–200). Following Uni Wikan, I define narratives as "stories or talk that have intention, characters, and plight" (Wikan 1995, 263). Although many forms of narrative are told in L'Arche,[5] Wikan's definition aptly describes the form that this essay focuses on: everyday, informal narratives shared regularly among L'Arche assistants in the course of their interactions. I argue that these narratives constitute productive activity insofar as they serve to create a positive, alternative social and moral reality and cultural environment within the organization. Narratives shape local knowledge and health care in L'Arche by replacing conventional, homogenizing, deficit-focused conceptions of developmental disability with a humanized notion of individual people who have abilities and gifts, with distinct personalities and care needs.

During one afternoon, for instance, I was to be in the L'Arche home making dinner with one of the community members, Oscar, for our housemates. I happened to meet up beforehand with caregiver Gord in the family room. Gord sat with Oscar, who, as was his usual habit, was lying on the couch after his day at a workshop. I mentioned to Oscar that he seemed unsettled and that I wondered why, but Oscar clearly did not feel like talking. One thing about Oscar is that while he may understand a range of conversations, he is either uncomfortable, unwilling, or unable to respond to just any old question. Questions to Oscar must be phrased in particular ways, and often require one to have substantial prior information already in order to get the questions right. Seeing this impasse, Gord jumped in, initiating a short story:

> GORD: Today was not a routine day at the workshop, was it Oscar? (*silence*) You were expecting to work on the vacuum parts today, weren't you?
>
> (*Oscar shoots a glance at Gord but remains silent*)
>
> GORD: Was it Jen's birthday? (*silence*) (*now to me*) The workshop decided to hold a birthday party for Jen this morning so they did not get around to working on the things that Oscar had been looking forward to. They said that they forgot to let him know the day before, so he was quite disturbed by this change in schedule. (*now to Oscar*)—You wouldn't even eat lunch, eh, Oscar? Now that's big!
>
> OSCAR: Nooooooo. Not hungry, eh? Not want to go to party.
>
> GORD: Well it's OK, you guys will be back on vacuums tomorrow, right? (*Oscar wrings his hands as he considers this*) (*now to me*) You may want to reconsider tonight's activities or something …

Gord's attempt at co-storytelling served several functions that are both particular to Oscar's personality and to his experience that day, and to the more general purpose of training me. The narrative format was a way of letting me in on Oscar's probable frame of mind without imposing any definitive judgements on what exactly that was (he was often thrown off by changes in routine but the effect was variable), or prescribing what that had to mean in terms of what came next. Gord's hints that the plans may need revisiting and the narrative just expressed suggested implicitly that making dinner together may be too stressful, but it was left open for me and Oscar to negotiate. This acknowledges Oscar's varied ability to handle his anxieties depending on his relationship with the caregiver.

Importantly, the narrative also attempted to keep Oscar's voice privileged over other interpretations (which are kept tentative), and cued Oscar that his concerns were being acknowledged and passed on to the next caregiver. Such transitioning was important to him so he could continue to process his upset through the rest of the day.

While these functions were somewhat specific to Oscar and that day, the narrative form also allows room for transferable lessons in the importance of routines to some people in the community, the anxiety that can result from changes, the need to inform and coach people through changes, and the potential for hidden upsets to be behind people's behaviours at any given time. This last item is vital for caregivers since there is often this particular type of narrative gap in understanding when working with those with limited ability to use words. It suggests a need for trusting that someone is not simply being difficult or "non-compliant" but instead has reasons for what they're doing that you may never know. If Gord had not been there to share the story for instance, I could have worsened Oscar's strain by pressing him to help with dinner, assuming he was just seeing if he could get me to give in as he often did on other days.

In order to avoid a reductivist interpretation or oversimplifying the actors' intentions, I should acknowledge that these informal narratives can fulfill other functions alongside the enculturative one.[6] Everyday narratives in L'Arche also function for sociability—either in relationship building, as humour, or as a way to give or elicit support from others. Another less explicit function of telling stories is to craft one's identity for others (Wikan 1992, 464) through the "ambiguity of reference" (Bruner 1996, 140).

In this essay, however, the central use of narrative being considered is in its teaching and enculturative function when used in everyday, informal settings. Aspects of the L'Arche ideology, such as considering differences as valued gifts, and caregiving as a two-way process, are counterintuitive for most new caregivers. As such, most are uncertain about how to translate these ideals from formal training into practice. This is not surprising, given anthropologists' findings that understanding difference and "the other" is not a natural impulse for people in any society, but rather is a skill that must be learned and worked at continuously (Geertz 1994). It is important, therefore, to provide caregivers with alternative imaginative frameworks to adopt. Such tools can help caregivers to recognize and articulate the mutually beneficial dimensions of work and relationships with people with developmental disabilities. Narratives can be a useful tool in this respect because they create a space for recognition of *commonality* amidst difference. Naming areas of common humanity heightens mutual resonance and understanding (Wikan 1992, 476). These sorts of narratives in L'Arche do not erase difference, but rather work towards reframing and revalorizing difference. This encourages caregivers to live with difference in new ways, effectively expanding their moral imaginations.

THE NARRATIVE GAP

This practice at L'Arche is significant because such informal, positive storytelling about clients is hardly common in the landscape of busy, mainstream healthcare systems and support agencies. There, the lack of resources and institutionalized taboos on intimacy with patients often result in a substantial loss of relational engagement (Chambliss 1996). One striking example of this loss comes from research showing that a majority of American state hospital nurses could not recall *any particular stories* about any specific patient in the preceding month (Benner 1994, 58). Other research suggests that when specific stories are told, they are often about *incidents* or *non-compliance* with section rules (Phillips and Benner 1994; Chambliss 1996). Thus, stories in this context often function solely to justify further constraints or, indirectly, the lack of attention given or rehabilitation achieved (Rhodes 1993; Young 1993).

This tendency creates a harmful narrative gap, or lack of shared stories, which is particularly problematic for clients with developmental disabilities. Typically, these people are in some form of long-term care arrangement (residential or supported living), and many have a limited ability to articulate their history, needs, or desires verbally. This communication challenge is exacerbated by very high staff-turnover rates and burnout in the field (Braddock and Mitchell 1992; Ungerson 1999). This results in large gaps in individualized understandings of how to support a particular person well in terms of techniques and relations. Informal storytelling has become a key tactic through which L'Arche works towards holding, adding to, and passing on such aspects of a person's history. To elaborate more upon the story discussed earlier, Oscar is highly sensitive to particular nuances of language and ways of talking, and so his well-being is tied directly to ability and willingness of his caregivers to learn these intricacies. Here, narrative complements experiential learning to achieve knowledge transfer and flexibility (since Oscar changes too) that would be very difficult and labour-intensive to capture in written training reports.

NARRATIVES CONSTRUCT MORAL WORLDS

In order to talk about how narratives can be useful in constructing this alternative moral subculture, I will relate a story that occurs in part due to the turnover just discussed, and the difficult disruption in routines and relationships that this often causes. Neil is a L'Arche director. He often tells new assistants a story about a significant conversation he had years ago with his friend, Frank, who has lived as a member of L'Arche since he was a teen. Many assistants leave for school at the end of the summer and, one year, Frank found this mini-exodus particularly trying. Frank is thoughtful and expressive, and he and Neil had a good conversation about how this situation made them both sad. Neil relates, though, that he also wanted to encourage Frank to see not just the loss but the other side of the coin—"what gifts had been given," by Frank during the year:

> "You know there is also the good side. You really changed those assistants' lives by welcoming them to share your home. Many assistants have told me how much they learned from your observations, how you choose to live, and what a character you are."
>
> Frank paused to reflect on that for a moment. Then he looked up and said, "Well if that's true, Neil, then how come no one has ever thanked me?"

This was years ago, and L'Arche is now more conscious of cultivating a spirit and practice of gratitude among assistants. Still, the narrative contains lessons that Neil feels continue to be instructive. The story conveys particular details about Frank, and his response to staff changes, that are important for those people who live with him to anticipate and be aware of in order to support him well at these times. It also evokes a way of perceiving a person with developmental disabilities that is not obvious to new assistants. It is, after all, only since the 1970s that professionals actively recognized that people with developmental disabilities had feelings and senses as well-developed as other people (Trent 1994). The story illustrates the depth and complexity of Frank's emotions, and hints at his sensitivity and his desire to be recognized for what he gives to his relationships. Given that this is a desire many of us have, the narrative creates a sense of common ground. Finally, the narrative highlights the unavoidably moral nature of engaging in dependency relations (Kittay 1999), especially with people known to have impoverished social networks (Lunsky 2002).

This story also reveals *how* narratives can teach. How we interpret our experiences and evaluate them in moral terms is neither natural nor obvious. Philip Reiff tells us that Freud believed that what "is moral is not 'self-evident' … [but] becomes and remains self-evident only within a powerful and compelling system of culture" (1966, 261). In this way, L'Arche is a cultural system that prescribes alternative moral norms to the mainstream, and provides categories of thought that construct *how* we experience life, and how we make sense of it. This, in turn, influences what parts of the flow of our lives we come to consider narrative-worthy, or *meaningful* experiences: in other words, what aspects will stand out from the continuous flow of daily life to be noted as "an experience" (Turner 1986, 35). "What *counts* as experience is neither straightforward nor self-evident" (my emphasis; Scott 1992). So even experience is not "natural" but always is itself already an interpretation through pre-existing cultural and personal lenses. These interpretive lenses are shaped over time partially by listening to stories, and are thus contingent and changeable.

Narratives teach through indicating what is culturally significant and relevant about a scenario, which also reproduces the norms and parameters of a particular cultural system.[7] Narrators choose to include certain experiences or events and not others in stories, which tacitly teach new caregivers *what counts* as experience or moral behaviour and what does not count (in a particular moral world). A culture is partly constructed through ongoing, changing stories (Gubrium 1999, 567). For example, hospital culture is influenced towards a scientific bias and away from humanistic concerns by the narratives doctors tell each other in medical school (Good and Good 1993), on rounds, and in case accounts (Poirier 2002, 48). Attending to silences, or what themes are *not* included in stories, is also important (Wikan 1995, 266). At L'Arche, people's medical histories or conditions are considered off limits for informal narratives.

Jerome Bruner wrote that "what people do in narratives is never by chance" (1996, 136). I take his words to mean that people tell stories *to let you know* that things could have been otherwise; other choices could have been made, but were not, and both the rationale and moral lesson are embedded in the narrative. Informal narrative thus conveys normative lessons about the subculture in which the story is produced and shared.

Same Narratives, Different Outcomes

Here I will introduce the stories of two assistants, Jack and Liam, to show both the advantages and limits of how narratives teach and do moral work. Both entered the same L'Arche home within six months of each other, and were similar in age, level of education, and class, but the outcomes of their experiences differed significantly. We move from Jack's successes to Liam's dissent, and examine what this tells us about informal narrative forms of teaching.

Jack entered L'Arche at nineteen after a semester of university and a year of odd jobs. He became an assistant in a home with a full complement of experienced assistants, so he received solid modeling by observing and practising with them, listening to their narratives, training, and retreats. By all accounts, his time as an assistant was fruitful for him and those he lived with and cared for. We had a casual discussion when he had been there for about a year. He mentioned hearing the story about Frank, recounted previously. I asked him whether that story affected how he supported or understood one particular resident named Jeremy. Jeremy is in his mid-thirties and loves country music, dancing with a partner who wheels his wheelchair about, and being with friends. His body is significantly underdeveloped and his muscles are very tense due to a condition he has experienced since birth. He often vocalizes but does not use words to communicate.

> JACK: Sure it did. Well, not just that one story, but lots of stories that I've heard from different assistants about the people with disabilities here. Looking back, I'd definitely say that together it all made me realize that Jeremy is a lot more than just a guy who can't eat by himself and yells a lot. You don't think about that at first because you are just a bit overwhelmed by him. He's so different than anyone I've ever hung out with obviously, so to be honest, it was hard to connect with him at first. Like in the bath, it sounds bad, but honestly I just sort of did the bare minimum that needed to be done because it feels odd to be in there with someone who's naked and who can't talk either to let you know what he wants or doesn't want.
>
> But after a few months Chris [another assistant] told me a story about a time when he noticed how incredibly relaxed Jeremy's muscles and body got when he stayed in the bath longer, because the water relieved the constant pressure on his joints. Since he told me that, I've tried to make the time to stay in longer with him, and do different things to make it fun like playing guitar or reading, or even prayer. I love music and he seems to too—he likes Sarah Harmer anyway! You figure out how to make that bath time more respectful of Jeremy. For sure, others' stories have helped me to tune in to him and other folks in the house in a different way.

Jack's thoughts illustrate how informal narratives can provide a different perspective on disability and alter the *attitudinal* conditions within which disability is conceived, and what people consider to be part of caregiving. For Jack, narratives supplied particular details about caring for and relating to a particular person well (in this case, Jeremy), but also provided transferable lessons for supporting others. The scenario also demonstrates how teaching through stories can give caregivers a sense that *they* are an important element in the often morally ambiguous caregiving mix, and not just doing routine physical labour. Stories allow for interpretive latitude which helps caregivers to feel that their interpretations, moral choices, and creative agency can make a difference to a person's wellbeing. Jack's narrative reveals his internal moral negotiation with what is "due" Jeremy beyond basic physical care; a question also grappled with by philosophers of the ethics of care (Kittay 1999).

After high school and his summer job, Liam came at the age of eighteen to work in the same community and home as Jack. Liam's parents, like

Jack's, lived far away. In spite of experiencing similar conditions in the home and hearing roughly the same narratives from the same people, Liam never seemed to take up the L'Arche ideology embedded in the stories passed on to him. It is difficult to determine if he chose not to embrace it deliberately, or if he simply never grasped it. Liam performed the basic labour of care competently, and was friendly with those he supported. The issue, however, was that he did so without appearing to grasp or believe that caregiving could be about more than supplying a one-way service for meeting people's physiological needs; the care he provided, therefore, seemed shallow and mechanical. Liam's performance lacked what you might call "soul" or moral conviction, and his case is important in how it illustrates certain limits to the didactic efficacy of narratives.

First, it shows that although everyday narratives are often credited with conveying moral lessons, it is also the case that informal narratives can be *morally ambiguous*. In other words, they gesture at the appropriate behaviour they hope to evoke, but they usually do not provide specific guidelines and provide instead interpretive autonomy to listeners to decide what is "morally sufficient" care. This can be a pro, as illustrated in the creativity Jack used in interpreting the ambiguity, or a con, as it allowed Liam to perform only the minimum level of physical care required at L'Arche. Liam's skeptical personality and greater interest in the social opportunities with other caregivers meant that his energy was often directed at satirizing the stories, undermining the possibilities they gesture at. As he reported to me in one interview,

> People here are so PC [politically correct] about everything—I just think it goes too far. Of course I want to be respectful of Elias and Tyler and Jeremy, but I just don't see a bath or a meal as such a huge event in their lives that I need to spend an hour extra on making it special every day. It seems like overkill and honestly I don't have the energy for it.

Perhaps Liam has a point in that the idea can be taken too far, or perhaps his resistance comes from knowing at some level that if he acknowledged the validity of the idea, it would require much more of him, as a moral agent, than he was prepared to give at that time. He made it clear in the home that he would not defer his other priorities for these reasons, and others allowed this in the short-term to see if he would adapt.

Second, the fact that Liam (intentionally or not) did not undertake or undergo the subjective transformation in outlook on disability that most assistants there do, suggests that everyday narratives are not necessarily binding. Their efficacy is often based on the assumption that the listener is ready and willing to accept the particular moral system that supports that reality. As Michael Ignatieff put it while explaining the limits of the human rights model, you cannot legislate someone to care (1984, 13). Furthermore, there is rarely only one narrative option at play for people to adopt: competing narratives offer different ways of viewing a situation. Liam, for example, appears to have found other narratives outside the L'Arche approach more compelling: "I want to do a good job, but I am not looking to be Vanier; I have other priorities that I care about like figuring out what to do with my life. So what I do at the house has to fit around that kind of thing."

Closing

Narratives shared by caregivers about everyday life and relations with people with disabilities teach largely by igniting and enhancing the moral imagination of new caregivers. While there are only a few principles to the relational kind of care approach in L'Arche, the stories allow the principles to be retold, relived, and reproduced daily without seeming clichéd or worn out because they are regularly refreshed with new characters and particulars. It is more often in the particulars of individual relationships that genuine compassion is forged than in general and diffused concerns about oppressed groups (Taylor 1994).

Notes

1 Recognizing the WHO typology of impairment, disability, and handicap, I will use "disability" herein given its international prevalence. Further, I will use the term "developmental" to encompass intellectual impairments such as Down syndrome, as well as other conditions like autism (Braddock and Mitchell 1992).
2 People with disabilities are also active storytellers at L'Arche, but that is outside the scope of this paper.
3 I.e., both those with disabilities and those who are there to support them. Some support people who now live out of the home due to family commitments and government restrictions on numbers in the home.
4 A L'Arche "community" is a collection of two to seven homes with varying numbers (two to ten) of residents and degrees of support; caregivers and people with disabilities live together, full-time. The homes are interspersed in regular neighbourhoods and connected through activities. They are not isolated retreat communities.
5 Other narrative forms discussed in the thesis include: self-narratives (life stories) of assistants in interviews, organizational metanarratives, and narrative in formal training.
6 See Pamela Cushing (2003a) for elaboration of this point.
7 Patricia Benner discusses similar revelations of narrative in her work in hospitals (1994, 58).

JANET MACARTHUR

DISRUPTING THE ACADEMIC SELF
Living with Lupus

> *Illness is a real loss of control that results in our becoming the Other whom we have feared, whom we have projected onto the world ...*
> —Sander Gilman, *Disease and Representation* (1988, 2)

Accounts of chronic illness, including this "autobiocritical" discussion of living with Systemic Lupus Erythematosus (lupus), often confirm the observation cited above: the social and physical impositions of chronicity or disability confront the self with something that the self resists. I see this as an encounter with the face or gaze of the Other, which can involve losing one self and finding another—a master narrative only retold because it is hard to hear. As an English professor, I was suspicious of such narratives; and because I saw myself as an entitled Western subject, gender notwithstanding, I could not envision citizenship in an "other" domain. (Here and elsewhere, I employ Susan Sontag's widely cited spatial conception of illness as its own kingdom, now a major trope of autopathographical studies. In illness, she states, we carry a different passport and become "citizens of that other place" [1978, 3]). Moreover the othering process of chronic illness can only be recognized retrospectively, often via testimonial—and SLE's retrospective is particularly attenuated because it is an "exacerbating-remitting" condition (Toombs 1995, 7), taking seven years, on average, to diagnose. Furthermore, one is shunted from "self-in-illness" to "self-in-life" (Hawkins 1999, xviii) by SLE's active and dormant phases (called "flares"); it therefore takes longer than it might with an unremitting condition to let go of the triumphal narrative of the "old self" beating the adversarial other of lupus. Nor does it help that everyone wants to hear this story of triumph, inured as everyone is to modern "medicine's single-minded telos of cure" (Frank 1995, 83). Lupus is not a battle to be won; it is an estrangement from self, an othering produced by the arbitrary shunting back and forth from remission stage "self" to active phase "Other."

Poststructuralist analysis asserts that Western culture constructs the Other as a "lack" of essence, presence, or autonomous identity. The body and its functions have often been situated in this lack. (Arthur and Joan Kleinman have attempted to address this discursive lack in their term the "body self" [1994, 716]). Illness and other extreme experiences confront—indeed, inhabit—consciousness with the body's presence; in cases where life is lived in extreme privation or pain, the body's needs press in and become identity. Trying to convey life lived *in extremis*, where body is sovereign over spirit/reason, is difficult, however, for expressions of the materiality of pain, viewed as inessential, are taboo, and therefore to be shamed, denied, or euthanized. Our discourses only grant legitimacy to an experience of pain where intellect, reason, and spirit are represented as transcendent over pain. Life lived *in extremis* is, therefore, life lived as other.

In 1997, I was diagnosed with lupus, a treatable but incurable autoimmune condition. Lupus flares, often characterized in language drawn from the battle myth of illness (Hawkins 1999, 61–77), occur when antibodies that fight "foreign" viral and bacterial "invaders" begin to "target" the body's connective tissue, producing a kind of somatic civil war. I no longer find this allegory useful in relating the psychosocial and physical course of lupus, which I now see not as an adversary in an agonistic narrative of struggle but as a mutation or remapping of self, a rerouting of self and its itineraries, the body's networks, and the body's terrain. Unlike military metaphors more suited to acute illness, a spatial/geographical, and therefore imagistic, conception of lupus enables me to acknowledge the othering effects of lupus as part of me. The chronicity of lupus and the unpredictability of its flares and remissions mean that one's "true self" or the "self-in-life" does not eventually emerge from behind some inauthentic sick self and go on, but that the "self-in-illness" presses for integration into self.

Julia Kristeva's notion of abjection as a liminal space between self and other is useful here: the abjection of lupus refuses to respect the culturally constructed boundary between self-in-health and self-in-illness. The abject is, for Kristeva, that which "disturbs identity, system, order. What does not respect borders, positions, rules." The abject is "filth, waste, pus, bodily fluids, the dead body itself" (Kristeva 1984, qtd. by Childers and Hentzi 1995, 1), substances clearly related to the shamed presences of chronic illness and disability. Kristeva suggests that art (here I would include autopathography) often expresses abjection, the "not-quite not-other [or] taboo excreted bits of the self" (1984, 308) which allow one to remake the self, or to locate blind spots in cultural logic. I associate these taboo excretions, these liminal presences, with the abjection of chronic illness that voicelessly calls for acknowledgement. For example, disabled or chronically ill not-quite not-others have called attention to the presumptuous binary thinking (in an oxymoronic inversion) of some of the "healthy" and "able-bodied" by designating them the "temporarily able-bodied (TAB)." The notion of the TAB participates in the ongoing poststructuralist challenge to the normative humanist concept of self as stable and "in control of itself." Jacques Lacan asserts that this is a presumptuous self who "presumes to know, but who is, unknown to himself, mired in misapprehension and delusion" (Anderson 2001, 64). A person with lupus confronts this presumptuous libertarian subjectivity within and without.

I began "losing control," witnessing the abjection and otherness of lupus, long before I was diagnosed. My lupus "presents" with symptoms of chronic exhaustion, cognitive dissonance, depression, and a generalized malaise. Here, I confront an inverse, oxymoronic reality where the pleasures of life are painful, the affirmations negations, and so on. This produces a slow but radical rupturing of identity which I see as a form of trauma. During a flare, I feel suspended from time, from life—exhausted by nothing, I spend a great deal of time surviving until my next nap or until bedtime. Lupus fatigue for me is the texture of otherness, not just its apparel but its heteronomous presence. This experience is hard to convey to those who dwell within the normative precincts of the kingdom of the well. During lupus flares, sleep is not murdered but stillborn. One awakens to the frayed edges of the unravelled, unrestored sleeve of care, something akin to but not the same as a sleepless night. I now acknowledge this hopeless sleep and waking as a form of suffering.

Moreover, lupus flares are as capricious as fate; they disrupt "you." People with lupus have no idea when their visitor's visa to the kingdom of the well will be revoked—this also results in their feeling suspended from time. Fecklessness, abjection, cussed survival through days of suspended time which one has no energy to redeem; all cancel the now, and the future involves so much contingency that it also seems to have been revoked. Many autobiographical accounts of incarceration, torture, and slavery attempt to convey the dehumanizing effect of living in a static, futureless present and the damaging psychic accommodations one makes to this. The vicissitudes of lupus can also cancel the future, completely disrupting any stability and predictability in the workplace and relationships, thereby eroding and altering identity. As Arthur Frank points out, "the changing physical capabilities caused by sickness require ongoing renegotiation of social obligations and personal identity" (1995, 82).

Lupus, described by Lupus Canada as the "disease with 1000 faces" (http://www.lupuscanada.org) presents itself ambiguously and often refuses to leave traces that can be verified by empirical tests. During this time, people with lupus usually struggle with a faceless (or overwhelmingly multi-faceted) and therefore anomic state by adapting to a number of provisional identities: a critical stage in the othering process of this illness, particularly if one is suspected of malingering and/or of psychosomatic illness. Rather than accept the socially shaming identity categories of "lazy" or "crazy," I attributed lupus malaise to something I had produced and something that I could therefore control. As the product of libertarian culture, I was only too willing to take responsibility for the unnamed symptoms of lupus. They were a result of choices I had made in diet, exercise, stress and time management, vitamin supplements, and so on, resulting in more self-blame than self-congratulation (another lupus inversion). When I had "good days," I would forget all about this other that had been me and attribute what I saw as the restoration of self, again, to my self: to my agency. Gradually, however, these movements between "good" and "bad" sites of self began to rot out the trusses of the material and ideological conditions that I assumed would always support me, and to create a growing mistrust of signs as symptoms of anything. This polyvocality was nothing to celebrate.

Another aspect of lupus which contributes to its creeping, othering malaise is its lack of stigmata, which relates directly to the role of other people in chronic illness. As a mostly invisible disability, there is little evidence that one is sojourning in the kingdom of the ill, no evidence of what Erving Goffman (1963) in his study of stigma and illness has called a "spoiled identity." An insider anecdote among people with lupus concerns the experience of being sick but being told that you look great. In my experience this can imply a number of things, some of them well-intended. In fact, a colleague recently spoke to me of someone whom s/he described as having "played the disability card." I must confess I did not disclose the fact of my dual citizenship in response to this TAB myth of disability as a deceptive game played for special dispensation. (Incidentally, numerous studies proclaim the workplace well-supported by the chronically ill and disabled). Clearly, the blessing of being able to "pass" in the TAB world is a mixed one. In the years of coping with lupus before it was diagnosed, as well as now, other people's responses contributed to the erosion of trust in what I feel; part of the estrangement from self that is lupus. It is important to remember that the Other can also be other people, who too can structure perception and consciousness. Arthur Kleinman observes that we undervalue the processes of social delegitimation, which are part of the social course of an illness or disability. This can intensify suffering (1995a, 181), whereas legitimated suffering often serves "to critique social structures and to inspire social reforms" (182), and to produce improved coping and self-efficacy.

However, TAB blind spots and assumptions can be enabling: lupus invisibility, for instance, allows me to "pass" among TABs. Without a ticket, I often drag myself onto the commuter train of the well and get from the A to B of my day without indwelling on the sick speak of my lupus other. (Note that I have developed my own language for this inverse reality.) This phrase captures the inward self-focus of lupus malaise, when the body's needs threaten to overwrite all other consciousness. As anyone with chronic pain will tell you, these put the lie to the old adage that it's merely "mind over matter." (Chronic illness inverts this and a lot of other conventional wisdom.) However, I am careful not to use my forged visitor's visa too often: it is disrespectful and unempathic to a part of me which others deny. Still, at the same time as I do not want to consecrate myself to the bad faith of modernity's denial of death, I do not want to make other or completely reject the simple robust pleasure of the self-in-life, its ebullient blindnesses, its quick, bright things and progressivist convictions. Part of this is life itself; part of this is still me.

As an academic, I have found cognitive dissonance (called lupus fog or fugue) particularly disabling. This includes memory lapses such as aphasia, problems with sequential thinking, and (particularly disabling) dissociation. In a lupus fog, the face of my lupus other is exposed: I can't find the right word, spell, explain, extemporize, write, or debate. To reduce these problems, neurologists suggest that one reduce distraction, avoid time pressures and busy places, limit taking on new and unfamiliar tasks, avoid speeded and timed tasks, use plenty of post-it notes, and avoid situations that divide one's attention (Kosaka 2002, 25–26). This advice, however, is the equivalent of throwing paper airplane sticky notes at the cognitive dysfunction targeting my career. The logical (but counterintuitive) thing to do has been to give up, to surrender, to fail. With lupus, giving up is an important part of maintaining self-efficacy.

By accepting limitations, by letting abject presences seep into my public life, I began to acknowledge the face and hear the voice of the not-quite not-other of lupus. This is part of a traumatic process which Emmanuel Lévinas has also equated with othering. For Lévinas, the self-absorbed, self-interested ego, what Arthur Frank calls the "cognitive-ethereal I" (1995, 33), is the starting point for discerning the other. The face of the Other disrupts this I; it is more than this I can grasp or appropriate. It transports you before you know you are in its sealed boxcar or its dark hold, before you know it as trauma. Rudi Visker paraphrases Lévinas:

> The Other divides me, "denucleates" and beleaguers me, does not leave me alone but instead obsesses me and persecutes me, takes me hostage and traumatizes me, brings me to hate myself, to abdicate my place at the center of my own concerns, to give everything up, to give nothing more to myself, and thus to hemorrhage ceaselessly ... (2000, 248)

For me, this is the physical, psychological, and social course of lupus, a recognition without meaning at first which produces a retreat into self, an attempt to salvage the space and entitlements of the cognitive-ethereal I, while falling into the solipsism of believing that your pain is unique. This is the heteronomy of not-quite not-other, the "subjection to an other law (Greek, *heteron*, other + *nomos*, law)" (Robbins 1991, 102) that Lévinas contends can be a call to responsibility. In Lévinas' view, to force this other to be the same by appropriating it to our own paradigms, or by indifferent recognition of alterity as isolated and incommensurable, is not ethical, for "the self is non-indifference to the other" (Lévinas 1981, 171). From such empathic witnessing in the space of abjection, one may become responsible.

What can a responsible academic not-quite not-Other presume to relate to the temporarily able-bodied academic from this place? First of all, that academics work too hard. I think that we need to acknowledge more often than we do that the academic workplace is similar to other workplaces in our society where, in the name of a very destructive and antisocial conception of professional achievement, work consumes most people's time and energy. Workplace has become the single site of adult identity and self-worth in our culture; hence, it is delegitimating to be outside the institutions of work in North American society. While I do not mean to be disrespectful to the enormous vocational energy involved in much professional achievement, I believe that present-day professional expectations have taken a toll that we are not consciously acknowledging. The escalation in the tempo of academic life over the past few decades is having a profoundly disturbing impact. I would suggest that, at present, the demands of the academic workplace are geared to the stamina and available discretionary time of a driven, robust, well-supported thirty-year-old graduate student without dependents. Evidence of this more frenetic professional pacing of academic life is showing up in the academic body-self: in higher rates (even when controlling for more sophisticated diagnostic techniques and more contractual entitlements for leave) of sick leave and long-term disability, unpaid leave, stress-triggered disease, various autoimmune diseases, reproductive dysfunction, sleep disorders, depression, and the socially shamed "stress leave," for example. To paraphrase Arthur Frank, the academic "body [knows] the story already" (63).

Part of the problem is that academe remains monadic, in spite of feminism, employment equity, discussions of diversity, and deconstructions of certain forms of meritocracy, and academe strives to maintain itself as such because many of us assume that the mind is its own bounded place. Monadic workplaces, like monadic philosophies, tend towards exclusivity and exclusionary practices. I can tell you that they are not good places in which to ask for help. Now academic life is a wonderful entitlement for most of us who feel fortunate to have this intellectual space and place of our own, especially for women, who have finally been allowed to live the life of the mind legitimately. I sometimes think, however, that what we see as entitlements are based on an intellectual myth that the body may become infirm but the mind is self-renewing. (Though, at the same time, I have heard many of my colleagues express their fear of Alzheimer's and other cognitive impairments, never physical ones; this is surely the return of the repressed.)

The ideal of autonomous academic selfhood and the reality of the monadic workplace exclude the body. This is evident in the structure of the academic year where teaching, evaluation, institutional service, and research are perceived as an eight-month, isolated, heroic quest that far too many survive through the compensations of bad diet, lack of exercise, and social isolation. The rhythm of our academic lives is based on accepting exhaustion as part of the seasonal cycle. We allow this because we have put such a premium on the monadic (but also enervating) solitude of the non-instructional period, or sabbatical. Like the culture at large, we exclude respite and rest from academic life. Having lupus means making time and space for rest, but these times and spaces have been eliminated from our lives and our institutions. Similarly, maintaining a high level of academic performance while child-bearing and rearing small children was considered extraordinary thirty years ago, but has now become industry standard. I have no answers to any of this, but think it is important to assert that this is unethical to the body self. Why should the body pay for professional increments in the currency of burnout, or arrive in the room of one's own in a state of exhaustion?

This escalated tempo of academic life has an impact on students as well. When workplace pressures increase, there is a tendency to become very focused on product, not process, and perhaps accounting, as Professor Harry Vandervlist notes (Craven 2002, 9), for the cyberplagiarism plague of late. As educators, we have failed to give students an alternative to the tempo of mass culture. Ironically, it was this alternative which initially attracted me to a career in the humanities twenty-five years ago.

Though the not-quite not-other academics have a responsibility to speak out about these barriers in the workplace, many do not "come out" because of rigid methods of social control. Citizenship in the monadic kingdom is subtly but easily revoked in destructive silences, marginalizations of one kind or another, in the widespread view that discussions of illness and disability are narcissistic taboo excretions, and in the retreat into the non-responsibility of policy and procedure. I believe that where postmodern academe has come to recognize difference, it has become respectful and proactive, for example, in terms of the specific alterities of race, ethnicity, gender, and sometimes class; but the otherness of disability and chronic illness remains largely invisible, flattened out as the same ("playing the disability card") or treated with detachment. This is disabling for everyone in the academic workplace, particularly for students with disabilities.

Moreover, it is difficult to express abjection in the objectifying language of the third person, or to ask for help in the discourses built up around a hermeneutic of suspicion (Frank 2002). Few illness narratives can survive a thoroughgoing deconstruction, an inquisitorial unmasking of essentialism; few cries for help can be heard by those inured to polyvocality, subversion, and subtext. As Arthur Frank has stated, ill people do not need their stories critiqued and decoded by an exalted interpretive community, as much as they require a body of empathic listeners (2002). Even in discussions of illness narrative, a pervasive fear of what I call the "Oprahfying" of academic discourse surfaces from time to time, of (shamefully) capitulating to the "emotional pornography" of confessional popular culture. Yet this response to the emotive abject may disable our ability to hear the voice or the chaos story (Frank 1995, 98) of chronic illness and disability. Similarly, many academics are nervous about some of the master narratives of illness: for example, the "journey" of chronic illness as spiritual recovery, as healing rather than cure, makes most cultural materialists cringe.

It is also important to remember, however, that materialist analysis of culture is a close cousin of rationalized modern medicine, which looks at illness and disability as a puzzle to be solved rather than as a mystery to be faced (Frank 1995, 84). From the site of lupus abjection, I have reread medieval and Renaissance accounts of illness and disability, noting how these writers at least had a legitimate site from which to express this mystery (which materialist analysis defines as false consciousness). In earlier times, self-in-illness was not the site of self-interrupted but a legitimate site of self, a place where one could legitimately "be," and not become a voiceless and muted abject.

I wish there were more legitimate fora for the discussion of disability and chronic illness in academe. At present, I often feel that my lupus is merely paperwork in the system. I know that my supervisors and colleagues attempt to protect my and their monadic intellectual sovereignty in their dealings with me: these are the conditions of respect in the academic workplace. My supervisors feel that they would be acting without respect to discuss this taboo, excreted part of me with me or anyone else. Many are, in Lévinas' sense however, indifferent to the alterity of chronic illness and disability, and do not see themselves implicated or responsible in any way. The "puzzle" that I am to the system must be left to the extrasystemic adjudicators: the specialists and the disability case managers. I think it is time for a reconstituted sense of respect.

In conclusion, I hope that I have helped in locating some of the forces within academe that are denials of access not only for the chronically ill and disabled, but for the temporarily able-bodied (TABs) as well. That I presume to make observations and recommendations, I attribute to lupus's improvisations, its shapeshifting, its deferrals, its reprieves, its revisionist remappings, and its redrawn boundaries, that have allowed me to see more clearly the crumbling coastlines and melting glaciers of the academic body politic.

SHARON DALE STONE

WOMEN SURVIVING HEMORRHAGIC STROKE
Narratives of Meaning

Stroke, whether hemorrhagic or ischemic,[1] carries the potential to disable survivors on physical, cognitive, and emotional levels. Although hemorrhagic stroke is not rare in children and young adults, there is little information available that is relevant to the lives of relatively young survivors of hemorrhagic stroke. Popular discourse does not distinguish between hemorrhagic and ischemic stroke, and understands stroke as an experience of old age. Within this context, young survivors of hemorrhagic stroke are an anomaly, and their experiences cannot be easily inserted or made intelligible within that discourse. What is needed is an alternative discourse, which allows for a recognition that the traumatic event of stroke can and does happen at any age.

To challenge the notion that stroke is an experience of old age, and to create a contextualized understanding of what it can be like to survive a stroke at a relatively young age, I have been collecting and analyzing the narratives of women who survived a hemorrhagic stroke before the age of fifty and were left with residual, invisible disabilities. I also have been gathering data through in-depth and open-ended interviews with a convenience sample of women, as well as analyzing other relevant narratives written by interview participants. The open-ended interviews focus on issues such as the experience of disability, sense of self, relations with others, and how these women make sense of the experience of stroke.[2]

Despite the multi-faceted nature of my data, the focus of this essay is on what participants had to say as they reflected on the significance of their strokes. Relying on excerpts from the narratives of six women (including myself) that were collected at an early stage of the research,[3] I discuss

TABLE 1
Summary Overview of Participant Characteristics

	Age at Stroke	Residence at Stroke	Marital Status at Stroke	Current Marital Status	Current Education	Employment at Stroke	Current Employment	Stroke-related Disabilities
J	11	Quebec	Lived with parents	Common-law, same-sex	PhD	N/A	University professor	•Right-sided weakness •Poor balance •Slight aphasia •Cognitive difficulties •Easily fatigued
B	17	Ontario	Lived with parents	Recently married	MSW	N/A	Child welfare worker	•Left-sided weakness •Easily fatigued
D	24	New York City	Single, lived with boyfriend	Recently divorced	Law degree	Lawyer, municipal government	Lawyer, municipal government	•Left-sided weakness •Easily fatigued
K	25	Oregon	Common-law, same-sex	Common-law, same-sex	BA; graduate student	Videographer for a university	Videographer for a university	•Right-sided weakness •Easily fatigued •Aphasia
L	31	Ontario	Common-law, opposite sex	Common-law, opposite sex	High school	Bookstore chain publicist	Mostly unemployed; sometimes does contract work as a publicist	•Left-sided weakness •Poor balance •Easily fatigued
S	36	Ontario	Married	Married	High school	Bank customer service manager	Unemployed; has applied for disability pension	•Poor balance •Cognitive difficulties •No sense of smell or taste •Easily fatigued

how identity can be affected by the traumatic experience of hemorrhagic stroke.

Each of the six stories in this essay were narrated more than three years post-stroke, so that each woman interviewed had learned to accommodate for residual disabilities and was able to reflect upon post-stroke experiences. My discussion of their stories is not meant to suggest that they are representative of the larger population of women survivors of hemorrhagic stroke. Indeed, in some respects these research participants are relatively homogeneous. They are a privileged group in terms of skin colour, previous and/or current employment, and in terms of access to medical knowledge and supportive social networks. They are also an exceptionally articulate and thoughtful group of women. Nevertheless, an analysis of their narratives is suggestive of issues and themes that may well be found in the narratives of others. Table 1 provides a brief overview of participant characteristics.

AGE AS A PROMINENT THEME IN THE NARRATIVES

Looking at these narratives as a whole, it is striking to note how significant age is in affecting not only initial diagnosis and medical treatment, but also the meaning that participants subsequently attributed to the stroke.

The three participants aged twenty-four and under at the time of their stroke were initially misdiagnosed with maladies ranging from flu to hysteria, even though each of them presented classic signs of hemorrhagic stroke. The three participants between the ages of twenty-five and thirty-six, however, were correctly diagnosed very shortly after being examined by a physician. Significantly, those who were diagnosed in a timely manner made a speedier, and arguably a more complete, physical recovery than those were not.

Those who were children at the time of the stroke recall that they understood neither the seriousness of what had happened to them, nor the long-term implications. J, for example, had been looking forward to going to a new school when she had her stroke. She was not hospitalized until several days afterwards, and she recalls her concern that she might miss the first day at her new high school. When she was taken by ambulance to the hospital, her hopes of immediate recovery were ended. That disappointment, however, was soon forgotten as she spent seven weeks in the hospital, and several months after that, re-learning basic skills such as walking and talking. Through all of it, however, J does not recall understanding the life-threatening nature of what had happened to her, and she does not recall understanding that her life had irrevocably changed.

In a similar manner, B recalls being in intensive care, and being angry with her father for calling her summer employer to say that she would not be working. In her words, "I couldn't imagine that in three weeks I wouldn't be fine."

B also recalls her hospitalization experience:

> Once it was diagnosed, the only slot for me was that of an old woman and I should be glad to be in a wheelchair. But I wanted to walk ... As it was I was always the youngest by far in the neurology and neurosurgery ward and the fact that I wanted to and expected to walk, and so on, was hard for them to figure. The nurses were very kind to me, rather like I was a favourite pet but had no facilities for me in regards to rehabilitation with my needs as a young woman understood. I remember thinking that I knew what it was to be eighty-five, but not eighteen.

D also raises the issue of the salience of age. Speaking about her experience at a rehabilitation institute, she says, "There were no other young stroke patients and I felt as if, by some bizarre time warp, I had suddenly become elderly and ended up in a nursing home at twenty-four."

For those who were already adults, however, age was not a factor that they considered significant in shaping their experiences of recovery and rehabilitation. Moreover, those who were older could readily grasp the seriousness of what happened.

In Retrospect: Making Sense of the Experience

On an emotional or psychosocial level, each participant has felt the impact of the stroke differently. K, for example, suggests that she has a new sense of self as a result of the stroke. Whereas she used to feel driven to push herself or be an overachiever, she is now happy to take things slowly and appreciate the little things in life. In her words, "My life may have been changed considerably back in 1990, but I have to say, it has changed for the better in many ways. It just opened my eyes to a lot. It really reminded me of the little things we often take for granted. It helped me slow down, become more real and down to earth."

Similarly, L was also an overachiever in her work. She pushed herself hard, frequently working sixteen hours a day, and competed fiercely with others to be the best. L reflects that

I think that one thing that did come out of the stroke, you know, that I never used to do before is—I was a great planner in that, you know, when I do this or I will do this, I will be this in such and such. Set a time or whatever. And now it's ... one day at a time. I lived a lot in the future and I think that's one of the bad things about our society, is we live too much in the future ... and we don't live for now. And I think that *that*, out of everything, is one of the biggest and best things that I've gotten from my experience.

My career was my life for such a long time, controlling everything as much as I could. And now I'm ... maybe I just came to this realization earlier, you know, as maybe I would have come to it when I was in my fifties, but because as I say I "stroked out," you know, I came to it in my thirties. That you know there're a lot of things you have no control over and just, you do the best you can do, and that's all anybody can ask of you. No one needs to say "poor L," or "what a horrible thing." 'Cause it wasn't. It's actually been one of the best things that's ever happened to me. Ironically.

As these excerpts indicate, both K and L feel that their lives have changed for the better because of their strokes. They are able to enjoy life more, and they believe that they have learned important lessons that they may not have otherwise learned. K does not comment on the significance of her age at the time of the stroke, but L is grateful that the stroke happened when it did, so that she was old enough to have experienced adulthood but still young enough to be able to reorganize her priorities without great difficulty. She has, as she says, "a lot more laughing left to do," and she intends to relax and enjoy herself. It is interesting that L takes the word "stroke," which has negative connotations in mainstream society, and gives it a positive meaning to describe her own experience. In so doing, she emphasizes the life-affirming effects of the stroke.

D was also profoundly affected on a psychic level by the stroke, but regards its effects somewhat differently from K or L. For D, having a stroke at age twenty-four, as she was just beginning to embark on a professional career, meant that her life took a turn that she had not originally envisioned. In particular, her dreams of professional upward mobility were shattered. "There are days," she says, "that I feel really bad. Like the days that I get my Wellesley [College alumni] magazine and I see what other people have done ... I can be relatively philosophical but yeah, I haven't had the career that I might have had." Yet, she can still find positive aspects in the experience, saying that it has made her a more compassionate and spiritual person. "I needed more of a connection with God," she says, "than I think I would have gotten if I hadn't had the stroke. So for the most part it has changed me for the better."

D was divorced only a few years before the interview. She was not happy in the marriage and she says:

> I have gained a lot of self confidence since I left my husband ... And I'm starting to think about different things I'd like to do ... and in a way, you know, my experiences have given me a certain confidence that if I can survive a stroke and work and raise two children and then go and get a divorce and survive that, I can do anything.

Thus, D experienced the stroke as a traumatic "biographical disruption" (Bury 1982) that prevented her from following the path that she originally charted for herself. At the same time, however, she learned a great deal from her experience. She was able to create a new life for herself in which she became a compassionate, more spiritual person. Certainly, it was a pivotal experience at an early age, but not a wholly negative experience in terms of outcome.

The other participants who had this pivotal experience at an early age are J and B, neither of whom had reached adulthood when their strokes occurred. B in particular feels that age seventeen was the worst possible age to be for something like that to happen. She says:

> I think if I had been older it would have been easier. But also if I'd have been a lot younger, it might have been easier. I think that that age, because it interferes so much with social development and with education, and things like that. That, for me I suppose, it was a fairly big chunk of time where I had to take, um, really getting sick, and really getting better, and then rehabilitation and all that stuff. So it was a fairly long period of time. And when I sort of re-emerged, I was so far away from where everybody else was. You know, like everybody else I had gone to high school with, for example, had graduated and gone to university and were down that path. And I really didn't know, I always felt that I was, I hoped nobody thought this was where I was supposed to be, this sort of netherland of, of doing things! That I didn't really want to be doing for the rest of my life but didn't know how, how to get from where I was to where I'd want to be.

B continues by saying that, for a long time,

> I think I just felt really different ... Much of my life, since the aneurysm, I felt as if I didn't fit in. I always knew I wasn't rendered retarded, but it took a lot to learn again, to catch up. One time it was suggested that I be placed in a home "for other girls who were socially unacceptable." I wouldn't even go to look. And now, I don't feel like I have a lot in common with a lot of the groups I should, age and job-wise. It's like the quotation at the beginning of one of the Herman Hesse novels about the difficulty of going away on a journey is that when you come back nobody has been where you have. I have often

thought of my experience like having been away on a long journey and now that I am back there is nobody who shared it, had a similar journey.

B regards her experience of stroke and recovery as crucial parts of her biography, making her who she became. Thirty years after the event, as she reflects on her life as a whole, she says that if she could live her life again and selectively erase certain events, her stroke is not something she would choose to erase.

For her part, J says that, at times, she feels that even those to whom she is closest are not able to understand how her life has been affected by stroke, much as they might want to. J feels that because she was only eleven years old when she had her stroke, she was not old enough to have formed a clear sense of identity. Consequently, she feels that her identity was shaped within the context of her experiences of surviving stroke. She says,

> I spent my teenage years preoccupied with what I couldn't do. My parents really reinforced for me that I was "handicapped," that I couldn't expect to do the things my sister did or expect to be independent.... It wasn't until in my twenties, after I left home, that I was able to begin developing a sense of myself as an independent person with a right to take part in social life. I never really learned how to be with people my own age ...
>
> On the other hand ... when I reflect on my experience of stroke and rehabilitation, I don't see it as a horrible tragedy. Sure, it wasn't fun, but I get angry that so many people see it that way, because I see it as just part of my life. A very important part of my life, that in many ways has shaped me. My life might have been very different had I not had that experience, but I'm not unhappy with my life. I'm not unhappy with my disabilities either. I learned quite a while ago to accept my disabilities and just get on with it. They're part of who I am.

The only one who does not regard the stroke as a life-changing experience with positive aspects is S, who was thirty-six at the time of the event. On the one hand, S says that she realizes how fortunate she is to have survived her ruptured aneurysm, and she enjoys and values life more than she did beforehand. She used to be a workaholic, getting to the office before 8AM, not leaving before 7PM, and sometimes working weekends too. Now, she says, she tries to live each day to its fullest.

On the other hand, S's identity was intricately bound up with her work. "I always enjoyed work," she says. "That's part of my identity, is work." Now that she's not part of the workforce, she misses it terribly. She has investigated volunteer work, which she says she would like to do in order to keep busy, but she was told by her long-term disability provider that unless she wanted to lose her benefits, she was not even allowed to do volunteer work. Thus, S has a hard time finding anything positive about the outcomes of her stroke.

S also says that she "used to be more carefree" but now takes life more seriously: "I question myself more often, I guess. I second-guess myself ... I'm not as sure of myself as I was before." Though S does not say it in so many words, it seems that she, like D, sees her experience in terms of biographical disruption. Her life was supposed to have followed a different trajectory from the one that it currently follows. As she says, "you can try to get over it and move on and put it behind you, but it's always, it's part of your life now."

Who Creates Survivor Narratives: A Concluding Note

It is, as mentioned earlier in this chapter, unlikely that these women are representative of the entire population of relatively young female survivors of hemorrhagic stroke. Nevertheless, it is interesting that all six, each from different parts of Canada and the United States, and each embedded within different social networks, share a sense of feeling left out of popular discourse. Each feels, on a visceral level, that others cannot understand what it is like to have the experience of surviving hemorrhagic stroke at a relatively young age. In this regard, B's use of the journey metaphor is striking, along with her feeling that she cannot talk to others about where she has been because they do not understand. There is little information available in Western culture to allow others to make sense of what these women might have to say about where they have been.

Tentatively, then, I suggest that each woman has been motivated to tell her story, at least in part, to try to create a basis for understanding, and to try to insert themselves into popular discourse so that they do not feel so strange, so foreign. The point is not to emphasize how special they are, but to emphasize how ordinary they are.[4] They do not want their experiences ignored, objectified, or abstracted out of the context of their whole lives. Rather, they would like others to recognize that their experiences are inextricably bound up with their current identities. Indeed, for those who were children at the time, their experiences were central for shaping their adult identities and sense of self. For those who were adults, former priorities have been replaced with a new sense of what is important in life, and experiences have been taken into account as a new identity—that of survivor—has been adopted. As S says, "it's part of your life now."

Notes

1 Ischemic stroke occurs when the blood flow in an artery leading to the brain is somehow blocked and brain cells are deprived of oxygen and nutrients. Hemorrhagic stroke occurs when a blood vessel in the brain leaks or ruptures, and blood spills into the brain or surrounding tissues. This type of stroke is typically caused by a ruptured aneurysm (a ballooning from a weak spot in an artery wall) or arteriovenous malformation (a tangle of thin-walled blood vessels).
2 This research has received ethical approval from Lakehead University's Research Ethics Board.
3 The only narratives that had been collected when this paper was presented in May 2002. One of the narratives included here is my own, as I am myself a survivor of hemorrhagic stroke in childhood. Space restrictions preclude a full discussion of methodological issues, but it can be briefly noted that my identity as a stroke survivor who is also a researcher added to my credibility and trustworthiness for those I interviewed.
4 Related to this point, Bruner argues that one function of autobiography is "to present ourselves to others (and to ourselves) as typical or characteristic or 'culture confirming' in some way" (2001, 30).

BRETT SMITH AND ANDREW C. SPARKES

MEN, SPORT, AND SPINAL CORD INJURY
Identity Dilemmas, Embodied Time, and the Construction of Coherence

The realist tale presented in this essay invites you first to imagine, if you can, having a life story that in the telling involves being a fit, able-bodied, young man with a disciplined and dominating body, as described by Arthur Frank (1995), who loves playing sport, and rugby union football in particular. Also imagine a life story whose main themes, over the years, have centred on the development of a strong athletic identity and a sense of self based on a performing body. Now imagine, if you can, this story from a life history interview.

> In the second half [of the rugby match], we turned up the pressure. It must have been about five or ten minutes to go until the end of the match ... I remember they [the other team] were coming at us, they were in their own half, there was I on the wing and he [the centre] was outside ... Then, then, [silence—five seconds], then as he [the centre] got closer and closer, in a very split second I changed my mind, sort of changed my position, just fractionally. This was in a split second, he dipped his shoulder at the same time as I lowered my position and his shoulder hit me straight on the top of my head. It was a bang against a brick wall really ... And the next minute I was lying on the floor saying: "Can you put my arms and legs down on the floor?" ... It just never dawned on me that maybe I was paralyzed ... In that moment I went from being a big strong man, to something totally opposite; to being disabled.

The purpose of this essay is to present a brief overview of findings to date from a research project that focuses on the lived experiences of men in the United Kingdom who have suffered a spinal cord injury (SCI) through playing the contact sport of rugby football union, and now define themselves as disabled. Three fundamental themes to emerge from the data that underpin the SCI experience are discussed. First, drawing on a number of analytical concepts, the narrative identity dilemmas associated with interrupted body projects for sporting men are highlighted. Second, biographical data are utilized to illustrate the ways in which time is embodied and, in turn, framed and constructed within the restitution narrative as defined by Arthur Frank (1995). Third, utilizing the principles advocated by James Holstein and Jaber Gubrium (2000), we explore the manner in which coherence is constructed in the stories told.

The methodology underpinning this project has been described in detail elsewhere (see Smith and Sparkes 2002, 2004, 2005a; Sparkes and Smith 2002, 2003). However, several points are worth mentioning again. Discussion in this essay is derived from data collected on fourteen Caucasian, heterosexual men who have all been heavily involved in rugby football union, and each of whom has experienced a SCI through playing this contact sport. All were involved in confidential, thematic, life history interviews conducted in their homes by the primary investigator (Brett Smith). Each participant was interviewed at least twice over a one-year period. The total time interviewing each person ranged from seven to twenty-three hours. All interviews were tape-recorded, transcribed, and analyzed reflexively, utilizing multiple forms of narrative analysis (see Lieblich, Tuval-Maschiach, and Zilber 1998; Smith and Sparkes 2005b; Sparkes 1999, 2005).

Theme One:
Narrative Identity Dilemmas

Prior to SCI, the bodies of the participants, not uncommonly, were a largely absent presence in their lives. SCI, however, shakes previous taken-for-granted assumptions about possessing a smoothly functioning body, drastically disrupting any sense of body–self unity and familiarity. At the same time, the body becomes the totality of the participants' worlds. Thus, the body *dysappears* (see Leder 1990) and becomes *inescapably embodied*. As Jacob, who is forty-two years old and has been disabled for twenty-two years, said: "The body is there all the time; I can't escape it; and yet I'm still surprised when I see my body in the mirror; I just don't recognize it."

Furthermore, the majority of the men suggested that SCI as a turning-point moment led to devalued notions of themselves as people. In part, this was due to the rapid dissolution of five central aspects of their sense of self: the loss of the working body–self; loss of the physical body, including bowel and bladder control; loss of, and disruptions to family and sporting relationships; loss of athletic identities; and loss of embodied masculinities. As an exemplar, Max, a forty-five-year-old who had played county standard rugby football but, like the majority of the men interviewed, is not involved in disabled sports, commented on the loss of athletic identities: "Who I was, as a sportsman, has gone. I've lost that part of myself and I want it back. I want to play rugby again; I want to be an athlete again; but disability has taken it away. I'm no one now; I'm incomplete."

In the face of what is experienced as a major loss, the men often attempt to reconcile the self or cope with their disability by taking narrative refuge in a *restored self*, specifically an *entrenched self* (Charmaz 1987). The desire for a restored self is reflected in the following comment made by Rob, a thirty-six-year-old, who, like many of the men interviewed, received financial compensation from the Rugby Football Union and is now on disability benefit: "I'm disabled, but it's not what I want. For me, I want my old self back. I want to get back who I was and I'll keep trying to get back myself until the day I die ... I will make a comeback. A cure will be found and I'll walk again."

The themes we have focused upon in this essay can have many interpretations. For us, moments just described signal the difficulty some men have in re-storying a valued sense of self in the face of a major trauma and epiphany. In part, these difficulties are exacerbated by the participant's *reliance* on hegemonic forms of masculinity (Gerschick and Miller 1995), and the strength of the athletic identities they developed prior to SCI through their involvement in rugby and other contact sports. Many might presume that these men have the *narrative resources* to contemplate options with regard to re-storying their lives, but we would suggest that, for the majority of the participants, this might not be the case and that their opportunities to re-embody or reinvent themselves, so as to form a different body–self relationship, are often constrained. In considering this issue, we have found three of the four dimensions of narrativity described by Margaret Somers (1994) to be useful. These are the *ontological* (my story), *public* (cultural and institutional formations), and *metanarratives* (epic dramas). In relation to these dimensions of narrativity we would suggest that one of the ways in which the participants' ontological narratives are framed, and constrained, is by the combined forces of the public narratives of heroic masculinity and the metanarrative of restitution.

As part of their exploration of *heroic masculinity* in the recovery of men from SCI, Douglas Kleiber and Susan Hutchinson (1999) undertook a documentary analysis of three disability magazines in the USA. They found the plot, events, and characters in the stories about men with SCI to be orientated around three themes of heroism: *commitment to battle*, *heroic qualities*, and *heroic action*. Kleiber and Hutchinson further argued that these stories and themes act as narrative maps or scripts for newcomers to the world of SCI in ways that can be inspirational or constraining. However, to the extent that these magazines and stories reinforce, rely upon, and actively cultivate a traditional model of masculinity, they may act to hinder the transformative potential of disability. As Kleiber and Hutchinson suggest, "Portraying recovery as aligning one's actions with those of the physically heroic not only creates an unrealistic ideal that most individuals cannot live up to, it also directs the course of recovery in personally limiting ways" (152).

The limitations of hero narratives are themselves connected to the constraints and contradictions inherent in a very powerful metanarrative. Specifically, the disciplined and dominating body the participants previously inhabited and made investments in as able-bodied sportsmen, we would suggest, had an elective affinity for a *restitution narrative*, and this legacy remains with them as disabled men (Frank 1995). This should not, however, be viewed as a state of "false" consciousness, since this, with its correspondence-to-truth overtones, asserts a belief in a real world independent of people's interests, or knowledge of those interests. Likewise, this (dis)embodied affinity to certain kinds of narratives should not be seen as necessarily "living in denial," "bad," or "wrong." For one, what constitutes denial and a good or bad narrative can be defined only in relation to the social and political community of speakers and listeners. Yet, problems arise when people become fixated on one kind of body and sense of self in circumstances where the restitution and hero narrative are not appropriate. Under such circumstances, individuals find it hard to remind themselves that other body–self narratives might have to be found and told. This is particularly so in conditions or times that foreground moral images of disability, health, and illness simply in terms of what Frank (2000) calls *rides*. However, without an increase in their narrative resources, and by being denied alternative relations of reciprocity within a community that affords the self's need for the recognition of others, the space and opportunity for these men to craft who they want to be, and can be, remains constrained for the time being.

Theme Two:
The Body and Narrative Time

Lives, as Brian Roberts (1999) reminds us, have to be understood as lived within time, and time is experienced according to narrative. Equally, as the men in our study have told their life stories to us, at particular times in their lives, the issue of time has been implicit in their accounts. For example, some men's memories of being able bodied are situated in the past, while living as a disabled person occupies the present and shapes the future. Accordingly, in what follows, we seek to make explicit the ways in which these men experience biographical time.

Prior to SCI, time was taken for granted. The participants' memories of being able bodied also evoked a life that was often viewed as if it were a continuous line of chronological marks. This *linear* narrative model of time was, in part, cultivated, shaped, and maintained through the men's involvement in rugby and other cultural practices. Rugby, as a historically grounded sporting ritual firmly entrenched in a masculine world, also provides a context in which human bodies are *disciplined* in time (Seymour 2002). As Phil, a forty-three-year-old accountant commented, "When I played rugby, I trained, ran, put on more muscle, and ate a good diet. My life followed a pretty straightforward path. Y'know, A, B, C, work, home, training, then a game at the weekends, and so on—a very regimented lifestyle." Importantly, a linear narrative and disciplined time, associated with masculine views of time, is embodied. Here, the *disciplined* and *dominating* bodies the men cultivated, partly via sporting practices, are bodies in time, and time is felt within them. These bodies have linear and disciplined time in their flesh.

Becoming disabled through sport, however, disrupts the critical time–body relationship upon which the participants build their lives. The incident of SCI means that the body becomes *immortalized* in time. Now the body is "a perpetual memorial to the split second of time in which the spinal cord was severed" (Seymour 2002, 138). Moreover, as Seymour (2002) pointed out, time is *ruptured* during the initial period of rehabilitation that accompanies the first three to twelve months of SCI, as the reality of bodily frailty, vulnerability, and finitude confronts the previous, taken-for-granted manner in which time and life was storied. Other comments made also suggest that within the context of the spinal rehabilitation unit, the participants in this study experienced time as *waiting* (Charmaz 1991). For Dan, a twenty-seven-year-old who lives with his parents, "To become disabled means spending a lot of time waiting and feeling bored. And since it's frustrating, not being able to do what you want when you want, I end up waiting for everything to happen ... In rehabilitation, I'd wait to see the physiotherapist and the doctors. I'd also spend a lot time waiting in the corridors simply to try to talk to people; but people really get on with their own thing, or are still in shock and it doesn't feel as though anything is changing. It can be a very lonely time."

On their return "home," following the period spent in a spinal rehabilitation unit, the participants begin the process of re-storying the body in relation to its temporal implications so that meaning is given their experiences. Now, in everyday life post-SCI, the disciplined and the dominating body experiences time in complex and different ways that were, in turn, powerfully shaped by specific cultural narratives. For example, current experiences of time, for many of the men, are mediated and shaped by the body's affinity for restitution narratives. Here, the past is in the future as they wait for a cure that will return them to an able-bodied state of being: As Matthew noted, "My future is the all important thing in my life because it's there when a cure will be found. In that sense, I suppose that I think of myself in the future, walking again, and being the person I was in the past ... As I've said, I loved my life in the past, and I don't want this life now. So my time now is spent thinking about the future and being able to walk again."

Notably, such comments connect these men to the "time perspectives" of the *past in the future*, the *present in the future*, and the *future as the past* as identified by Brian Roberts (1999) and to a *philosophy of the future* ("temporal orientation") noted by Michele Crossley (2000). Other comments made by those who embodied restitution narratives also suggest that these men have experienced some of the different kinds of time identified by Charmaz (1991) and Seymour (2002), such as *waiting* time, *consumed* time, *ingested* time, and *disciplined* time. For example, talking about his current post SCI experiences of consumed and ingested time, Richard, a single forty-two-year-old, said: "There are only twenty-four hours in the day and unfortunately I spend most of it doing the most mundane, predictable things that I never thought twice about when I was able-bodied. Y'know, making a cup of tea or a sandwich can take an age whereas before it only took a minute and I never gave the process a consideration. But that's not a bad thing I suppose because I have to watch what I put in my body, although I still need a lot fluids, which means I sometimes wet myself, and that can be quite embarrassing I can tell you."

This discussion above has hinted at how biographical time is experienced by the participants when they were able bodied and involved in sport, and how they now experience time as disabled men, none of whom are involved in sport. It has also briefly noted ways in which this transformation is experienced by the disciplined and dominating body and how these experiences are mediated and shaped by specific cultural narratives (e.g., restitution).

THEME THREE: THE NARRATIVE CONSTRUCTION OF COHERENCE

The notion of coherence in the telling of life stories or life histories is a much-debated issue. For example, Elliot Mishler (1999) argues that coherence is essentially and intractably ambiguous, defying efforts at formal and precise definition. Accordingly, Mishler asks researchers to direct their attention, amongst other areas, towards examining the artful practices through which storytellers "do" coherence, and how "complex and differentiated ways narratives can be organized to serve their meaning-making functions" (110). In a similar vein, Holstein and Gubrium (2000), concerned with the practical production of coherence in life stories, call for a focus on *narrative practice* that, for them, lies at the heart of self-construction. We will apply some of the principles of these approaches, and draw on a number of analytical concepts provided by others, to parts of a life story told by one of the men in our study in an interview context.

Harry's Story: Composing Coherence within a Restitution Narrative

The following is an extract from an interview (July, 2001) done by Brett Smith with Harry, a former county rugby union player and farmer, who acquired a SCI nine years ago at the age of thirty-two. Unlike the majority of the men in this study, he remains married and has one young child.

> BRETT: How do feel about your body now?
>
> HARRY: It depends. Y'see, there are times when I'm battling against disability and I'm very determined to overcome what has happened to it [the body]. And I've had some success as well. As you can see, I'm able to move the fingers, which the doctors said would never happen ... I've had other victories as well, like leaving the rehabilitation centre before most people who have the same level of [spinal] injury as myself. So, y'see, I've overcome each challenge. And while I can't control the body, which is one aspect of disability that I've never been able to accept, I do think that I've made a lot of progress. I'm still not happy, though, and having no control only stokes me up. Knowing that, well, it frustrates you, and I can feel the anger rising, which again as I've said,

> I end up taking all my anger and everything out on my wife, brother, or whoever is around. And so I hate myself even more.
>
> But, as I say, it all depends. Because usually my mind is on walking again and regaining full movement. That's my main aim, and I do believe that I will walk again, which is something that I can have control over. I say this because medicine is advancing, and I visit a private physiotherapist occasionally so that I can keep it, the body I mean, well, the muscles and the body strong, for when a cure arrives. I've also tried acupuncture, which I'm thinking of having again since, while okay, it didn't help in any way the first time, I have to keep persevering. And I must keep the body in a good state otherwise it might not survive spinal surgery, or whatever the doctors will find to make me walk again. And waiting to walk again is something my family want as well, which is not surprising because I can be very distant with them. It a very lonely existence sitting in a wheelchair, and I do feel distant from much of what my family does. So, y'know, I concentrate all my efforts on trying to beat disability.

By the end of the extract, we might come to interpret Harry's prefatory remark, "It depends," as pointing his listener to the embodied, multivocal character of narrative composition. More specifically, Harry's initial *horizon meaning*, or pattern of *narrative linkages*, suggests that in order to help make sense of events and to tell his stories, he first draws upon a plot that echoes a *romance* narrative (Lieblich et al. 1998). We also witness that this public narrative or classic monomyth is embodied. In Harry's story, the body is *dissociated* from the self. The narrative linkages lengthen to compose a body that assumes the *contingency* of disability and impairment, but does not accept it. Notably, as Harry continues, and as the narrative linkages develop further, he also narrates a body that is *dyadic* in its relation to other bodies. Thus, in keeping with the pattern of composition, we might predict that if Harry had continued with this story he could have composed and made further linkages with what Frank (1995) calls a *dominating body*.

Mid-response, however, Harry *shifts* his body narrative, altering his story's *footing* and *horizon*, displaying *editing*. To be precise, the comment "But, as I say, it all depends," sets off a different pattern of linkages that come to form a *horizon of meaning* akin to a *restitution narrative*. As part of this, the body that is created in this kind of story shifts a dominating body into the background and foregrounds a *disciplined* body (Frank 1995). The narrative linkages make up a body that attempts to reassert *predictability* and is *dissociated* from the self. Importantly, the linkages now extend to a body that is *monadic* in its relation to other bodies.

Despite the brevity of this section, we hope to have provided an illustration of the manner in which coherence is embodied and artfully constructed in the stories told by one man on becoming disabled, and how the various narrative practices that inform this process are themselves framed by both the local and cultural conventions of telling (for greater detail, see Smith and Sparkes 2002).

Closing Comments

In this essay, we have attempted to provide at least a sense of the main themes to emerge from an ongoing research project that focuses on men, sport, SCI, and the reconstruction of body–selves. Clearly, space limitations restrict us from illuminating both the complexity of the participants' experiences and of the stories they tell. Certainly, our growing awareness of the diversity of the stories we are being told, and the contradictions and tensions contained within them, raise a number of issues that require further exploration and elucidation. For example, a small number of men in this study, in direct opposition to the dominant personal tragedy storyline of disability (Oliver 1996) and impairment, now appear to view SCI as an opportunity to reject disempowering identities (such as hegemonic masculinities) and, in turn, re-story a differently valued sense of body–self. Notably, these men draw on the social model story and what Arthur Frank (1995) calls a *quest* narrative. The data generated would also suggest that these public and metanarratives help create *developing* selves, bringing body and self together to form a communicative body-self (Frank 1995).

As part of our work in progress, we have aspired to highlight some of the (dis)embodied dilemmas and constraints the men encounter on a daily basis. We also hope that this work serves as an invitation to take up the different issues it raises, and to explore further the lived experiences of people who become disabled through sport.

PART III

The Larger Picture

THE EDITORS

Introduction
Metanarrative Politics and Polemics

In a paper on the "problems and prospects" of illness narratives given at our conference (a version of which has since been published[1]), Catherine Riessman re-emphasized the need to consider the social contexts of narrative production and reception. She reminded us that although experiences of illness and suffering may be viewed as "personal troubles," such experiences and the narratives they give rise to are always situated in specific historical settings. This section of the book, which includes essays stemming from the social sciences, the humanities, rehabilitation sciences, and interdisciplinary studies, directs attention to the broader socio-political contexts and ideological frames or metanarratives that influence the creation and exchange of stories of disease, disability, and trauma.

The particular contexts within which such narratives are constructed, along with the polemical and political "work" that they perform (Langellier 2001), was of interest to many members of the Wall project. Several were particularly concerned with documenting gender differences. One co-investigator, Isabel Dyck, engaged with Pamela Moss in research that produced the book *Women, Body, Illness: Space and Identity in the Everyday Lives of Women with Chronic Illness* (2002), and another colleague, Patricia Vertinsky, was working on the experiences of women with disabilities today, as a sequel to her 1990 study of perceptions of women's health in the nineteenth century. Margaret Dorazio-Migliore and Marsha Henry, who both held postdoctoral fellowships as part of the project, produced a report on the current intersections of gender, race, ethnicity, and health in Canada for the BC Centre of Excellence for Women's Health, entitled

Making Women Visible (2002). Their investigation documented how the experiences of racialized women are often ignored or trivialized in contemporary health research. Many other studies show that the marginalization of sectors of the population (such as Aboriginal groups and sex trade workers) has profound effects on their access to health care, and false assumptions are often made about the reasons for their ill health. Some of these groups wish to rediscover traditional, or complementary healing practices, but such alternatives to mainstream health care are rarely encouraged. State policies not directly related to health issues may also have an impact, as when questions of citizenship affect the treatment received by refugees who have survived traumatic experiences. Stories about the experiences of marginalized people can destabilize dominant views of health and illness, as well as attract attention to their needs.

The first three papers in this section highlight the intersecting roles of gender, race, class, and ethnicity in a Canadian context. Lyn Jongbloed begins by examining the stories of Vancouver women with multiple sclerosis in relation to policies governing disability income. Her essay points out how these policies have evolved unevenly over time and are maintained by powerful political interests, even though they perpetuate outmoded social values. Better policies will only be developed if policy makers are forced to acknowledge the difficulties experienced by persons with disabilities and society's ethical obligations towards them. Personal stories can be very effective in persuading those in authority of the need for change by providing concrete illustrations of the situations that individuals have to face. They also demonstrate the complex intersections of various types of "othering," based on gender, race or ethnicity, (dis)ability, age, and socio-economic status.

In recent years, autobiographical narratives by members of Canada's First Nations who suffered from residential school policies have received a good deal of attention. In their contribution to this volume, Robert Procyk and Christine Watson, both teachers at the First Nations University of Canada in Saskatchewan, examine the stories told by three graduates of First Nations University, who subsequently have been employed there. They show how, for these individuals, an education that recognizes historical injustice has served as a "path out of colonization," despite the fact that educational establishments historically have acted as instruments of colonization and trauma. While trauma cannot be removed or remedied, a supportive environment where the effects of such experiences are acknowledged and literally taken into account can allow a new story of healing to begin. The collective story told by First Nations people is evolving into one of resistance and recovery, countering earlier accounts based on acceptance of defeat and humiliation.

Racism is obviously a highly significant factor in stories of trauma told by people of Aboriginal descent. It has played an equally central role in the collective and individual experiences of immigrant groups of various ethnicities, particularly those of Jewish background who live with shared memories of attempted genocide. Bina Toledo Freiwald discusses Fredelle Bruser Maynard's serial autobiography, which conveys the anguish of growing up "Jewish and alien" in a small town in Western Canada in the 1920s and 1930s. Freiwald evokes changing definitions of trauma to juxtapose Maynard's gendered experience of racism with the social exclusion described by another serial autobiographer, Elly Danica, whose sense of exclusion as an immigrant is compounded by the experience of incest. In her case, there is no refuge from alienation to be found by identifying closely with her family of origin. Both these writers have produced serial memoirs that simultaneously serve a confessional / therapeutic and testimonial / emancipatory function, using individual experiences to represent the widespread and long-term traumatic effects of social discrimination based on race and gender. These autobiographical narratives can be compared with the filmic treatments of incest and collective trauma discussed by Finney and Chivers. Issues of authenticity and authority arise, as they did in Lauren Slater's serial memoirs Helen Buss discussed in chapter 4, since memory is central to the production of a series of re-collections that piece together a fractured self/story. The intersections of the physical and psychological are also prominent in all these accounts.

A number of papers in this volume deal with experiences of "mental illness" and psychiatric labeling and treatment. Richard Ingram situates narratives of such experiences as part of the "psych wars." Tracing first the post-World War II expansion of psychiatry and multiplication of the diagnostic categories that he regards as "simulation models," he goes on to question the role of narrative therapy in both mainstream psychiatry and the anti-psychiatry movement. The schizophrenic discourse discussed by Lourdes Rodriguez del Barrio has already raised the problematic issue, from a narrative perspective, of a "non-story." How much use can narrative therapy be for those who are deemed, by diagnostic definition, to be incapable of "making sense?" Can they, in turn, throw light on the potentially repressive nature of narrative by highlighting its limits?

The power of narrative is also discussed by Shelley Reuter, in a paper which examines shifts in the medical construction of agoraphobia through the late nineteenth and twentieth centuries. Reuter maintains that clinical discourse about the disease helped fix the boundaries of gender, race, and class. She points out that the presumption of "whiteness" as well as middle-class femininity in early studies of agoraphobics persisted almost until the present day, and delayed recognition that the majority of people in the United States who suffer from agoraphobia are poor African-American women. Such women are often not included in clinical studies because they do not have access to therapy, and the socio-economic determinants of their condition are overlooked by the biological approach currently favoured in psychiatry.

The role of class in the treatment of a medically defined condition is also considered by Joanne Muzak, who charts successive stages in the twentieth-century reconceptualization of drug addiction in the United States. She explains how a disease model emerged in the 1970s and 1980s as a reaction to changing patterns of drug use and abuse among the country's youth. Using Martha Morrison's 1989 memoir, *White Rabbit*, as a case study, Muzak shows how the new, putatively value-free understanding of addiction privileged middle-class addicts, protecting them from social stigma while perpetuating normative views of class and gender.

While Ingram, Reuter, and Muzak highlight changes over time in medical narratives of disease, J. Daniel Schubert reveals how the passage of time and advances in research can affect the experience of a specific illness. He examines the stories of people living with cystic fibrosis whose prognosis has changed; due to advances in treatment, their life expectancy has increased from two to thirty-two years. Nevertheless, like those living with AIDS discussed by Diedrich, people with cystic fibrosis live their lives under the shadow of death. How is their perception of time as a precarious present affected when they survive into adulthood? Stories of aging by people who were not expected to survive call into question the temporal structure of illness narratives and demand a more general rethinking of the narrative assumptions imposed on experience.

Part III concludes with a paper by James Overboe that also takes us back to some of the issues raised at the beginning of this volume. It uses the autobiographical mode to ask the ultimate question about the relationship between having and telling a life story and the ethics of personhood (a topic examined in a panel discussion with Hilde Lindemann Nelson and summarized in the introduction to Part I of this book): should those who are judged to be incapable of communicating a story be regarded as non-persons (and therefore without rights), or should old people with dementia be classified as post-persons whose lives are not worth living?[2] Overboe explores the concept of post-personhood, maintaining that it is a humanist construct that facilitates the mistreatment—to the point of death—of those who cannot "make sense" according to the dominant mode of expression. Like Heidi Janz and Julie Rak in their chapter and Joy James in hers, Overboe exposes the ableist perspectives that govern the reception and interpretation of narrative. Drawing on his own experience, he argues for the need to expand the concept of personhood in order to embrace those who may, at some point in their lives, be perceived as inarticulate.

The papers in Part III represent a range of narratives of resistance that are both individual and collective. While every specific experience of disease, disability, or trauma is unique, and each person has his or her own story to tell, individuals are also marked as belonging to intersecting categories (gender, race, age, class, etc.), which affect their access to resources such as health care, therapy, and a platform from which to proclaim their stories. Those who experience chronic physical illness, disabilities, or problems of the mind are also boxed into other categories, with diagnostic and prognostic labels that indicate what kinds of stories will be told about them.

Like Janet MacArthur and Sharon Dale Stone (both in this volume), or Arthur Frank (whose work is discussed in the introduction to Part II), Ingram and Overboe integrate their own experience of disease or disability into their research. By acknowledging their experiences in this way, they run the risk of being negatively assessed in their profession as academics. Yet for them, as for others, the danger of telling their personal story is outweighed by the benefits of sharing the experience. There is a greater danger if these stories are not heard by the temporarily able-bodied or the not-yet-ill, those whose support is required to improve services that we all may need eventually.

The three parts of this book focus on the intersections between three principal functions of narratives of disease, disability, and trauma: the aesthetic, the therapeutic, and the polemical. In the introduction, we explained that a functional analysis enabled us, as a multidisciplinary research team, to pool our resources, compare our methodologies, and address common ethical issues. This last section is followed by a final, separate essay: a collective analysis of Margaret Edson's play *Wit*. Rather than concluding our discussion, this essay demonstrates the difficulty of providing a conclusion when a narrative of illness is approached as a performance that may be interpreted in various, and ultimately incompatible, ways. Unlike scientific research, which aims to demonstrate a degree of certitude based on the replicability of results, the outcomes of narrative endeavors and narrative inquiry tend to provoke a sense of possibilities rather than certainties.

The result is a range of variable but viable contextualized reactions, rather than one "true" answer to a problem. Edson's play, about an academic woman dying of cancer, provides a final, dramatic example of narrative as co-constructed by narrator and audience. It illustrates how a personalized story can serve as a both a teaching tool and a meditation on the meaning of life and death as constructed through language; it also combines the pathos of empathetic identification and the comic relief made possible by aesthetic distance.

The discussion of *Wit* aims to demonstrate some of the possibilities and limits of cross-disciplinary exchanges. The postscript that comes after will attempt to weave together the threads that run through this volume, to assess the degree of "fit" that emerges between the three parts, to acknowledge the loose ends that do not fit in and force us, appropriately, to maintain a certain dis/ease and dis/ability in our efforts to reframe and refocus our approaches to un-fitting stories.

Notes

1 It was also presented at a conference held in May 2002 at the Commonwealth Communication Research Centre, Cardiff University, and appeared in the conference proceedings. See Riessman 2002c.
2 Janice Graham, a medical anthropologist and one of the co-investigators for the Wall project, conducts research on communicating with persons suffering from dementia. She organized a CIHR-funded workshop on that topic during our project, and is now continuing this research at Dalhousie University.

LYN JONGBLOED

Disability Income
Narratives of Women with Multiple Sclerosis

People's daily lives are conducted within a context, and persons with disabilities encounter social, political, and economic environments that both enable and limit their daily activities. This paper focuses on the impact of one aspect of these environments, namely disability income policies, on the lives of women with multiple sclerosis.

Multiple sclerosis (MS) is a chronic disease which affects women at about twice the rate of men (Poser, Paty, McDonald, Scheinberg, and Ebers 1984). Its typical onset is during the late 20s or early to mid 30s, when women may be training for a career, working full-time, staying at home to raise children, or combining part-time work with domestic responsibilities. The disease has an unpredictable course (Confavreux, Aimard, and Devic 1980) and manifests itself in a range of ways, from little apparent incapacity to severe paralysis, with fatigue, motor symptoms impairment, and sight disturbance as the most common problems.

Women with MS who no longer have income from employment need some form of income security to compensate for their lack of earnings. Income support programs are described and analyzed in the literature, but there is little documentation regarding the experiences of income program applicants or recipients, or how particular disabilities influence this experience. This paper aims to identify the primary income support programs available to women with MS who are no longer in paid employment, and to document the impact of the programs on their lives.

Methods

This essay is based on a subset of findings of a larger study with a qualitative and quantitative phase on employment and women with MS (Jongbloed 1996). Fifty-four women diagnosed with MS participated in the qualitative phase. They were contacted either through a MS clinic in western Canada or a local chapter of the MS Society. Of these women, thirty-one were employed and twenty-three were not employed at the time of the interviews. The mean age of those no longer employed was forty-four. The amount of time the unemployed women had been out of the paid work force ranged from several months to fourteen years. Six women had professional educations; thirteen had been employed in clerical and retail sales jobs; four had been employed in semi-skilled or manual jobs. Nine of the women were married, eight were divorced or separated, and seven had never married, and all the women lived in the Greater Vancouver area of British Columbia. This essay is based primarily on interviews with the twenty-three women who were no longer employed.

Two investigators and a research assistant conducted semi-structured, in-depth interviews with these women to explore different aspects of their lives, including work experiences, income issues, housing, and personal relationships. Interviews took place in the women's homes, ranged from one to two hours in length, and were tape-recorded, transcribed, and computerized to facilitate data coding and categorization. Intermeshing of data collection, analysis, and problem definition is an integral feature of qualitative research (Glaser and Strauss 1967; Hammersley and Atkinson, 1983). The two investigators and the research assistant identified and discussed emerging themes from the interviews they conducted and organized the themes into categories.

Findings

The income sources of women who were no longer employed were disability benefits from the Canada/Quebec Pension Plan (C/QPP), long-term disability insurance (employer and private), social assistance (disability benefits), and other personal income. Many women derived income from more than one source. Data analysis revealed some common themes, showing that a large proportion of the women interviewed experienced difficulties related to accessing benefits, the adequacy of benefits, other constraints, and fatigue. Each of these themes will be discussed further.

Accessing Benefits

To access benefits from the C/QPP, long-term disability insurance, or social assistance, applicants had to meet certain eligibility criteria and be assessed by a physician. The restrictiveness of the definition of disability in order to be eligible for C/QPP benefits was problematic for ten of the twenty-three subjects who received money from the C/QPP. A woman of twenty-six who had been working at a car rental agency said, "I've been getting brainstem attacks, and they affect my vision, my speech, my balance, and they make me tired and weak. At work I couldn't take a rest if I wanted to and when I have an attack I'm supposed to stay in bed for a month or two." The doctor told her that he didn't want her to work any more. She tried to get C/QPP disability benefits, "but the government says that I'm not disabled enough. They told me to get an easier job. Well, the job I had was as easy as you can get. I mean, I'm just sitting behind a desk and writing out forms." She was in the process of appealing her eligibility.

The experiences of the ten women who applied for long-term disability benefits varied. Four reported problems accessing benefits, while the other six did not. Some women felt victimized by the requirement that after two or three years they had to prove themselves incapable of working at any job (not just their previous jobs). One woman said:

> There is a problem with the long-term disability people. Of course, it's their business, and I understand, they want you off the plan ... After two years, in order to stay on long-term disability, you have to prove that you are not able to do ANY form of work whatsoever. So if my doctors say I can sit in my electric wheelchair on the corner, one hour a week, and sell pencils, I will be cut off all my benefits. If they find out about my volunteer work, I'm cut off all my benefits ... I want to enroll in a time management and stress management course, but I can't. As soon as I take that, I'm cut off all my benefits—I can't risk the rest of my life without any income. So you're totally victimized.

In order to access social assistance disability benefits, applicants have to demonstrate financial need and disability. Financial need is assessed through a needs test in which income and required expenditures are determined. Most social assistance recipients experience the assessment of financial need as intrusive. One person said, "they look at your bank statements, and because they have my bank account number, I assume that they could go in and check my balance any time."

An individual is allowed to access disability benefits once a physician has issued a medical certificate indicating that he/she is unable to work. Fatigue, a central symptom in multiple sclerosis, is invisible but potentially debilitating, and it can be difficult for some physicians to understand the impact of something that they cannot see. This situation further adds to the complexity of and discretionary elements in the assessment process, and has caused problems for six of the twenty-three participants. According to one woman, her first neurologist asked her,

> "Do you want to go to work?" And I'd said, "Well, you know, basically it's not up to me. I might want to go to work but I'm not able to right now." It was mainly fatigue. And he had me seeing the unit social worker, and why it was I didn't want to work ... And meanwhile he would only sign my letters for the insurance company, for like a month at a time, so the money keeps stopping.

She said that, in contrast, her second neurologist was completely different. He said "Look, this is it; it's not going to get any better, it's not going to change, this is the story. She is disabled." Physicians exercise considerable discretion in the assessment process. Some physicians were much more liberal in their evaluation of the impact of disability than others.

Adequacy of Benefits

Some of the women had individual income, and nine lived in households in which there was an additional source of income. However, others had to cope with reduced income. The level of income replacement from long-term disability programs is typically in the range of 60–75 per cent of pre-disability income. The C/QPP benefit consists of a flat sum plus an earning-related component which equals 75 per cent of the retirement pension to which the individual would have been eligible (Government of Canada 1996). The fact that benefits are based on employment earnings works against women with MS who may have worked part-time because of fatigue and other MS-related symptoms, combined part-time work with domestic responsibilities, or taken time off work to raise a family. One woman explained it this way: "I stayed at home and raised my family. I did tailoring and house painting on my own. So I wasn't a contributor for sixteen years, and that greatly affected my C/QPP disability pension."

Social assistance benefits are below the poverty line (Government of Canada 1996), and the activities of women on social assistance are severely curtailed by lack of income. One woman, describing her situation, said:

> How can you be healthy if you don't have the money to be healthy? On social assistance, you're on the poverty line. I'm just existing. If I was working, I'd be able to visit and go and do a few things. This way I can't do anything. I don't even have the bus fare, you know.

Another said, "The MS Society sent me information. In fact, they sent me the whole book, because I haven't got the money to go there."

One woman explained how being on social assistance disability benefits constrained her social activities: "If I want to go somewhere friends are going, I have to sit down and say, 'Is this going to be worth it to me?' because if I go and do this event, am I going to be short for the rest of the month?"

OTHER CONSTRAINTS

Insurance companies do not cover clients for conditions which pre-existed their insurance coverage. This means that the women interviewed who had long-term disability insurance when diagnosed with MS felt unable to change employment. One woman applied for a new job and was told that since she had MS, she could not receive short or long-term disability coverage through that employment. She said,

> So, I was really upset. It makes me feel like a prisoner where I work. Not that I don't like what I do, but my opportunities are limited, very limited. In fact, I'm probably going to be where I am forever. I don't have a choice.

Because the course of MS is uncertain, some women were afraid to return to the work force once they had established eligibility for disability payments. Fifty-four per cent (N = 88) of the women in the quantitative study who were no longer in paid employment identified loss of current income as a factor that discouraged them from looking for work. They felt they could not afford to lose the financial security they had. This dilemma kept some women with MS unemployed.

The structure of disability benefits provided through social assistance in BC creates disincentives for work for some women. Some people with MS have significant drug costs, and the costs of these drugs is covered while they receive social assistance disability benefits. However, they are not allowed to work while receiving these drugs. Since drug coverage is worth several hundreds of dollars per month to some women, it is a better financial decision to remain on benefits than return to work.

DETERMINATION OF DISABILITY

Deborah Stone (1984) points out that, in all societies, workers are regarded as more deserving than non-workers. Each society has two distributive systems: one based on work and the other based on need. Most people have their needs met by working. However, society has to decide when people are in need, and how much money to give those in need. Those with disabilities may be in need, but disability has always been problematic because it can be feigned. Since the nineteenth century, physicians have been assigned the role of determining when someone should qualify for disability benefits. This was because advances in scientific medicine offered new diagnostic techniques such as the stethoscope and x-rays, which could distinguish between "genuine disability" (an inability to work) and "feigned disability" (Stone 1984).

The three disability programs most frequently used by women with MS require a physician's report to establish eligibility. Agencies want to allocate benefits only to those with "legitimate disabilities." Symptoms are generally viewed as legitimate only when their parameters can be defined and tangibly displayed in the form of test scores (Monks 1989). A woman may have a combination of invisible disabilities (such as weakness, incoordination, and fatigue) which limit her ability to work, while her visible disabilities do not do so on their own. Because fatigue, one of the major symptoms of MS, is invisible, disability benefit claims by people with MS are likely to be subjected to more scrutiny than the claims of people who have entirely visible symptoms.

Structuring of Benefit Programs

To be eligible for benefits from a disability income program, the applicant has to be declared unemployable. Fatigue is a common symptom in MS, and many of the women surveyed who had moderate physical impairments consequently wished to work part time. Their wishes were also influenced by responsibilities such as child care and housework: work primarily performed by women. At the time of the study, these women were unable to access income support from the C/QPP, social assistance, and most long-term disability programs unless their disabilities rendered them completely incapable of employment. Their choices were to continue working full-time, under considerable strain, or to work part time and forego half their income. Women living in households with another source of income and women with high individual incomes could more easily afford to choose the part-time option. Single women in low-paying jobs had fewer options.

In our study, only one of the twenty-three individuals was permitted to combine part-time work with receipt of partial benefits. This embodies a view that people are either totally disabled or totally able-bodied. In reality, however, people fit on a continuum of work ability (Lonsdale

1990). By not allowing those with disabilities to receive partial benefits as well as employment income, disability programs deny people the satisfaction and economic self-sufficiency that they might gain from participating in the labour force part-time.

Adequacy of Benefits

Long-term disability insurance generally provides greater income protection than the C/QPP or social assistance. However, it is not mandatory for employers to offer their employees long-term disability coverage. Consequently, less than half the population has this benefit. Those in management positions and unionized workers in the public sector and larger manufacturing operations are more likely than other employees to have long-term disability insurance as an employment benefit (Torjman 1988). Benefits provided by the C/QPP are extremely low; consequently, some recipients also require social assistance. Those who depend entirely on social assistance for their support live below the poverty line (Fawcett 1996). Currently, the income of persons with disabilities depends on whether they became disabled at work, in a car accident, had contributed to the C/QPP before becoming disabled, or are war veterans. The majority of people with disabilities are not eligible for benefits from Workers' Compensation, automobile insurance, the C/QPP, or war veterans programs, and consequently receive provincial social assistance benefits, which are so low that many recipients live in poverty (Government of Canada 1996).

There are several barriers to the development of a comprehensive disability insurance system. First, it is not a priority of the federal government. Second, most reforms in this area require agreement of the federal, provincial, and territorial governments and consensus is not easily achieved. Third, the legal profession and the private insurance industry benefit from the current system, and oppose the move to a comprehensive scheme. Both groups have strong input into the political process, and government is reluctant to antagonize them (M. Prince 1991).

Principles Underlying Disability Policies

In order to analyze issues of accessing, structuring, and adequacy of benefits, one needs to ask what it means to have a disability and what society owes to people with disabilities. Disability is multidimensional and is associated with medical and economic challenges as well as issues related to discrimination. However, each of these models of disability uses a different normative base to answer the question of what society owes persons with disabilities. Also, because the models and their normative bases are not conceptually linked, no one model can be used as the basis for disability policy development (Bickenbach 1993). The medical model focuses on medical needs and suggests the normative principles of charity and accommodation. It does not raise questions of justice, nor does it emphasize rights of people with disabilities. The economic model stresses participation in the form of economic integration and the principle of welfare maximization. The thrust of the socio-political model is the attainment of rights and equality, and here disability becomes part of the moral and political sphere where issues of justice and entitlement have to be addressed.

According to Jerome Bickenbach, questions that need to be answered include:

- Should the goal be to foster participation in education, employment, and community life?
- Many kinds of benefits may be given to people with disabilities. Should benefits be viewed as rights which can be legally enforced, or as privileges?
- Are benefits intended to produce particular results, such as increasing the employment level among persons with disabilities, or are they a means to an unspecified end, such as a skills upgrading program?
- Should policies benefit everyone in society or just those with disabilities? For example, should a program improve the employment situations of people with disabilities or improve the economic conditions of people with disabilities and of society? (1993).

Acknowledgements

I wish to acknowledge the women with MS who participated in this study. The research on which this paper is based was funded by grants from the British Columbia Health Research Foundation and the Social Sciences and Humanities Research Council. The principal investigator of the study was Isabel Dyck, School of Rehabilitation Sciences, University of British Columbia.

ROBERT PROCYK AND CHRISTINE CROWE

Narratives of Trauma and Aboriginal Post-secondary Students

Introduction

The experience of collective trauma by Aboriginal people manifests itself as an underlying but insidious influence on the success rates of Aboriginal students in post-secondary education. As faculty members in a First Nations–controlled post-secondary institution, we see the effects and legacies of communal trauma on a daily basis. Although not all of our students may be cognisant of the impact of colonization on their own lives, it is clear that their own individual struggles with securing funding, housing, child care, and support systems derive from historical and unresolved traumatic experiences with relationships within their families, communities, the province, and the nation as a whole.

The creation of the Saskatchewan Indian Federated College (now First Nations University of Canada) in 1976 became a means of dealing with trauma and building a bright new future for Aboriginal people and their subsequent generations. SIFC was founded on the belief that education was to become the "new buffalo" for Aboriginal people. After years of residential schools, lack of Aboriginal content in school curricula, institutional racism, and the invalidation of traditional Aboriginal knowledge and teachings in educational institutions, SIFC was created to validate the First Nations experience as equal to non-First Nations ways of knowing. Our first chair of SIFC, Ida Wasacase, explained the vision of SIFC in this way:

> We have to produce and develop the Indian way first, and secondly the non-Indian way. I have tried to institute in the curriculum of the SIFC the concept

of bilingual and bi-cultural education. We want our students to understand both the Indian and the White cultures so that they can move more easily from one to the other. It is important that our people be able to work and relate in a modern cultural setting, but it is important also for our people to understand their own culture. Similarly they should be able to work and apply methodologies used in traditional White institutions for social work, education, and administration within the Indian communities. (College document)

In keeping with this initial vision for the College, the SIFC mission statement identifies history, language, culture, and artistic heritage as the four pillars for the survival of Aboriginal identity in a post-colonial Canada. Indeed, according to its mission statement, SIFC was conceived "to preserve, protect, and interpret the history, language, culture and artistic heritage of First Nations." The SIFC mission statement acknowledges that these four facets of Aboriginal culture have been traumatized by colonization and are in need of regeneration.

Despite SIFC's best attempts over the past twenty-five years to use education as yet another means of healing First Nations communities, the college continues to struggle with the legacies of historical trauma, as we deal with decreasing enrolment and increasing withdrawal rates. While SIFC has graduated approximately sixteen hundred students in its twenty-five-year history, each term we lose many bright, creative, and intelligent students who cannot complete their programs for various reasons, many of which are associated with traumatic events within their own lives and those of their communities. Each semester, approximately one sixth (16.6 per cent) of our students are "required to discontinue" (RTD) their studies due to poor academic performance. The stories they tell are ones of struggles with institutional life, self-esteem, family, and community demands on their time, and the harsh realities of everyday living as an Aboriginal person in Saskatchewan. Many of these stories are never heard, as students drop out and carry on with their lives outside the post-secondary setting.

The stories we are going to tell are ones about Aboriginal men and women who have both struggled and succeeded as SIFC students. In these examples, themes of individual and communal trauma are woven throughout and continue to resonate in the halls and classrooms of our college. While we can be certain that SIFC does attempt to address these experiences of trauma through its institutional procedures, policies, and programs, the reality of our successful completion rates tells a different story.

The Stories

As a college, we consider a student to be "successful" at the moment of graduation. This definition of student success does not supersede other kinds of personal, social, emotional, or intellectual achievements, but it does identify the ultimate reason for SIFC's being: as a post-secondary educational institution, SIFC can only consider itself successful by the number of students it graduates. After considering a list of possible people to interview, we chose to contact three people who had been "successful" in this way: they have graduated from SIFC, and are now working at this institution in high-level academic and administrative positions.[1]

The choice to interview former SIFC students who are now employees presents an obvious advantage because these interviewees know the college from two perspectives, having had the very different experiences of both student life and administrative responsibility. These interviewees, working as closely with students as they now do, have the distinct advantage of being able to compare and contextualize their own individual narratives about being an SIFC student with those of past and present students, since they hear narratives of trauma every day in each of their offices. However, the fact that these former students have a high enough opinion of the college to choose to work at SIFC may have influenced some of their answers to our questions. To some degree as well, their narratives may be coloured by self-interest in their desire to place the college in a positive light so as not to appear critical of their own employer. That said, each of our interviewees is well aware of SIFC's problems with student retention, and each person was very willing to discuss areas that he/she sees as in need of improvement.[2]

John

John is a thirty-seven-year-old Status First Nations male originally from a reserve north of Regina. He left high school in grade ten, and worked in various maintenance and management positions in the construction industry until eventually finishing grade twelve. As John recounts, he knew by the age of twenty-five that he would have to go to school to "get a good job." He chose SIFC because he wanted to be a "team player," and "thought it was important to come to the college that was owned by the Indians of Saskatchewan." The fact that his mother had been one of the founding faculty members of SIFC in the 1970s also influenced his decision. He entered the college in 1989, and took ten years to complete his degree, graduating with a BA in 1999.

The biggest challenges for John in terms of completing his post-secondary education were money and self-motivation. Financially, John had always been self-sufficient and it was difficult to make the transition to what he calls the "meagre allowance" offered by Indian Affairs. Academically, John admits that school was the most difficult experience he had ever encountered because he was not, as he terms it, "academically inclined." As he stated, "I'm just not cut out to be a student, I understand that, but that didn't stop me from getting the post-secondary education that we need to get ahead."

Like many of our students, John was required to discontinue (RTD) at one point during his program. When asked what had contributed to being forced to withdraw from his program, John replied:

> I couldn't cope with the work. It was just too much. I had a death in the family as well ... I had an uncle who was close to me who died. It didn't register until about a month or so after he had died, and I felt a lot of guilt for abandoning him in his final month of life, because he basically drank himself to death. So, I just let it slip away. One assignment becomes two assignments, and I dug a hole that I just couldn't get out of.

When asked what the college could have done to help prevent him from being forced to discontinue his studies, John replied:

> I think what the College needs to do more is intervene with problem students. The semester is four months long, and the instructor knows if a student is struggling. There should have been some sort of mechanism, like there is now, to identify those students who are having problems. I was going through some issues when my uncle died, and it probably would have been a good idea to have taken a compassionate leave at that time rather than failing one semester and coming back for more torture. I didn't ask for help because I was getting pressure from family who questioned whether I could go to school and really accomplish it.

After being RTD'd, John spent four years working in the construction industry before realizing he was tired of being "an intellectually disgruntled carpenter," and applied to re-enter the college. Two years later, John graduated from SIFC. When asked what he had taken away from his experiences at SIFC after ten years, he replied:

> The Indian studies classes encapsulated long periods of history that made sense of why we are where we are today.... The culturally relevant curriculum at SIFC justified my pride in being an Indian. It gave me the information to feed back to others who questioned why Indians are even proud of themselves to begin with. There are a lot of ignorant people out there, and you have to learn

the history to change their minds. Education will be the mortar that holds the foundation of the next generation of Indian enterprises together. That's why I'm so proud to be working at the college today.

Anne

Anne is a forty-nine-year-old Métis woman with a BA Honours degree from SIFC and an MA from the University of Regina. She is the first person in her family to have graduated with a degree. The family background she described in our interview is not unfamiliar to many of the stories we hear from our students:

> I grew up in a dysfunctional home, like many Aboriginal people. There was alcoholism, I saw a lot of violence in my youth, a lot of gory violence. My Dad's an alcoholic, my Mom is a binge drinker, and I married an abusive alcoholic. When I think back about why I did that, it was my world, I didn't know there was anything better. That kind of dysfunction was normal to me.

Unlike most of our students, Anne graduated from high school and had always known she wanted to go to university. However, her intentions to go directly from high school to university were interrupted by an early marriage and a full-time government job. She suffered physical and emotional abuse until she left her marriage at the age of twenty-eight. At that point, she was thinking about going to school, but had two small children and debt to pay off from the breakup of the marriage. Three years later, she married another man and had four years of relative financial and emotional security with him. After her second divorce, at the age of thirty-four, and with two kids aged ten and eleven, she applied to attend SIFC. Anne remembers the transition from working mom to student:

> It was traumatic for all of us. We were living in relative comfort, financially, and all of a sudden I was a single parent again. We had to move back to the ghetto. So, I packed up my kids and moved into Gabriel Dumont low-income housing. In fact, that low-income housing saved my life, and this is so important for students. Because had it not been for Gabriel housing, where my rent was $50/month when I was a student, I wouldn't have made it through.

Along with financial support from student loans and the opportunity to live in low-income housing, Anne believes she was successful as a student because she came in as a mature student and "knew what I wanted." As she recounts, "I had these two kids, so it wasn't an option of this being unsuccessful. I came in with the mindset that I couldn't fail, so I did whatever it took to get through."

Anne chose SIFC because of the cultural component. She also identified a sense of community at SIFC and immediately began to form connections with her professors and the other Aboriginal students in her classes. As she explains,

> I think that what's really good for our students is that community. You get to know people and you feel kind of looked after. I know I certainly did. It's so different because of that community. Coming to the college changed my life. As students, we all worked so damn hard and were all in it together and doing something really important. It really bonds people together.

Anne's educational experience and success have led her into a senior level administration position in the college, and she deals directly with students on a daily basis. In our interview, she talked at length about the stories she hears from students, and how they often ring true with her own experience. When asked to comment on the relationship between these stories of trauma and the importance of education, Anne had the following reply:

> I think education is the tool to get our people into a place where they can be healthy, because you can't be healthy if you are poor. You can't be healthy ... if you don't feel in control of your own life. I think education is a path out of colonization, because you have to know what colonization is first before you can combat it. We are all in pain, we've been there, and we can help our students find their way through just as others helped us with our own success. But you have to find that balance between being a caretaker and doing everything for the students and empowering them to take on the responsibility of their success themselves.

Brenda

Brenda is a Métis woman in her mid-forties. She earned a BA from SIFC and an MA from the University of Regina, and is currently in a senior-level administrative position at the college. Brenda grew up in a working-class neighbourhood in a family she describes as "dysfunctional and alcoholic." Both of her parents have a grade eleven education, and, given that history, it is perhaps not surprising that Brenda dropped out of her commercial high school in grade eleven as well, and left home at age seventeen to move to Saskatchewan. In fact, Brenda did not have contact with her family for over twenty years after she left home, and therefore received no family support or encouragement to return to school.

In 1978, she enrolled in the SIFC Indian Social Work program in Saskatoon, but only lasted two months. She attributes her lack of success to various personal issues, such as her recent separation from her husband and a lack of adequate housing in Saskatoon for herself and her children. The trauma of moving to a new city and beginning a new life took its toll on Brenda's children; as she remembers,

> My kids were upside down, their whole lives were turned around. They changed cities, daycare, parents, everything. They got kicked out of daycare, they were acting up, and I wasn't managing to pick them up until six o'clock at night. Life was not in a manageable state. I decided to stay home with my kids until they were in school. I had to go on welfare, which I had never done.

After dropping out of the Indian Social Work program, Brenda remarried and had another child. Her second husband, an alcoholic, was murdered in a bar fight, and she remained on welfare in Saskatoon. However, Brenda was motivated to return to school when she saw the effects of the poverty cycle on her children:

> My daughter asked, "How old do I have to be before I can get my own welfare cheque?" and I thought, "Oh my God," and went the next day to welfare and said that I wanted to go to school, and I was in school within a month because I didn't want my girl to grow up thinking that way.

When she returned to SIFC in 1988, Brenda found encouragement from faculty and staff, many of whom came from similar backgrounds and experiences. As she comments about one faculty member, "I knew her back when she was on welfare. She was my deceased husband's cousin. I know what she has been through, and I thought that if she can do it, I can do it." This sense of community, along with encouragement from fellow students, allowed Brenda to continue her studies. In addition to peer support, Brenda also received financial support by moving into the same Gabriel Dumont low-income housing project as Anne. Like Anne, she believes that low-income housing was instrumental in allowing her to continue her education, and eventually to earn a graduate degree.

After completing her MA, Brenda became a faculty member at the college and has risen to a senior administrative position. She asserts that education has given her influence, and recounts meeting with the vice-president of the CBC and the president of SSHRC. However, Brenda acknowledges that the legacies of trauma are always apparent in Aboriginal post-secondary education. As she notes,

> Narratives of trauma don't go away and they don't get fixed. It's a lifetime of continual work trying to strive for a balance. Nothing has changed. Our students still come here thinking they aren't bright enough to be here, they don't have realistic goals, they have no models, and some can't imagine themselves

with an education and jobs. Most students come here with children, and most come here across the board poor. Almost 100 per cent carry narratives of trauma, and how do we handle this?

Conclusion

Brenda's question, "How do we handle this?", cuts to the very heart of the matter of Aboriginal student success at the post-secondary level. These stories present some of the challenges that many of our Aboriginal students face when coming to post-secondary education. Our interviews with these three "successful" students, who have completed their degrees and graduated despite huge barriers, compels us to ask why these students have been successful as post-secondary Aboriginal students when so many others, faced with similar challenges, have not. Where does SIFC's responsibility lie in relation to encouraging student success? How can we, as an administrative body, take steps to ensure that we are holding up our end of the educational deal? On the other hand, when do we step back and encourage the student to take responsibility for his/her own success?

The answers to these questions reside in the stories themselves, for it is clear that it is not the student, SIFC, or the government alone that can ensure the success of Aboriginal students in post-secondary education. Instead, as each of our interviewees identified, success results from the effective combination of a variety of factors coming together—housing, funding, family support, child care, and a sense of belonging—to provide an environment that is conducive to successful educational endeavours. As a First Nations-controlled institution, we are especially interested in how we can best create that kind of nurturing environment and, according to our interviewees, it seems as if we have been at least partly successful in achieving that goal. For instance, all three of our subjects identified SIFC as a place of comfort, a place of belonging, and a place without shame. In his interview, John described the sense of community among the Aboriginal students at the university by telling this story:

> There was a student who would go to his locker and get out his quart of milk, his loaf of bread, and his little package of bologna. And he'd go and eat it in the student lounge. You would never see an Indian student picking up his food and taking it into the cafeteria to eat. It made me understand that the SIFC lounge and the students who went there formed more of a community where people could be themselves if they were too poor to buy a packaged lunch or a prepared meal. They could just bring their odds and ends here and assemble them in the student lounge.

It is clear from this story that SIFC's success as a First Nations institution resides in its ability to provide a safe and supportive environment in which students can feel comfortable being themselves, and in which narratives of trauma can openly be shared and acknowledged without fear or shame. But, it is also important to remember that our three subjects represent those students who have not used trauma as a crutch, but as a starting point instead. For our interviewees, education became a tool for healing personal trauma; the halls and classrooms of SIFC became a place of hope and positive energy of the kind not found at the soup kitchens and welfare offices they had known previously.

In order to achieve this dream, there remains much work to be done. As Brenda reminds us, "Narratives of trauma do not go away and they do not get fixed. It's a lifetime of continual struggle to find a balance." Narratives of trauma told by Aboriginal post-secondary students indeed may not "get fixed" by coming to a First Nations educational institution, but the acknowledgement and validation of those narratives in a First Nations setting may at least make the journey a little less frightening. The road to healing may be long, but every graduate represents a transformation from a narrative of trauma to a narrative of success. In other words, narratives of trauma may not "go away," but they can be and often are used as a means of personal motivation for educational achievement. So, even as SIFC continues to struggle with low retention rates, and even though we lose many bright students every semester, it is those transformed narratives—the narratives of success—that we find comfort in and gather together to celebrate in greater numbers every year at convocation ceremonies. Those narratives of success, through the work of our graduates in the larger community, are slowly but surely encouraging others to envision their own narratives of trauma as beginnings rather than endings.

NOTES

1 For reasons of confidentiality, we are unable to use our subjects' real names or identify their positions. For the purposes of this paper, we also chose three subjects who have English as their first language in order to eliminate the additional struggles associated with being an ESL student in a post-secondary institution. John was interviewed on 7 December 2001, Brenda on 9 January 2002, and Anne on 31 January 2002.
2 In the next phase of our study, we will be interviewing former students and graduates who do not work at the College and who may, therefore, offer stories about their experiences at SIFC (now FNUC) that differ quite dramatically from those recorded here.

BINA TOLEDO FREIWALD

Social Trauma and Serial Autobiography
Healing and Beyond

> *The problem with mapping distress in the mind of the individual is that such a cartography tends to overlook the fact that the causes, locus, and consequences of collective violence are predominantly social.*
> —Arthur Kleinman (1995b, 181–82)

> *I believe that most Jews, even the most assimilated, walk around with a subliminal fear of anti-Semitism the way most women walk around with a subliminal fear of rape.* —Evelyn T. Beck (1991, 22)

The serial self-representational practices of two Canadian immigrant women autobiographers, and the insights their narratives offer into the vicissitudes of self-construction in the face of social trauma located at the intersections of gender and race/ethnicity/religion, are the focus of this essay. In 1972, Fredelle Bruser Maynard published *Raisins and Almonds*, an account—she would belatedly acknowledge—of "the anguish, the deep sense of exclusion" (1989, 133) she experienced "growing up Jewish and alien" in the small towns of western Canada during the 1920s and 1930s (1985, xix).[1] It was followed in 1989 by *The Tree of Life*, a volume focused on her adult life and introduced as "tougher ... [and] truer" than the earlier memoir (xxi). Elly Danica's 1988 incest narrative, *Don't: A Woman's Word*, also set in western Canada and speaking (however obliquely) to the immigrant experience, is a text composed of numbered fragments that opens with the abused child's crushing pain and closes with the adult survivor's defiant "I am" (94). It was followed in 1996 by *Beyond Don't: Dreaming Past the Dark*. In each case, I want to suggest, the second volume does more than take up where the earlier one had left off, and the return to (and of) the past is governed by a logic that partakes of (but also exceeds) a traumatic wound that is "not available to consciousness until it imposes itself again, repeatedly" (Caruth 1996, 4). In each case, the first autobiographical foray—the first attempt to work through trauma—both succeeds and fails, preparing the way for its sequel.

The autobiographers themselves tell us the measure of their success. *Raisins and Almonds* had its genesis, Maynard explains, in "a small painful experience of anti-Semitism" that triggered "a flood of memories ... [releasing] sorrows long held in check" (1989, xx–xxi). The incident, retold three times over the course of the two volumes, captures Maynard's experience of abjection as both a woman and a Jew. The incident occurs during a work trip to Atlantic City where Maynard—a prize-winning PhD graduate married to a non-Jew and living a thoroughly assimilated life in a New England university town—has to grade college entrance examinations (work she was able to get, ironically, on the recommendation of a former student), having lost her university teaching position when she became pregnant with her first child. The crushing moment comes when a fellow examiner reports to her what he thinks is an amusing conversation he overheard between two college board officials discussing minority-group pressures for representation: "'Well,' said No. 1, 'we've got our token black.' 'Oh?' said No. 2, 'Who?' 'Fredelle Maynard,' said No. 1. And No. 2 said, 'Fredelle Maynard's not our black. She's our Jew'" (1989, 133). The incident leads to a "volcanic eruption" of feeling for Maynard (1985, ix) and the writing of *Raisins and Almonds,* a book that she recognizes in retrospect fundamentally changed her life: "I realized, after long confusion, who I was and wanted to be" (ix). Shortly after its publication in 1985, her marriage of twenty-five years to (the gentile) Max Maynard ends, and the self-questioning provoked by the autobiographical project culminates in the recognition that "my essential nature ... was intimately involved with my Jewishness" (1989, xvii).

Danica, too, describes the writing of the first volume of her autobiography as an enabling process of self-recovery, a re-membering of a self shattered by her father's abuse of her from the age of four until she left his house (never a home) at eighteen: "the daily writing was where and how I worked towards a re-integration of the aspects of Self which had been fragmented" (qtd. in Williamson 1993, 80–81). Although not Jewish, Danica also experienced rejection and marginalization as a non-English-speaking immigrant. Here, however, I am primarily interested in the comparability of the trauma she experienced as a woman (incest as a type of gendered violence) and that experienced by Maynard as a Jew (anti-Semitism as a type of racialized violence). Like Maynard, Danica returns to her experience in spite of the apparent therapeutic success of her first account. Why, then, if the first writing process was so effective, do these autobiographers need to revisit the past and re-enter that scene in which "a subject-in-process is constructed" (Gilmore 2001, 97)? Perhaps, as the remainder of this essay will seek to argue, it is because for those subjected to the "'normal' insidious traumata" suffered simply for being "a woman, a Jew" (Brown 1995, 109), recovery remains elusive and healing proves an insufficient idiom with which to dream past the dark.

These two serial autobiographies can serve to engage trauma theory and autobiographical practice as mutually illuminating explorations of individual and social worlds in distress. Of particular interest to my project are recent developments in trauma theory that challenge two key aspects of earlier definitions of Post-traumatic Stress Disorder (PTSD): the designation of the trauma-inducing stressor as an event that is "outside the range of usual human experience" (American Psychiatric Association [APA] 1994, 783), and the exclusive focus on the pathology of the patient. The work of Judith Herman and Arthur Kleinman, among others, has been instrumental in offering both a critique of this model and an alternative vision. Herman's *Trauma and Recovery* (1992) shifts the focus of analysis from the impact of exceptional, circumscribed, traumatic events to the effects of prolonged and all-too-common social traumata. Kleinman's *Writing at the Margin* spells out the insidious consequences of a medicalizing and pathologizing discourse of trauma wherein "social problems are transformed into the problems of individuals" (1995b, 177). The call for an approach to trauma that would recognize the pervasiveness of stressors that are not accidental but "of human design" (Herman 1992, 7)—such as the social traumata of prejudice and exclusion that find their expression in racism, classism, sexism, and ageism (Adams 1990; Sanchez-Hucles 1998)—has not gone unheeded. One is heartened by changes to the American Psychiatric Association's most recent *Diagnostic and Statistical Manual of Mental Disorders* (*DSM-IV-TR*, 2000), indicating a willingness to broach the issue of social traumata. While the *DSM-IV-TR* still identifies the exposure to an extreme traumatic stressor involving a threat to one's *physical*, but not *psychic*, integrity as a primary diagnostic feature of PTSD, it does acknowledge the role played by psychosocial stressors, noting that PTSD "may be especially severe or long lasting when the stressor is of human design" (464). It is "trauma of human design" that shapes the lives and autobiographical projects of Maynard and Danica. Their narratives, in turn, enable us to explore not only "the faces of oppression" (Nelson 2001, 108) that harm subjects, but also the range of strategies employed by such subjects to (re)gain agency.

Psychosocial stressors, P.L. Adams reports, "are now known to weigh heavily on several population groups": topping the list of groups with known heightened risk or vulnerability are "Females" and "Discrimination-oppressed minority groups" (1990, 379). Two aspects of the analysis of the social trauma suffered by such groups are of particular relevance to the present discussion: the recognition that the *severing of attachments*—the experience of "alienation" and "estrangement" from self and others (367)—is a defining feature of the traumatic experience, as is the acknowledgment that the *pursuit of belonging* is a crucial component of the process of healing and recovery. The damage inflicted by *social* trauma—understood as the sanctioned and pervasive betrayal of affiliative bonds affecting the full range of human interactions, from the most intimate to the institutional—is, therefore, particularly acute. Experiences of social betrayal make healing difficult if not impossible since all three stages of recovery—"establishing safety, reconstructing the trauma story, and restoring the connection between survivors and their community" (Herman 1992, 3)—depend on the possibility of envisaging a world in which one can attain a sense "of familiarity, of being known, of communion" (1992, 236). Racism and sexism are the traumas that shape the lives of Maynard and Danica, and their autobiographical practice attests to both the severity of these assaults and the formidable challenge that recovery-as-belonging poses for such subjects.

It is perhaps no accident that Freud's foundational theorization of trauma emerged in the context of his own intimate familiarity with destructive gender and race ideologies. Although Freud would eventually repudiate his earlier insights into trauma being a response to *actual* experiences of violation, opting instead for a theory of "intrapsychic reality and subjective experience" (Van der Kolk, Weisaeth, and van der Hart 1996, 55), his *Autobiographical Study* suggests (obliquely, symptomatically) that psychoanalysis itself has its roots in, and is a response to, exactly these types of external violence. *An Autobiographical Study* is framed by the two forms of persecution that gave Freud's life its shape: the anti-Semitism that precipitated the family's migrations over the centuries, and continued to dictate his status as "an alien because I was a Jew" (1948, 14), and his effective banishment from the Society of Medicine, early on in his career, because of his work on *male* hysteria. Freud would recover from the gender-related blow by finding/founding his professional community of belonging in psychoanalysis and its acceptable study of female hysteria. His far more sinister fate as a racialized subject, however, is captured in a laconic comment he made at the conclusion of his 1935 Postscript to *An Autobiographical Study*. Referring to the Goethe prize awarded him in 1930, Freud writes, "This was the climax of my life as a citizen. Soon afterwards the boundaries of *our country* narrowed and the nation would know no more of *us*" (1948, 135; emphasis added). The pronominal slippage here is poignantly revealing—this is Freud's primal scene of trauma as a secular, assimilated, German Jew: the banishment from the collectivity, the brutal denial of belonging.

Fredelle Bruser Maynard, too, would long in vain to say "our country." Growing up as the daughter of Russian Jewish immigrants, she was the only Jewish child in the small prairie towns the family would move to in a series of failed attempts to integrate socially or economically. She would long to escape the "small playground persecutions" (1989, xiv), the schoolyard taunts of "*you lousy kike*" (1985, 102) and "you *killed* Christ" (1985, 21); the teachers rewarding her correct answers with "We don't need your kind to tell us what's what" (1985, 76); the persistent sense that the world around her was "alien if not actively hostile" (1989, xiv). Such anti-Semitism, the adult autobiographer recognizes, "must have been less crushing to those of my friends whose Jewishness was an active, positive force ... For me, so ambiguous, so ill-defined a Jew, anti-Semitism was peculiarly painful" (1985, xiv).[2] The title of *Raisins and Almonds* seeks to evoke the sweet promises of the Yiddish lullaby sung to her as a child: "The goat goes tripping down the street/ To buy raisins and almonds for my sweet/ ... / Goodness and health are the best things to own,/ Freidele will read Torah when she is grown" (1985, epigraph), but the opening of the autobiography leaves a distinctly sour taste on the tongue. The autobiographical narrator recalls, "Being Jewish, I had long grown accustomed to isolation and difference. Difference was in my bones and blood, and in the pattern of my separate life ... All year *I walked in the shadow of difference*; but at Christmas above all, I tasted it sour on my tongue" (1985, 19–21; emphasis added).

Read as a symptomatology of "complex post-traumatic stress disorder" (Herman 1992, 119), *Raisins and Almonds* and *The Tree of Life* tell the story of a subject who has walked in the shadow of a *double* difference: her racialized difference as a Jew, and her gendered difference as a female within both the Jewish and non-Jewish worlds. Although Maynard did not intend it to be so, the lullaby's reference to the Torah is ironic, for its promise that "Freidele will read Torah when she is grown" is belied by a millennia-old tradition in which "the equation of Jewishness with maleness is supported not only by women's exclusion from those traditional religious practices central to Judaism—prayer and study—but by the absence of positive images of women as holy" (Heschel 1991, 34).[3]

To the question "*Who am I?*" (1985, ix), Maynard's response at the conclusion of the first volume is "Woman and Jew, I am also my parents' child" (1985, 196). This, in turn, becomes the lens through which the past is reconstructed in the second volume. Maynard presents *The Tree of Life* as a narrative of self-discovery culminating in a self- and life-affirming identity as a Jew and a mature woman in charge of her life. Nevertheless, what the two autobiographical volumes demonstrate most compellingly is the extent and impact of the traumas she suffered—as a Jew, a woman, and her parents' child—and the difficulties of acceding to personal and social agency under such conditions. From the beginning, the Freidele of the lullaby is a child of survivors, born into a world in which the violence against Jews and against women that marked her parents continues to define the parameters of her life. She grows up with "tales of pogroms" (1989, 25), and her mother's repeated "tales of affliction" (138) about growing up in a household "where boys were kings and girls scullery maids" (193–94), and of her rape at the age of nine by a Russian soldier (139).

Although Maynard seems unaware of her father's part in perpetuating a damaging gender ideology, her observations about his sexualizing view of women (his daughters included), defining them exclusively in relation to men, are telling (1985, 194). Little wonder, then, that with her sense of self so severely undermined she would seek validation from a male and a gentile, only to find herself betrayed again. The marriage becomes a site of repeated trauma, but Maynard's narration of it in *The Tree of Life* suggests an even more complex psychosocial reality (which space constraints prevent me from exploring here), raising difficult questions about the price of identity and/as difference. Maynard recounts the many hurtful ways in which Max Maynard's "unease with a Jewish wife" (1989, 69) manifested itself, but she also reflects on her own (and her family's) ambivalent attitude towards gentiles and their entrenched "stereotypes of the non-Jewish world" (68).

The world of her adult life offers Maynard no respite from the traumas of gender and race, and when there is little change in the external trauma-inducing reality, there can be little hope for change in the internal psychic condition. Maynard's two autobiographical volumes are framed by descriptions of the prairie landscape of her childhood (1985, 199–200; 1989, xx). These descriptions foreground her sense of powerlessness and of being alone in the world, evoking the psychic landscape of trauma: a feeling of being "utterly abandoned, utterly alone," trapped in a situation where "neither resistance nor escape is possible" (Herman 1992, 52, 34). Objective reality makes escape impossible: learning and knowledge, for example, are the young Fredelle Bruser's first lines of defence and the adult Maynard's still-hoped-for means of escaping her "outsiderness" (1989, 78), but they prove of little use in a world where teachers can be racist (1985, 76) and the academy openly discriminates against women (1989, 78).

Resistance, too, proves beyond reach, as the possibility of social critique eludes Maynard, who fails to make the connections, necessary for recovery, between one's experiences and "the social and material conditions engendering these experiences" (Profitt 2000, 103). She remains, for example, virtually silent on the Holocaust (1985, 155); the trauma of gender remains unexamined as both volumes conclude with an uncritical portrayal of a male figure as saviour, showing the mature woman to be still driven by the neediness of the young girl who was taught to "worship the father" (Buss 1993, 157). Maynard's experience as an economically disenfranchised, classed subject (Rimstead 2001, 195) remains equally unexamined. Such distancing, in turn, mitigates against any sense of solidarity or identification with others in a similar predicament. Finally, even the Jewishness Maynard reclaims later in life seems to offer little comfort. A combination of factors—the legacy of anti-Semitism, her parents' own isolation as Jews, and her secular upbringing (see Schaub 1997)—leaves Maynard with little more than superficialities from which to form a meaningful sense of Jewishness. At the close of the second volume, she responds to her granddaughter's question "What's Jewish?" by talking about "Jewish food, Jewish holidays ... [and] the solemn bar mitzvah procession, following the Torah in its tasselled, filigreed silver case, that celebrates a Jewish male's coming of age" (1989, 243). The irony of trying to attract her granddaughter to Jewish life by telling her of a ritual that excludes her as a female seems to escape Maynard, but here, as elsewhere in the two volumes, the autobiographical text seems to speak a truth—about the impasses a traumatizing social world creates—that its narrator cannot fully voice.

More overt about the effects of trauma, Elly Danica's autobiographical narratives also offer a more hopeful trajectory. Like Maynard, Danica too struggles with the aloneness that is the condition of collective racialized and gendered trauma. As "an immigrant, a foreigner, a woman" she knows the feel of multiple blows and the taste of defeat:

> When I was a child, denial became a way of life. At school—if I wanted to get home without being waylaid by bullies and beaten up for my difference—I was required to deny that I had been born in Holland, spoke Dutch as my first language and was an immigrant. At home denial was how I learned to see the abuse I endured as normal or inevitable. (1996, 21)

Having given voice in *Don't* to the abused child who will always be a part of the grown woman,[4] Danica seeks to find her adult voice in *Beyond Don't*. The second volume puts the autobiographical act to many uses: reclaiming those other parts of her self that could not have been brought into the incest narrative; resisting the new ways in which her childhood experiences seem to rule her life now that she has come to be perceived solely as an incest victim; reinventing herself; and continuing to work through her relationships with her family of origin. Danica's second volume, like Maynard's, revisits her relationship with her mother, while also rethinking the very terms of kinship: "I'm learning that family need not be the collection of people into which you are born ... but it is hard to give up entirely on one's family of origin" (1996, 92).

Ultimately, Danica both acknowledges that restoring ruptured attachments is imperative if healing is to proceed, and recognizes that, for her, kinship will remain unattainable: "It is possible that, as an immigrant child, bookish, odd, sad and depressed, and further distanced by the abuse I was experiencing, I made isolation a habit" (1996, 90). Unlike Maynard, however, Danica does succeed in voicing a meaningful "we," as she resolves to make the transition from speaking personally to speaking politically in order to address "the social and political causes of child sexual abuse" (1996, 95). At the conclusion of *Beyond Don't*, Danica writes, "We need to build communities in which the priority is the care, protection, nurturance, needs and rights of children and other vulnerable people" (1996, 151). Her second autobiographical volume is indeed an active gesture towards the creation of such a community. In Danica's case, the autobiographical return is for the purpose of moving beyond healing in pursuit of personal and collective transformation, with the goals of "self-recovery, social analysis, and collective action" (Profitt 2000, 102).

As a practice that allows a plural present self to grapple with its past(s), serial autobiography is both a symptom of and an antidote to the rupture that is trauma's aftermath—that "breach in the mind's experience of time, self, and the world" (Caruth 1996, 4). As a genre that draws on both the confessional and the testimonial, autobiography is particularly well suited not only to assist in the process of individual recovery but also to contribute to a "project of social change" (Alcoff and Gray 1993, 283). Ultimately, what writing in a public form can accomplish that the private journal or the therapy session cannot is *intervention in the public sphere*, by creating, for example, "an alternative jurisdiction" (Gilmore 2003, 715); by daring to contest oppressive master narratives (Nelson 2001, 169); by militating against—and compelling the reader to reconsider—the social and material conditions that engender trauma. Narratives like Maynard's and Danica's can, and should, lead us to ask "whether we need healing or non-violent, but far-reaching, revolution" (Horsman 1999, 45).

Notes

1. This pattern of delayed re/cognition—constitutive of the belatedness of trauma—resonates with the larger historical context within which Maynard's experience is embedded. In 1934, the year Fredelle Bruser turned twelve, a Canadian Jewish Congress study "uncovered such extensive anti-Semitism, most of it relatively legal, that the report was never released lest it prove demoralizing to Canadian Jews and help legitimate anti-Semitic expressions" (Weinfeld 2001, 322).
2. Waddington, a contemporary of Maynard's who also grew up on the Canadian prairies as a daughter of Jewish immigrants, describes a similar response to the prevailing anti-Semitism (1989, 6).
3. Norma Joseph offers this succinct overview: "Debates concerning the propriety of teaching women emanate from early rabbinic literature. The Talmud states that women were considered exempt from the obligation to study Torah ... In fact, the Mishnah in *Sotah* 3:4 and the ensuing Talmudic debate posit the question of whether women were even allowed to study" (1995; 207).
4. For discussions of Danica's *Don't*, see Warley (1992) and Winter (1996).

RICHARD INGRAM

Reports from the Psych Wars

What are the "psych wars"?[1] Two references help to provide a context for this concept. On November 19, 1999, the *New York Daily News* ran a headline on its front page that read "Get the Violent Crazies Off Our Streets."[2] This headline conflates "craziness" with belligerence, and demands that a certain minority be removed from public spaces in which they are seen as dangerous trespassers. Ron Coleman, a prominent member of the Hearing Voices Network in the UK, coined the slogan "psychotic and proud" as a gesture of defiance against such exclusionary practices (James 2001, 110). Instead of protesting the negative effects of being labelled "psychotic," Coleman affirms an identity that is generally believed to be among the least desirable of all social identities.

This "report" is tuned to the "psych wars," to the sounds of shots ringing out. The first section explores a few of the dimensions of psychiatric imperialism since World War II, invoking the work of Baudrillard to develop an understanding of the unifying text of American—and, increasingly, global—psychiatry, the *Diagnostic and Statistical Manual of Mental Disorders* (or *DSM*). The second section critically appraises the concept of "narrative" as it functions in the context of the psych wars.

Hyperreal Psych Wars

It was the Hollywood mogul Samuel Goldwyn who observed, "Anyone who goes to a psychiatrist ought to have his head examined," yet most people do not opt to become psychiatric patients. If the psychiatric profession were to rely on voluntary recruits alone, then its scope would be considerably smaller than it is now. As a disciplinary apparatus, therefore, psychiatry has relied on a steady stream of recruits who are press-ganged into service as patients. From the perspective of the state apparatus, the use of coercion has been justified as an essential component of what is sometimes called "the war on mental illness."

The narrative of fighting to overcome this enemy, however, has been challenged by a counternarrative that considers the very concept of "mental illness" to be fraudulent. By the 1970s, books such as E. Fuller Torrey's *The Death of Psychiatry* (1974) suggested that the profession was itself on the verge of collapse. Looking back, however, it is clear that, far from expiring, psychiatry was undergoing a fundamental transformation. Indeed, the profession emerged strengthened from its breakdown by entering into a Faustian pact with the pharmaceutical industry. The condition of this pact was that psychiatry was obliged to renew theories of biologically determined behaviour that had been discredited by the events of World War II. Psychiatry's rehabilitation was achieved by resuscitating theories of innate defects in order to shore up the concept of "mental illness," and to gain a more secure position within the medical establishment.

The success of the counternarrative that rejects the concept of "mental illness" could be measured in terms of the dramatic reduction in the number of institutionalized patients. By re-inventing itself as psychopharmacology, though, psychiatry has become less dependent on the mechanism of confinement. Not only has it managed to integrate the critique of the "stigma" of mental illness, psychiatry has also produced the category of "consumer" to supplement the category of "patient." This shift from "patient" to "consumer" enhances psychiatry's claim that it operates on the basis of consent.

Nevertheless, the process of de-institutionalization is being re-evaluated, and there are signs that it may be reversed. I have referred to the prominent American psychiatrist E. Fuller Torrey because he embodies this reversal, having mutated from a dissident within his profession into a leader of the new press gangs. Torrey states, "For a substantial minority ... de-institutionalization has been a psychiatric *Titanic*" (1996, 11). It appears that the main reason behind the great push for de-institutionalization in the 1960s and 1970s is being forgotten, and that we need to have our memory jogged. David Gonzalez, a "mad movement" activist,[3] arrived at the following striking comparison by employing information from the *World Almanac and Book of Facts* on the number of Americans killed in combat (Famighetti 1994, 163), together with figures from the US Substance Abuse and Mental Health Service Administration's Center for Mental Health Services:

Between 1950 and 1964, more people died in United States federal, state and county "mental hospitals" than the number of Americans killed in the Revolutionary War, the War of 1812, the Mexican War, the Civil War, the Spanish-American War, World War I, World War II, the Korean War, Vietnam, and the Persian Gulf War combined. (Gonzalez 2005)

In short, the "war on mental illness" has been the most lethal confrontation in which the United States has ever been engaged.

At the heart of this confrontation lies the text that is regularly referred to as the "psychiatrist's Bible," the *Diagnostic and Statistical Manual of Mental Disorders* (the *DSM*). Since the publication of the first edition in 1952, this text has grown exponentially. One indicator of the rapidity of its expansion is the number of pages needed to list and define the diagnostic categories in successive editions. For the second edition, published in 1968, the number of pages was fifty-one; for the 1987 revised version of the third edition, the number was 350; and for the enigmatically named "text revision" version of the fourth edition that emerged in 2000, there are 742 pages of lists and definitions.[4]

One way of approaching the *DSM* is to treat it as an ideological text in which the traces of battle have been inscribed. Louise Armstrong, a journalist who has written about one aspect of the psych wars that she describes as "the psychiatric policing of America's children," summarizes the militaristic manoeuvrings in and around the *DSM* with these observations:

> Reading about the evolution of the *DSM* ... is somewhat like reading the history of the Balkans: ongoing border wars, eruptions, skirmishes, the odd assassination, uprising, overthrow ... To read about the evolution of the *DSM* is to know this: It is an entirely *political* document. (1993, cited in Caplan 1995, ix)

Although I do not doubt the productivity of this approach, the drawback is that it aims to diagnose psychiatry's underlying traumas by identifying textual symptoms, which entails the embrace of some of psychiatry's own methods.

In an effort to avoid making truth claims about the psych wars, I am going to utilize the concepts of "simulation" and "deterrence" as they are articulated by Jean Baudrillard in *Simulacra and Simulation* (1994). There is a parallel, I want to suggest, between the nuclear arms race and the stockpiling of diagnostic categories. The connection between military and psychiatric expansionism is that, in each instance, the simulation of an extreme threat triggers a proliferation of security systems, spreading out in a chain reaction to cover all social relations. For psychiatry, any situation in which a mad person remains anonymous to the authorities is a danger to be averted. With this simulated threat as its alibi, the American Psychiatric Association has assembled the vast diagnostic machine of the *DSM*. Aside from being a perfect example of what Deleuze and Guattari (1987) call an "apparatus of capture,"[5] the diagnostic machine of the *DSM* functions as a security system that dissuades the population from behaviour that risks being identified as symptomatic of "mental illness."

A typical response of "anti-psychiatry" and the "mad movement" to this vision of threat is to argue that the mad are less violent than the general population, and positively docile in comparison with psychiatrists who practice "involuntary commitment" and "involuntary treatment"—also known as arbitrary incarceration, forced drugging, and electro-shock. However, this strategy of rationalist critique will be ineffective if, as Baudrillard asserts, "we are in a logic of simulation, which no longer has anything to do with a logic of facts and an order of reason" (1994, 16). Following Baudrillard, then, will lead us to the conclusion that the figure of the "psycho" can be neither proved nor disproved because it surpasses the oppositions of "real" and "imaginary," "true" and "false"—in short, it is "hyperreal."

As for the *DSM*, its diagnostic categories have long ceased to represent realities that precede them, and have instead become simulation models that generate hyperrealities. The *DSM* may once have been compiled from "case studies," or narratives of investigation into the aetiology and trajectory of "mental disorders." However, a threshold has been crossed so that it is the lives of patients that are now expected to conform to the models of "mental disorders," rather than the other way round.

Posters from a project known as the Early Psychosis Initiative illustrate how diagnostic categories operate as simulation models. Towards the end of April 2002, four posters started appearing on lampposts in the Vancouver-Richmond area of British Columbia, Canada, each of which showed a figure said to be between the age of seventeen and twenty-four. One of the posters read:

> Mary used to be really popular. Now she won't talk to her friends because she doesn't trust anyone. Psychosis is a treatable medical condition that affects thinking and perception. Three out of 100 people will get it. Worried about yourself or a friend? Visit [website provided] or call us at [phone number provided] for confidential help.

On the website, there is a particularly chilling request that promises to usher in a wave of psychiatric McCarthyism: "The Early Intervention Program would like to hear from you if you or someone you know in the

Vancouver or Richmond area is showing early signs of psychosis. Please email us at [email provided] or call [phone number provided]." This evangelistic project, which was co-ordinated by the Department of Psychiatry at the University of British Columbia, preaches a script into which we are invited to write ourselves, or those we know, as actors. Its simple narratives precede and have priority over the lives into which they will insert themselves, which is why I consider them to be simulation models.

The Order of Making Sense

I now turn to the theme of "narrative" to raise some concerns about the problem of "making sense," for which "narrative" is so often prescribed as the solution. The previous section began by referring to the decline and subsequent recovery of a psychiatric narrative based on the concept of "mental illness," and to an anti-psychiatric narrative that rejects this key concept. Gayatri Spivak has argued that "we need a commitment not only to narrative and counternarrative, but also to the rendering (im)possible of (another) narrative" (1999, 6). In this section, I challenge the assumption that there are only narratives, counternarratives, and (excluded) other narratives, by asking what is rendered impossible by the form(s) of narrative.

Madness can evade capture by inhabiting "the desert of the real" (Baudrillard 1994, 3) for only so long before it corrodes into models that substitute for the real. When the real recedes, a desperate search for authenticity ensues. "When the real is no longer what it was," Baudrillard contends, "nostalgia assumes its full meaning" (6). The current popularity of autobiographical texts that recount the "lived experience" of madness could testify to what Baudrillard designates as a "panic-stricken production of the real" (7).[6]

My doctoral dissertation focused on the testimonies of psychiatric consumers, survivors, and ex-patients, and particularly on those published since the introduction of Prozac in the late 1980s (Ingram 2005). Instead of relegating these texts to the realm of nostalgia, I considered them to be strategic interventions in the psych wars. They could be read as attempts to reclaim authority and authorship in lives that have been organized to fit with the simulated narratives of psychiatry's diagnostic machine. There is a comment in a 1972 interview by the dissident psychiatrist Félix Guattari that supports this interpretation. Asked if radical critiques of psychiatry could transform the discipline into the leading human science, Guattari replied, "Rather than psychiatry why not the schizophrenics, the mad people themselves? I don't believe that those who work in the field of psychiatry ... are really the ones in the avant-garde" (Guattari 1995, 83).[7]

Unfortunately, the goal of re-appropriating one's life from the apparatus of psychiatric capture is, I think, impossible. One explanation of why this objective is unattainable was proposed by Jacques Derrida in his 1963 lecture, "Cogito and the History of Madness," which is a critique of Michel Foucault's book, *Folie et déraison* (Derrida 1978).[8] Foucault had done his utmost to avoid writing a history of psychiatry, and had instead framed his project as an archaeological investigation that sought to excavate the silence of a madness that has been buried beneath psychiatric language. Derrida argued that the decisive flaw in this approach was that the silence of madness could only be evoked in the language of reason. No one who resorted to the language of reason, even if they were, like Foucault, contesting reason, could avoid being complicit with psychiatry as the delegate of state apparatuses that uphold the rule of reason, on which their argument depends:

> All our European languages, the language of everything that has participated, from near or far, in the adventure of Western reason—all this is the immense delegation of the project defined by Foucault under the rubric of the capture or objectification of madness. Nothing within this language, and no one among those who speak it, can escape the historical guilt ... which Foucault apparently wishes to put on trial. (1978, 35)

This debate manifests one of the dilemmas faced by the psychiatrized. The concept of "making sense" of illness, which has gathered all the force of a regulative ideal for people with all types of illness, is particularly oppressive when it comes to hold sway over people who are judged to be "mentally ill" on the basis of their alleged failure to "make sense."

However, the "order of making sense" is by no means limited to psychiatrists and psychoanalysts. The anti-psychiatry movement often promotes holistic approaches centred on talk, writing, or art therapies as alternatives to the reductionism of psychopharmacology. In her study of the psychiatric survivor movement, Barbara Everett maintains that

> from the perspective of the actual patient, psychiatry and anti-psychiatry may not be as far apart as they appear to the protagonists. Each identifies the patient or client as a victim, either of disease or environment. In both cases, rescue is achieved only through professional intervention. (2000, 35)

I would add that psychiatry and anti-psychiatry believe that the condition from which "victims" should be "rescued" is one in which they have either lost or been deprived of the ability to "make sense."

Moreover, a growing convergence of the regulative ideals of "making sense" and "redemption through creative work" is leading to the elevation of "narrative therapy" to the status of a moral imperative. "Narrative therapy" is not a homogeneous concept: variations on the theme can be found in psychotherapy;[9] in some of the recently published memoirs by psychiatric consumers, survivors, and ex-patients; and in many disciplines across the humanities, social sciences, and health sciences. For an example of narrative therapy as moral imperative, I am going to cite the conclusion of Naomi Schor's essay, "Depression in the Nineties." She counsels:

> Narrative, however contested by currently dominant forms of criticism, must be retained lest storytelling be lost as an essential meaning-giving and, I will risk the word, universal means of making sense of one's hopes and desires, one's ideals and despair, not to say one's depression. (1995, 163)

My view is that by preserving the order of making sense, the kind of endorsement that Schor gives to narrative therapy colludes with the simulation models of psychopharmacology.

By juxtaposing two contrasting images, a 1997 advertisement for Prozac suggests a narrative of recovery. In the first image, an object barely recognizable as a vase lies in pieces above the slogan "Depression shatters." In the second, the vase has been reassembled and contains a vibrant flower. Two slogans accompany the restored vase: "Prozac can help" and "Welcome back." Prozac can come to the rescue, we are encouraged to believe, whenever fragmentation, multiplicity, dispersion (the shattered vase), and "the blues" (the colour surrounding every piece of the vase) have broken us apart. We will understand that life itself had receded (the former absence of the flower), as warmth and vivacity (the red flower) are restored. Prozac enables wholeness, unity, and coherence to return (the intact vase), and so puts Humpty Dumpty together again.

What I am highlighting here is the continuity between, and the inseparability of, Prozac and narrative. As was the case with the poster of "Mary" that was plastered on BC lampposts, the simulation model integrates a diagnostic label with a specific treatment to produce psychiatric patients. A distinctive feature of this narrative is the transformation of the psychiatrized person into a consumer. Whereas the victims of "psychosis" are presumed to be in such a serious condition that informants are needed to turn them over to the authorities, this advertisement persuades us that consumers choose Prozac, and therefore that psychiatry operates on the basis of consent.

Conclusion

Contrary to Schor, therefore, I think that the category of "narrative" is not receiving sufficient critical attention, and that the part played by narrative in the psych wars is predominantly pernicious. A triple critique of narrative needs to be developed, whose combined effect should be to erode the idea that madness is an illness consisting of a deficit in the capacity to "make sense." First, we need a critique of narrative as an injunction that results in those who fail to bow to the order of making sense being judged to be "mentally ill"; second, a critique of narrative as a technology or "mode of enframing" that positions psychiatric patients as senseless bodies, dependent on mental health professionals who are presumed to know the true nature of their patients' "mental disorders"; and third, a critique of narrative as a commodity, which would analyze the role of narrative in psychopharmacology's pill-pushing campaigns, building on Roland Barthes' insight: "Why do we tell stories? For amusement or distraction? For 'instruction,' as they said in the seventeenth century? Does a story reflect or express an ideology, in the Marxist sense of the word? Today all these justifications seem out of date to me. Every narrative thinks of itself as a kind of merchandise" (Barthes 1991, 89).[10]

To sum up: what I am proposing is an interrogation of the ways in which the psych wars are structured by the moralities of "production," "meaning," and "narrative." I want to emphasize that my aim is not to supplant them with counter-moral values of "anti-production," "anti-meaning," and "anti-narrative." Instead, it is to affirm that which comes before, between, and beyond the oppositions of production and non-production, meaning and non-meaning, narrative and non-narrative.

Notes

1. The first part of this chapter has been published. Please see Richard Ingram, "Reports from the Psych Wars, Section 1: Hyperreal Psych Wars," in *The Stigma of Cinemania*, <http://www.cinemaniastigma.com/pages/9/index.htm> (last accessed December 5, 2005). It is reprinted with the permission of David Gonzalez.
2. The front page bearing this headline is reproduced on David Gonzalez' website, *The Stigma of Cinemania*.
3. On the "mad movement," see Shimrat (1997).
4. Some of this information is taken from Patchen Barss (2002).
5. Deleuze and Guattari state that the mark of an "apparatus of capture" is "that very particular kind of violence that creates or contributes to the creation of that which it is directed against, and thus presupposes itself" (1987, 448). For example, the violent creation of the problem of "mental illness" by a discipline that justifies its existence in terms of the need to target this very problem.

6 Lauren Slater remarks on "the huge proliferation of authoritative illness memoirs in recent years, memoirs that talk about people's personal experiences with Tourette's and postpartum depression and manic depression, memoirs that are often rooted in the latest scientific 'evidence'" (2001, 221).
7 Guattari's remark was made at a time when critiques of psychiatry from within the profession would have been viewed by many as the basis for transforming the discipline. Hence the significance of Guattari's insistence that it is schizophrenics rather than dissident psychiatrists who constitute the avant-garde.
8 Jacques Derrida, *Cogito et l'histoire de la folie*, Collège Philosophique, March 4, 1963, translated as "Cogito and the History of Madness" (1978, 30–63). A comprehensive analysis of this debate between Foucault and Derrida can be found in Roy Boyne's *Foucault and Derrida* (1990).
9 In the field of psychotherapy, Michael White and David Epston's *Narrative Means to Therapeutic Ends* (1990), has been followed by such titles as *Narrative Therapy: The Social Construction of Preferred Realities* (Freedman and Combs 1996) and *A Different Story: The Rise of Narrative in Psychotherapy* (Beels 2001).
10 The critique of narrative as commodity has been developed in Jonathan Metzl's *Prozac on the Couch* (2003).

SHELLEY Z. REUTER

Agoraphobia, Social Order, and Psychiatric Narrative

Taking its name from *agora*, the Greek word for public square or marketplace, "agoraphobia" is the term given to the fear of public or open spaces. This phobia develops in response to previous experiences of overwhelming anxiety in everyday situations such as in crowds, on buses or trains, or even while driving—situations from which a person may be unable to escape or get help, and where they are at great risk of embarrassment. These symptoms can range in severity, of course, but "attacks" may include rapid heartbeat, chest pain, shortness of breath, gastrointestinal distress, faintness, dizziness, sweating, fear of losing control or going insane, fear of dying, or a sense of impending doom. People who experience these feelings avoid phobic situations—places where they have experienced anxiety—and in extreme cases they rarely leave their homes without a trusted companion. The prevalence of agoraphobia has been estimated to include as much as five percent of the population (Rosenbaum et al 1995, A4). In the US, this translates to approximately twelve million people—most of whom are women.

Although there are a few references to these kinds of symptoms in early nineteenth-century writings, and general references to phobias that appear as early as the fourth century BC (in the writings of Hippocratic physicians), agoraphobia was first described formally in 1872, in an article written by German neurologist Carl Otto Westphal (1833–90). His article described the symptoms of three Berliners, all of whom were male, who complained of the difficulty they had walking through open spaces, crossing streets and squares, and of being in crowds and enclosed spaces. After Westphal published this article, the written clinical discourse of agoraphobia developed a life of its own, and continues to thrive today. Indeed, a recent search on Medline turned up nearly two thousand references published in the last three decades alone. Together these publications have provided a forum for physicians to theorize about the phenomenology (signs and symptoms), causation, and treatment of agoraphobia, and many authors still cite Westphal's report even today.

Contained within this clinical discourse is what I refer to as the "psychiatric narrative." Specifically, while the disease describes very real physiological experiences of suffering, a socio-cultural account of society is implicit in this discourse. Taking a genealogical approach, this article examines the literature on agoraphobia with a view to disrupting the assumption that psychiatric knowledge does not itself constitute a type of narrative. Several themes emerge: these include the relationship between urbanization, social change, and mental life at the turn of the nineteenth century; the relationship between agoraphobia and gender, "race," and class; and the shift in recent decades within psychiatry from an emphasis on biopsycho*social* explanation for mental diseases to an emphasis on strictly biological explanations. Together these themes demonstrate that the question of what it means to be "normal" underpinning psychiatric accounts of agoraphobia has historically signalled a more fundamental and normative question of what it means to have social order.

The City and Social Change

In the late nineteenth and early twentieth centuries, an expanding medical profession led many doctors to specialize in psychological medicine (Porter 1997, 498), and it was not uncommon for physicians to describe modern urban living as a dangerous strain on mental health. Urban living itself increasingly came to be pathologized, and a "generalized fear of [the] metropolis" manifested in many physicians' writings (Sutherland 1877, 266). As Sigmund Freud wrote, for example, a tension existed between "living in simple, healthy, country conditions" as the "forefathers" did, and living in "the great cities," which caused "increasing nervousness of the present day and modern civilized life" (1963, 21). An American physician, Dr. Charles Atwood, argued similarly that "our rapid and over strenuous life," unaccompanied by sufficient rest, caused an "increase in nervous and mental derangement" (1903, 1070–2).

A parallel discourse developed among some classical social theorists such as Karl Marx (1964 [1884]), Emile Durkheim (1933 [1893]), Max Weber (1958 [1904–05]), and Ferdinand Tönnies (1957 [1887]); each, in his own way, was concerned about the changes of modernity and its associated social problems. Georg Simmel especially focused on mental life and the metropolis, observing that life in the modern (capital) city, with all its "nervous stimulation"—the crowds, the intensity, and the rampant individualism—produced the ideal conditions for the development of mental problems. Life in this context was so fragmented that people had to distance themselves from each other in order to protect their fragile psyches, developing what he called a "blasé attitude" just to cope. In the most severe cases, he surmised, people experienced agoraphobia (1950 [1903], 1978 [1907]).

Echoing the concerns of physicians and social theorists, many architects and urban planners were also convinced that city living caused poor physical and mental health. As one wrote, "Recently a unique nervous disorder has been diagnosed—'agoraphobia' ... a very new and modern ailment" (Sitte 1965, 45). He also noted that "numerous people are said to suffer from it, always experiencing a certain anxiety or discomfort, whenever they have to walk across a vast empty place" (45).[1] In light of this and other "fashionable" ailments, as Sitte called them, architects and planners strove to design social space to minimize disease and promote a healthy (social) body (Rose 1994, 65). From this concern to promote health arose the idea of the need for separation between private and public spaces, and the subsequent construction of the home as a refuge from the filth and immorality of urban streets. Retreat into the private home also provided another means of coping with the pressures of modern urban life. It is interesting that all of these urban critics mobilized the concept of agoraphobia as both a diagnosis *and* a metaphor for the widespread estrangement, or alienation, endemic in modern urban society.

Gender, Race, and Class

Today women comprise over 80 per cent of diagnosed agoraphobics, but up until the First World War, agoraphobia was far and away more prevalent in men—affluent "adult men of education," as one doctor put it (Van Horn 1886). That this was so calls attention to the rare occasions when women were diagnosed with agoraphobia. When they were, their symptoms were interpreted in terms of the female reproductive system. One woman's agoraphobia, for example, was believed to stem from excessive lactation and frequent childbearing (Suckling 1890), while in another, whose agoraphobia was always much worse in the week prior to her menstrual period, it was believed to be related to a cervical laceration.[2] In contrast, diagnoses in men were usually made in terms of problems with their nerves. As an American physician named Dr. Webber wrote, in this "pathological group the entire nervous system ... may be thrown into extreme commotion" (1872, 446). Still, with nerves and nervous problems commonly seen at this time as being essentially feminine (Theriot 1997), it seems that, one way or another, regardless of whether it was women or men being diagnosed, agoraphobia, like other modern urban mental diseases, was conceptualized as a feminine disorder (Vidler 1993).

There is another sense, however, in which this disease became gendered. If the thesis put forth by Georg Simmel, the physicians, architects, and urban planners of the time is correct—that the stresses people experienced in the metropolis led individuals to develop agoraphobia—then the question becomes why, for the first fifty years of its history, were agoraphobics predominantly men? Wouldn't both genders have been exposed to the perils of modern city living? Further, why did the trend shift from men to women after World War I?

It is important to consider that although women were encouraged into public space through new forms of employment (for working and lower-middle-class women) and a seductive market consumerism that included exhibitions, department stores, refreshment rooms, rest rooms, and reading rooms—places bourgeois women could go unchaperoned (Wolff 1989)—there were also restrictions on women's movement, at least at an ideological level. In this context, staying home for a bourgeois woman signified *normality* insofar as the ideology of "separate spheres"—evident in nineteenth-century deportment manuals—declared a "True Woman's" primary roles to be those of wife and mother (see Welter 1966). The accuracy of the concept of separate spheres has been disputed in recent feminist historiography but, with the symptoms of agoraphobia mapping directly onto *what was expected* of bourgeois women, perhaps their staying home "passed" as appropriate feminine behaviour rather than making them candidates for psychiatric diagnosis like their male counterparts (who, incidentally, were in effect behaving like women in accommodating their fear, thereby feminizing agoraphobia in yet another sense).

After World War I, agoraphobia came to be diagnosed more prevailingly in women, and it appears that what was previously considered normal bourgeois feminine behaviour—domesticity—became something to see as pathological: as agoraphobic. There are at least two possible explanations for this change in perception. First, during the war and in the absence of their male partners, women achieved some measure of independence, but with this independence came increased public responsibilities that not all women necessarily wanted to assume. With modern urban life apparently so difficult for everyone, it is possible that not all women could face their own emancipation, and agoraphobia may have provided a legitimate means to avoid gender politics.

Second, as a result of the war, a discourse of "war neurosis" or shell shock emerged, and this diagnosis was frequently invoked by doctors in their assessments of men's anxieties, whether or not the men had been anywhere near an exploding shell (Shephard 2000). This suggests that a diagnosis of agoraphobia called male patients' masculinity into question in ways that a somewhat more heroic diagnosis of war neurosis would not have done. This would not necessarily have saved men from disgrace, but the point here is that, in these early days, agoraphobia helped demarcate gender and gender roles.

Another thing worth noticing is that the patients in this literature are rarely described in racialized terms, even though, historically, many mental diseases have been racialized (Grob 1985). This silence on matters of "race" suggests that the typical patient presenting symptoms of and diagnosed with agoraphobia historically has been white, since in western discourse—medical and otherwise—whiteness tends not to require qualification or even articulation. It is taken for granted.

This thinking is manifest in a manual used by early twentieth-century mental health professionals called *The Statistical Manual for the Use of Institutions for the Insane* (American Medico-Psychological Association 1918), which provided instructions on how to classify incoming patients not only by symptoms, but also according to socio-cultural measures such as "race." The manual took its classification criteria from another manual known as the *Dictionary of Races or Peoples*, published by the US Immigration Commission (Dillingham 1911). There, the so-called English are described as "the principal race" with higher evolutionary status, as compared with the so-called "Negroes," who are said to belong to "the lowest division of mankind from an evolutionary standpoint" (100).

To the extent that this racial classification derived from notions of evolutionary progress, it follows that the normalization of whiteness evident in both this *Dictionary* and in the *Statistical Manual* can also be linked to ideas about civilization and modernity, as Laura Briggs has demonstrated in her study of hysteria (2000). Like hysteria, agoraphobia was also constructed as a nervous "disease of overcivilization" and, as such, was the almost exclusive prerogative of affluent whites. In other words, in addition to gender, agoraphobia demarcated the boundaries of race and class: with the well-heeled English as the normative standard against which all the other so-called "races" were measured, only affluent, white people were seen as viable candidates for these kinds of problems. Hence, there was no need to articulate any racial criteria in the psychiatric literature because patients' normative whiteness was tacitly understood.

The normative white (medical) subject has persisted in the discourse of agoraphobia throughout the twentieth century, making a relatively recent discovery by American epidemiologists (Boyd et al. 1990; Weissman 1990) that the prevalence of agoraphobia (and other phobias) was higher among African-American women with the lowest socio-economic status quite surprising. This unexpected observation can be explained in part by the fact that most agoraphobia literature is based on clinical populations (as opposed to community populations), which for economic and historical reasons are over-represented by whites. With less economic access to therapy (US Census Bureau 2000; US Department of Health 1986, 1987), minority groups are commonly excluded from clinical studies (Gamble 1997). As well, there is a longstanding legacy of distrust of the medical establishment among African Americans, which makes them much less likely to see doctors with their problems (Gamble 1993). This finding also reflects the related possibility that agoraphobia may have passed undetected in African Americans until recently because the official criteria for this diagnosis (taken from the American Psychiatric Association's [APA] *Diagnostic and Statistical Manual of Mental Disorders* [*DSM*]) are based on a normative white experience that excludes the issue of racism as a possible—and legitimate—reason for not going out into public spaces. It appears, then, that just as agoraphobia offered commentary on urbanization and modern social change, it also had something to say about gender, race, and class.

From Biopsychosocial to the Strictly Biological

Let us turn now to psychiatry in its contemporary context. Another dimension of the psychiatric narrative of social order derives from the resurgence of biological positivism in psychiatry in recent decades, especially since the APA's (1980) third edition of the *Diagnostic and Statistical Manual of Mental Disorders* (*DSM-III*). *DSM-III* coincided with the marginalization of psychoanalysis from mainstream psychiatry after decades at its forefront, for failing to conform to the APA's new standards of validity and reliability.[3]

Returning to the narrative theme of this discussion, it is interesting to note that, prior to this neo-positivist transformation, psychiatric literature really did read like "narrative" in the conventional sense, with characters (patients) that experienced and felt and did things. This was particularly true of the psychoanalytic case literature that tended to focus on one patient and his or her analysis over the long term. Contemporary psychiatric literature, however, has a very different tone, reading more like lab reports with capital S's (for Subjects) rather than people in them, and heavy with statistical measures and the jargon of psychiatric expertise. This transformation to biological neo-positivism has had important sociological implications: first, the exclusion of psychoanalysis has also meant the exclusion of overtly social explanations for mental disease. The elimination of the concept of "neurosis," for example, demonstrates this above all. Second, the *DSM* was intended to guide psychiatrists in their diagnoses, but it has also served historically—like structural-functionalism—as a kind of moral and ideological prescription for how people *should* live if society is to operate smoothly. The eminent sociologist Talcott Parsons, for example, wrote nearly fifty years ago that to be "the main 'breadwinner' of his family is a primary role of the normal adult male in our society." The "'corollary of this role' is that of his wife, who is responsible for 'the internal affairs of the household.'" Housekeeping and childcare constitute the "primary functional content of the adult feminine role in the 'utilitarian' division of labor'" (1954, 187–91).

It is interesting to compare this with the following criterion only recently added in *DSM-IV*: "Individuals' avoidance of situations may impair their ability to travel to work or carry out homemaking responsibilities (e.g., grocery shopping, taking children to the doctor)" (APA 1994, 396). This criterion is clearly a gendered one, especially given that by the time this criterion was added to the DSM in 1994, it was already established that most agoraphobics are women. Indeed, in its implicit Parsonian conception of social order, the notion that the measure of health is one's ability to work or carry out homemaking responsibilities must be called into question. It is significant that the *DSM* defines the agoraphobic by her decreased productivity and consumption, and it is equally revealing that behaviourist therapy programs—which flow out of *DSM* criteria—incorporate shopping into treatment plans. When doctors sanction shopping as a goal of therapy, they transmit a cultural imperative to their patients, an imperative that reflects a dominant ideal that links normal femininity with consumption and, in one case, normal masculinity with paid work (Lim 1985), thereby pathologizing the possibility of living outside the imperatives of patriarchal capitalism. Indeed, agoraphobia is bad for the economy (Edlund 1990), but while some may consider not working (for pay) ideal feminine behaviour, the implication of this *DSM* criterion is that interested economic assumptions help constitute the lens through which psychiatrists gaze at their patients. One also cannot help but suspect a link between this criterion and resistance to the increasing presence of women both in the paid work force and in professions traditionally occupied by men.

Finally, the shift from psychoanalysis to biopsychiatry is also important because it reveals a very particular interpretation of social order; or rather, disorder. Social disorder—represented by diseases like agoraphobia—results from the rejection of "normal" society, and this rejection is implicit in agoraphobia's very symptoms. Consequently, the discourse of this disorder, including the literature on agoraphobia and the *DSM* criteria, have depicted society in regulative terms such that the literature and the *DSM* criteria on which it is based are more than simply accounts of a disease, its symptoms, causation, and treatment. Together they tell a story about what kind of psychiatric explanation shall count, and about the relationship between psychiatric disease categories and the society *in which*, and the individuals *to which*, these categories are assigned. Finally, they tell a story about social order and its normative social dimensions; namely gender, race, and class.

Notes

1 Credit for the discovery of Sitte's text goes to Vidler (1991, 35).
2 After her physician, Dr. Potter, "made local applications," this patient was still unable to travel without trepidation so she took matters into her own hands, keeping "a flask well filled with brandy" in the right hand and "her Bible in the left ... presumably the one counteracting the influence of the other" (Potter 1882, 474).
3 Psychoanalysis, it should be noted, has drawn extensive criticism as a normalizing episteme. Michel Foucault, the most well-known proponent of this view, characterized psychoanalysis as a "regime of truth" infused with power relations (1978, 5). Although psychoanalysis challenged dominant biogenic notions of normal illness, it was nonetheless a discourse (and practice) of normalization in its own right. In alleviating "the effects of repression" and allowing "individuals to express their incestuous desire in discourse" (129), psychoanalysts became the arbiters of lifestyle, and the self-inspection of psychoanalysis, like the Catholic confessional, a way of life. "Bio-power" turned everyone into self-normalizing subjects, with each person striving to ensure that all their actions and thoughts conformed to what science had shown to be normal, healthy, and productive (Dreyfus 1987, 319–20).

JOANNE MUZAK

"THEY SAY THE DISEASE IS RESPONSIBLE"
Social Identity and the Disease Concept of Drug Addiction

Prompted by demographic changes in drug use during the 1960s and 1970s, most notably an explosion of drug use by America's middle-class youth and heroin addiction among returning Vietnam veterans (Musto 1999, 247; Kandall 1996, 143), older, stigmatizing views of addiction began to give way to notions that promoted the reintegration of addicts into acceptable social roles (Acker 1993, 202). By the 1980s, addiction had been reconceptualized as a disease in which genetically inherited biochemical abnormalities in the brain and liver cause compulsive cravings and "out-of-control" behaviour (Acker 1993, 202; Morrison 1989, 184). This disease model of addiction not only explained drug use and abuse in dominant culture without demonizing the addict, it also accommodated white, middle-class addicts by offering them the possibility of recovery.

In this essay, I will read Martha Morrison's 1989 memoir, *White Rabbit: A Doctor's Own Story of Addiction, Survival, and Recovery*, as a case study of how this newly reconceptualized disease model of addiction operates in the narrative reconstruction of one's life as a "new" addict—a white, middle-class drug addict. As a young, white, middle-class woman, Morrison represents a segment of the drug-using and drug-addicted population that most troubles society by upsetting not only stereotypes of the addict, such as the urban black man, but also constructs of femininity and normality. I explore the emergence of the supposedly non-stigmatizing disease concept of addiction as a historically specific response to the changing demographics of drug use. Examining Morrison's representation of class and gender in relation to her addict identity, I argue that what is at stake in this apparently non-punitive concept of addiction as disease is the maintenance of middle-class privilege and heteronormativity.

I begin with a brief historical overview of the disease models of addiction, followed by a contextualization of the demographic shift in drug use that encouraged the reconceptualization and popularization of the disease concept in the 1970s and 1980s. Turning then to *White Rabbit*, I will consider Morrison's use of the disease concept to reconstruct her identity as a white, middle-class, female drug addict. Throughout, I shall engage in ongoing critical debates over the utility of the disease concept of addiction. My goal is to identify the disease concept as reliant on normative notions of class and gender, despite its claims of indiscrimination.

In her article "Stigma or Legitimation? A Historical Examination of the Social Potentials of Addiction Disease Models," Caroline J. Acker traces the shifts in the formulation of opiate addiction as a disease in the twentieth century, and identifies three distinct changes in the disease model in the United States since about 1900. Before 1920, "a diversity of views regarding the nature of opiate addiction as a scientific or medical phenomenon coexisted and competed" (1993, 194). During the late nineteenth and early twentieth century, bacteriologists and public health workers developed knowledge about infectious diseases, and declining rates of epidemic diseases like cholera and chronic diseases like tuberculosis favoured biological research as the most productive approach to comprehending and controlling disease, which included opiate addiction (197). One group of medical professionals, therefore, sought to demonstrate that addiction was a "definite physiological disease condition with definite uniform manifestations … and definite understandable causation" (C.F.J. Laase, cited in Acker 1993, 198). Louder voices, however, postulated the "vice theory," which understood addiction as a "moral lapse" and called for a punitive rather than medical response to opiate addiction (Acker 1993, 198). Variant theories interpreted addiction as a psychiatric disease, and others asserted that addiction was a condition "between a vice and a disease" (198). Although these proposed models depended on scientific observation, they were highly influenced by prevailing cultural attitudes towards addicts, which held that addicts were weak-willed, morally corrupt, and often psychiatrically disturbed (198). The mixed message that emerged was that "addiction was a disease but not a respectable one" (199): an addict may be sick, but he still carries a social stigma.

According to Acker, a dominant disease model of addiction emerged after 1920 concurrent with punitive federal drug legislation (200).[1] Sociodemographic changes at the turn of the century contributed to growing fears over drug use and, in turn, pushed America toward a national antidrug policy (Kandall 1996, 44). As Stephen Kandall explains, "the number of drug users among the black and Chinese populations was on the rise; urban addicts were beginning to outnumber rural addicts; drug use was increasingly associated with poverty; and the press began reporting links between drug use and crime more frequently" (1996, 44). By the time the Harrison Anti-Narcotic Act was passed in 1914, America had come to perceive drug addiction and addicts themselves as a threat to the nation (Jonnes 1996, 49).[2] The Harrison Act, which effectively criminalized the possession of opiates, reflected the popular punitive attitude towards addicts.[3] Physicians who were perceived to be prescribing opiates improperly (i.e., providing narcotics to addicts for addiction maintenance) were swiftly prosecuted, and soon became afraid to treat addicts as patients (Kandall 1996, 76; Acker 1993, 201). The prosecution of physicians eliminated community-based outpatient treatment for addiction (Acker 1993, 201; Kandall 1996, 85). Addicts were also vigorously prosecuted for possession of narcotics; by mid-1928, violators of the Harrison Act constituted the majority of federal penitentiary inmates (Musto 1999, 184).

Consistent with federal policy that criminalized the possession of opiates, and thereby criminalized addiction, the post-1920 disease model of addiction further stigmatized addicts as deviants and criminals. The Public Health Service–sponsored research of psychiatrist Lawrence Kolb shaped attitudes towards addicts for much of the first half of the twentieth century (Acker 1993, 201). Kolb posited a psychiatric disease model that claimed addiction was caused by a character defect in certain kinds of people—"delinquent types," as he called them (Acker 1993, 201; Courtwright 1982, 115).[4] In effect, addiction was defined as a kind of deviance and addicts were treated accordingly, sent to federal "hospital-prison-sanitariums" (Jonnes 1996, 111) like the infamous US Narcotics Farm at Lexington, Kentucky.[5] Research on the physiology of addiction was discouraged throughout the first half of the twentieth century, and physicians remained reluctant to treat addicts as anti-drug laws increased in severity from the 1930s well into the 1950s (Acker 1993, 202; Musto 1999, 246).

The next chapter in America's history of drug use is well documented as a cultural phenomenon. The 1960s witnessed, in David Musto's words, "an astounding increase" (1999, 247) in illegal drug use. This increase was all the more "astounding" because, for the first (highly publicized) time, white middle-class youth represented America's drug users and future addicts.[6] New patterns of drug use among "new population groups" (Acker 1993, 202), or perhaps more accurately, newly recognized population groups—primarily white, middle-class men and women—continued to emerge throughout the 1970s and 1980s. Heroin-addicted Vietnam veterans of the 1970s and cocaine-addicted young white urban professionals of the mid-1970s and early 1980s (Jonnes 1996, 306), for example, presented a new and unsettling picture of addiction. Addiction among the dominant culture not only challenged prevailing narratives of addiction as a problem restricted to ethnic minorities, the poor, and the otherwise deviant, it also represented a notable market opportunity in the private health care sector (Acker 1993, 202).

Unable to accommodate the notion of such widespread "deviance" in dominant culture and unwilling to address the socio-political aspects of the changing demographics of drug use, society had to reinvent addiction, at least as it applied to the "new" addicts. After all, these "new" addicts, otherwise "normal" and "successful" people, did not deserve to be locked up or outcast. A conceptual shift in the disease model away from the psychiatric toward the physiological and biological fit the bill. The reconceptualized disease model emphasized the addict's "out-of-control" behaviour as a consequence of physiological reactions to repeated drug use, and genetic inheritance, psychological, and social environments were cited as predisposing factors (Acker 1993, 202). Despite a postulated physiological basis, this model stressed behaviours—loss of control, compulsiveness, continued drug use despite negative consequences—as diagnostic signs of the disease (203). This seemingly paradoxical formulation of disease, which continues to dominate contemporary interpretations of addiction, has several implications. First, the model is no longer drug-specific,[7] and the emphasis on behaviour "justifies early treatment intervention" (203).

By the early 1980s, a reconceptualized disease model was generally accepted by treatment professionals as well as the public (Frans 1994, 71). This model holds that drug addicts are sick and unable to control an illness with which they were most likely born, but are able to recover from this illness under proper medical supervision. Proponents of the disease concept argue that it relieves the overwhelming guilt and moral stigma of living with addiction (Driscoll 1993, 257). This message, I would argue, however, does not apply to all addicts. It has a special resonance for white, middle-class addicts, as those most likely to be able to afford treatment and be most easily reintegrated into society.

As the disease model shifted from punitive and stigmatizing to non-punitive and legitimating to accommodate (and profit from) addiction in white middle-class America, Martha Morrison entered a treatment program at Ridgeview Institute in Atlanta for doctors with drug problems. Acquiring her drug habit during "the psychedelic sixties" (Morrison 1989, 18), Morrison, a twenty-nine-year-old, white, middle-class, female professional, exemplifies the new face of addiction. As such, she experiences the disease concept as simultaneously liberating and protective. She is able to use the disease concept to legitimate her experience of addiction, and to construct a socially acceptable addict identity because she occupies a privileged socio-economic position. Her representations of class, as well as gender, reveal the normative assumptions and functions of the disease concept of addiction.

I would like to begin my analysis of Morrison's autobiography with a brief description of the role the disease concept plays in the book's organization. The disease model provides a narrative framework for Morrison's life story. Because it presumes a genetic predisposition to addiction, or in Morrison's words, "the *inherited potential* [for the brain and liver] to respond in an abnormal or allergic fashion to mood altering chemicals" (emphasis mine; 1989, 184), the disease model suggests that addiction is an always already, although invisible, condition for some. From a position of "recovery," the disease concept insists on the retrospective reinterpretation of one's life as an always already addict (Warhol and Michie 1996, 355). As a subscriber to the disease concept, in other words, Morrison reinterprets even her earliest childhood behaviours as signs and symptoms of her disease and as characteristics of an addict. Early on in *White Rabbit*, for example, Morrison recounts taking her mother's prescription painkillers apart, instinctively knowing at age twelve to collect and ingest the potent pink balls from the capsules (19–20). She recalls her behaviour as a clear sign of the addiction to follow:

> Later I learned that this was what heroin addicts used when their drug of choice was scarce. They'd break them down and shoot them up. At the age of twelve in Fayetteville, Arkansas, I'd never heard of the expression "breaking something down," and in the early 1960s I doubt anyone in town knew much about "shooting up." But I didn't need to be shown; *I came by the urge naturally*. I didn't shoot up for quite some time, but *I had the right instincts*. (emphasis mine; 20)

Morrison recalls childhood and adolescent behaviours, emotions, and events chronologically as symptoms of her addiction.

In addition to demanding recourse to the symptom, which pathologizes behaviour by encouraging "what might have been experienced as 'normal' ... behaviour to be reinterpreted retrospectively as signs of [addiction]" (Warhol and Michie 1996, 335), the disease concept produces a prophetic addict identity. That is, because addiction is popularly understood (and promoted by groups such as Alcoholics Anonymous and Narcotics Anonymous) as a treatable but incurable disease, addicts remain addicts for life (Cain 1991, 214).[8] Morrison understands that this disease has always been and will always be a part of her life, and she structures her life story and identity accordingly.

Although the disease concept is ubiquitous in the narrative framework of Morrison's life story, we learn late in the book that Morrison did not always accept the notion of addiction as a disease. In excerpted letters that she wrote to friends at the beginning of her treatment, Morrison in fact emphatically rejects the disease concept:

> I have a biochemical/genetically-based disease, or so they say. Horseshit. This goes against everything I've known from the street angle, patient angle, and professionally ... I can't buy this disease bullshit ... They want me to "surrender" to a "higher power"—God, or whatever, they're not specific. In other words, give up the little control I've got left. What shit ... how could I have let this happen? They say I'm "not responsible." ... They say the disease is responsible. What B.S. (159–64)

Morrison's suspicions echo critics' concerns over the utility of the disease model. Feminist critics find the notion of giving oneself to a "higher power" and admitting one's powerlessness especially problematic. As Charlotte Kasl points out, many women who abuse drugs do so because they feel powerless in their lives (qtd. in Berenson 1991, 68). The disease concept not only requires women to give up what they never had (Driscoll 1993, 254), but also reinforces women's internalized oppression (Berenson 1991, 78; Frans 1994, 79), thus maintaining oppressive gender roles. Furthermore, the powerlessness implicit in the disease concept "erodes human capacity for taking responsibility for one's actions" (Acker 1993, 193). This erosion of human responsibility leads to a reduced sense of culpability for social inequities and institutional oppression that cause, or at least contribute to, addiction, while the remedy simultaneously is affixed "at the level of individual intervention" (Frans 1994, 77). According to this critique, then, the overall effect of the disease concept is a depoliticization of addiction (Frans 1994; Bepko 1991).

Morrison's skepticism about the disease concept is short lived, however. A few weeks into her treatment program, she describes listening to a lecture on the disease concept. Morrison recounts with epiphanic zeal the moment she comprehends addiction as a disease:

> The first time I heard Dr. Doug Talbott give the "disease concept" lecture, I was in shock. This man might as well have been telling my life story—the pro-

gression of the illness, the loss of control, the denial, the confusion, the paranoia, the guilt, the embarrassment, the withdrawal, and the terrible loneliness. He had answers to some of the "whys' that I had never understood, like why I continued to take drugs despite the horrendous consequences. (184)

When "disease" is manifest in behaviours and emotions, and when it becomes the impetus of a narrative, a "life story" with which she can identify, as it does here, Morrison accepts the disease concept of addiction as a valid scientific explanation for her seventeen-year polydrug addiction. She also experiences liberation from the painful and puzzling thoughts and emotions she associates with her addiction.[9]

Morrison's socio-economic status facilitates this enthusiastic embrace of the disease concept. Insisting on the normality of her background, Morrison suggests that her class necessarily precludes addiction. When she finally recognizes herself as a drug addict, the disease concept allows her to retain the bourgeois privilege of invisibility and to maintain a socially acceptable role as a "sick" person. Following the introductory chapter with an excerpted diary entry which depicts Morrison injecting herself with seventy-five milligrams of pure methamphetamine hydrochloride (1), Morrison describes her familial and class background. Born and raised in Fayetteville, Arkansas, "a small, relatively quiet town" (8), she recalls a childhood full of "material comforts" and a "stable, happy" and conflict-free family life (9). She describes her family as "fairly well off," "middle-class ... staunch southern Baptists" (9). Although her adolescence coincides with "the psychedelic sixties" and rejection of "all the values and morals [she] had been raised to cherish" (18), Morrison, as is expected of her and as she desires, proceeds to college and, eventually, to medical school, where she becomes a self-described "hot-shot resident" (109) as well as a wife. Because Morrison's white, middle-class, small-town background, secure family life, and academic achievements stand in contradistinction to cultural expectations of "the drug addict," they allow Morrison to cultivate a severe drug addiction without being a suspected and stigmatized addict. Morrison's adherence to normative assumptions about class and addiction likewise prevent her from imagining her drug use as problematic. Analyzing the introductory diary excerpt that portrays her injecting methamphetamine, Morrison writes,

> Clearly, at the time I wrote this account, I had no idea whatsoever that I was an addict. Despite an extremely troubled history with drugs, despite my training as a physician, the fact that I was addicted eluded me completely. How could I be a junkie? I had been an exceptional student and was now an award-winning medical resident. I lived in a nice house, had a respectable husband

and a reasonably happy family life. I had my shit together. Moreover, I was a star in my particular stratosphere. (6–7)

The relation Morrison constructs here between her class identity and her addiction presumes the inadequacy of socio-economic explanations of addiction. Unlike the majority of American female drug addicts, Morrison cannot cite poverty, an abusive family environment, childhood trauma, or lack of access to education as the causes of stresses that lead to addictive drug use (McCaul and Svikis 1999, 432). Without this socio-economic narrative of causation, Morrison turns to a narrative of causation that conceptualizes addiction as a result of inherited, uncontrollable internal conditions, and conceptualizes the addict as a blameless and socially acceptable victim of these conditions.

While Morrison is quick to establish her class and familial background as "terribly normal" (17), she is just as quick to identify characteristics of her gender as unusual. She describes herself as "something of a tomboy … tough and athletic … I always played to win" (10) and "learned early on that I could manipulate men" (16). As characteristics of her childhood gender identity alone, these traits are not particularly remarkable. They resonate later, however, during Morrison's stay at Ridgeview when she is derided for being competitive, manipulative, tough, and outspoken. Part of her supposed predilection for addiction, these gendered characteristics must be neutralized in order for her to recover. With these violations of female gender roles as provocation, a male counselor informs Morrison of her proper position and cultural offense: "you're powerless, and you have no control … I'm going to clean out your mouth, make a lady out of you" (197). When Morrison recollects "always [being] one of the boys" (11) at the beginning of the book, then, it is with a sense of diagnosis. Like other early behaviour and emotions, violations of gender norms seem to signal an underlying illness.

Nonetheless, until her counselor promises to "make a lady out of" her, Morrison does not consider her gender identity problematic, and successful recovery is signaled by her pledge to be a loving wife to Dr. Talbott's son (243). Morrison recovers this femininity, however, only after she has been "clean" for months. In the early stages of her treatment program, she recognizes herself as an addict by identifying with the men, "old hippie, street-shooting dope fiends who rode up on their fat hog motorcycles … hard-core guys" (176), at Narcotics Anonymous meetings.

Upon entering twelve-step meetings, Morrison also reconceptualizes the relationship between her class identity and her addiction. She describes herself as a "street junkie" and recalls feeling uncomfortable "around all these doctors, with their uppity professional bullshit" (175). "I fit in better," she writes, "with the degenerates ... I'd been forging scripts, ripping off drugstores, and firing up dope for eight years before I entered medical school ... I was a bottom-line street junkie" (175). These moments in which Morrison employs stereotypes of the addict to conceptualize her own addict identity do not only illustrate the persistence of gendered and classist narratives of addiction. Morrison's white bourgeois privilege also allows her to take up this rhetoric, to take on the identity of "street junkie," and to identify with minority culture while still enjoying the privilege of invisibility and the possibility of recovery. She has recourse, after all, to the disease concept as the "real" explanation of her addiction.

White Rabbit ends conventionally with Morrison marrying Dr. Talbott's son and returning to work, this time as an addiction treatment specialist. Morrison's successful recovery, then, is signaled by heteronormative romance and the attainment of white middle-class notions of productivity and expertise, narratives that both shape and are facilitated by the disease concept of addiction. As a white, middle-class addict seeking treatment in the early 1980s, Morrison falls under the newly sheltering effects of the disease model. Encouraged to hold the disease responsible for her addiction as part of the "new" population of drug addicts, she is able to construct her social identity as a "sick" person, and, as such, recovery reassures the renewal and maintenance of her class privilege and heteronormativity.

Acknowledgements

Research for this paper was supported by a Social Sciences and Humanities Research Council of Canada Doctoral Fellowship. I would also like to acknowledge the Sarah Nettie Christie Travel Bursary at the University of Alberta, which enabled me to travel to UBC to present a version of this paper at the 2002 "Narratives of Disease, Disability, and Trauma" conference. And, for their helpful comments on earlier versions of this paper, I would like to thank Daphne Read, Julie Rak, Melisa Brittain, and Marino Eliopoulos.

Notes

1 For a comprehensive history of American domestic and foreign drug policy, see David F. Musto's *The American Disease: Origins of Narcotic Control* (1999).
2 The belief that drug addicts threatened the nation is, of course, wrapped up in a complex set of ideologies and historical circumstances that cannot be addressed in the space of this essay. I will say, however, that addiction historically has been associated with the

intersection and interarticulation of a range of differences, including class, ethnicity, race, gender, and sexuality, which always circulate in the discourse of the nation (Friedling 2000, 6). Many cultural historians have examined how these differences function in the rhetoric of drugs and in US drug policy. See, for example, Thomas Szasz, *Ceremonial Chemistry* (1974); David Courtwright, *Dark Paradise* (1982); Stephen Kandall, *Substance and Shadow* (1996); and Jill Jonnes, *Hep-Cats, Narcs, and Pipe Dreams* (1996).

3 For a detailed account of the Harrison Anti-Narcotic Act of 1914, refer to David Musto's *The American Disease*, specifically chapter 3, "The Harrison Act." Stephen Kandall also provides a chapter on the Act in *Substance and Shadow*: see, chapter 4, "The Harrison Anti-Narcotic Act," which focuses on the implications of the Act for female addicts.

4 Kolb's most influential research, conducted during the 1920s and '30s, was reprinted in his 1962 book *Drug Addiction: A Medical Problem*. Kolb's influence on psychiatry's conceptualization and treatment of drug addiction is still felt. Leon Wursmer, for example, cites Kolb heavily in *The Hidden Dimension*, Kolb's own influential psychiatric study of what he calls compulsive drug use.

5 Lexington was notoriously ineffective as an addiction treatment facility. Living conditions were oppressive and substandard. For a first-hand account of life at Lexington, see Janet Clark's *The Fantastic Lodge* (1961).

6 Drug use in the 1960s is well-traversed territory. While it is beyond the scope of this essay to provide a history of this period, I will note that, as in the beginning of the twentieth century, America experienced massive socio-economic and political changes during this time, which included unprecedented economic growth and the looming threat of nuclear destruction. For thorough accounts of America's socio-political conditions and their relations to drug use during the 1960s, see Musto (1999), Kandall (1996), and Jonnes (1996).

7 For an insightful discussion of the expansion of the concept of addiction, see Eve Sedgwick's "Epidemics of the Will" (1993). Sedgwick analyzes what she calls the "epidemic of addiction attribution" (131)—the recent phenomenon in which all human behaviours and emotions have come to be understood as potentially addictive.

8 On their website, Narcotics Anonymous addresses the question "Is addiction a disease?" with this response: "We treat Addiction [sic] as a disease because that makes sense to us and it works. We have no need to press the issue any farther than that" <www.na.org/bull17-r.htm>.

9 I do not mean to underestimate the value of relieving the guilt many women experience as drug addicts. As violators of powerful constructs in their roles as nurturers and guardians of morality, female addicts, including Morrison, express tremendous guilt and shame, and I think it is important to alleviate these often debilitating emotions. I am not convinced, however, that reconceptualizing oneself as "sick" is the best means to assuage these emotions. I would rather that women be given the tools to consider the impact of these oppressive gender roles in their emotional responses to their addictions.

J. DANIEL SCHUBERT

Temporal Assumptions
Aging with Cystic Fibrosis

> *Just as lived spatiality is characterized by an outward directedness, a purposiveness and intention, so time is experienced not as a static present but as a moving toward the future.*
> —S. Kay Toombs, *The Meaning of Illness* (1992, 68)

> We went to the ... orthodontist and he did a history and he said yeah, you definitely could do with braces. But why? You've got this, this CF, and I really think you are wasting your money. Why don't you hold on to that precious fund for your parents. It's like $3,000 and that would be better capital ... for burial expenses than it would be for getting your ... teeth straightened.
> —Lori, a thirty-six-year-old person living with CF, describing an event that occurred at about age eighteen.

In his description of the ethical potential of illness narratives, Arthur Frank (1995, 55) suggests that "the conventional expectation of any narrative, held alike by listeners and storytellers, is for a past that leads into a present that sets in place a foreseeable future." Among the many problems associated with chronic illnesses, then, and especially with life-threatening chronic illnesses, is that they threaten the ill person's temporality and their future directedness. Until recently, this has resulted in the silencing of those who experience such illnesses. The emergence and increasing legitimacy of the illness narrative, however, has begun to rectify this problem. Illness narratives have gone a long way toward providing a way for the ill to articulate what it means to be alive after the onset of chronic and life-threatening illness.

Narratives construct or reconstruct realities in particular ways (Bruner 2002; Lyotard 1984). Stories make worlds, and in doing so, they legitimate ways of storytelling and ways of being. However, any given story leaves out as much, perhaps, as it includes, and, in this essay, I will examine what the temporal structures of illness narratives leave out. I do so by asking a simple question: if a temporal dimension is implicit in all narrative, and if the self is a discursive category constituted through narrative, what does it mean to live one's entire life—and not just the life that takes place after the onset of chronic illness—at the edge of life expectancy? What is life like for those who have never had a foreseeable future, or at least not the kind of future outlined by contemporary life-course studies that describe the transitions that exist between childhood, adolescence, adulthood, and old-age?[1] There is a unique cohort of people alive today who can address this question: for the first time in history, there are significant numbers of adults living with cystic fibrosis (CF). Until very recently, CF has been a childhood disease. However, improvements in diagnosis and treatment over the last half century have increased life expectancy from less than two years to more than thirty-two years. What this means is that CF is no longer just a childhood disease. What it also means is that those adults living with CF have lived their entire lives near, at, or even a few years beyond their assumed life expectancy. This differs from the general population of industrialized nations, where it is the elderly who are living near life expectancy. For the most part, unless they are victims of accidents, suicides, or homicides, people in wealthy countries get old before they die (Nuland 1993), but those with CF are too young to be old. Those with the disease who die as adults die young in comparison to those without CF. Even with the dramatic improvements in the treatment of CF that have emerged in recent years, life expectancy is still less than half that of the general population. On the other hand, in the CF population until recently, just about everybody was young. Very few people with the disease lived to see adulthood, and most died while they were children or adolescents. Now, adults with CF are too old to die young.[2]

There is, of course, a vast literature of chronic illness that addresses end-of-life issues. However, as already suggested, most writers in the field focus attention on those for whom chronic illness arrives relatively late in life. Chronic illness for these people is, as Kathy Charmaz and many others have suggested, an interruption in what is otherwise a relatively non-ill life. Charmaz spends much of her book *Good Days, Bad Days: The Self in Chronic Illness and Time* (1991) describing the metaphors that give meaning to those whose lives are interrupted by illness. In addition to the interruption metaphor, in which becoming ill is understood in relation to having been not ill, Charmaz identifies the intrusion metaphor—where illness is like the relative who comes to visit for a few days and ends up moving in forever—and the metaphor of immersion, where individuals with chronic illness come to see more and more of their lives through the lens of their illness.[3]

While most of the literature on chronic illness and pain resembles that of Charmaz in its focus on the ways in which illness and pain interrupt the lives of the healthy and pain-free, many of those born with CF experience illness not as an interruption but rather as the only way of life they have ever known. I do oral history interviewing to try to understand what life is like for these adults. One of my narrators, David, a thirty-two-year old male, says of knowing only CF:[4]

> Of course, if you are born with something, you ... don't know it's ... different from what other people have ... it is not that you assume that other people have it, you just don't think in those terms. I probably didn't fully realize that ... something was different with me having CF until probably ... elementary school.[5]

If Arthur Frank (1995, 56) is correct that illness is a "crisis of self," then those with CF have led their entire lives not only with a time-, energy-, and life-consuming disease, but with a self that knows crisis before it knows normalcy. Or better, a self that knows crisis *as* normalcy. This requires, as Myra Bluebond-Langner (1996) suggests, a redefinition of normalcy. Frequent hospitalizations, daily therapy regimens, the ingestion of digestion-aiding enzymes prior to each meal or snack, and the threat of early death are not part of the normal routine for most people. Bluebond-Langner details the great length to which families of children with CF go to normalize their lives.

Living one's entire life at or near life expectancy also requires a rethinking of the temporal assumptions of illness narratives. Certainly this cohort of people with cystic fibrosis has not lived time in the ways that most "normals" do. Beyond that, however, adults with CF have lived time differently than even most "normal" ill people. Many have lived their entire lives in what Arthur Kleinman (1988) calls the "sheer exigencies of their problems" with chronic illness. This suggests that those with CF have a completely different relationship to time.

Contemporary illness precipitates a fall from timelessness into time, suggests David Morris (1998). Morris, however, follows Charmaz in the assumption that illness interrupts a non-ill life. Thus he must speak of a "fall" into time. Prior to the intruder that is chronic illness, the non-ill live a timeless existence. The onset of illness brings an awareness of, or a falling into, time. To be born with a life-threatening chronic illness, however, means that those with CF have always lived time. Indeed, rather than falling, they were born into it.

Cystic Fibrosis: The Disease Narrative

Readers need to know something about a disease in order to understand what it is like to live with an illness, so illness narratives invariably include a disease narrative. This account of the lives of adults with CF is no different. Cystic fibrosis is a genetic disease that affects approximately thirty thousand people in the United States and almost ten thousand people in Canada. Though CF is found in all populations, the disease occurs most frequently in Caucasians, being present in about one in every three thousand births. Most people with the disease receive their diagnosis during childhood or adolescence, although increasing numbers of CF patients are now receiving first diagnoses of the disease as adults (Widerman et al. 2000). CF affects a variety of organs, the lungs and pancreas most severely. The CF gene was identified in 1989, and the mutations that occur in this gene lead to the defective production of a salt-regulating protein in the body's cells. As a result, chloride ions and water cannot flow properly through cell membranes, leading to the production of thick, sticky mucus. The most threatening consequences of this are difficulties breathing because of effects on the pulmonary system and, for about 90 per cent of those with CF, difficulty in digestion because of effects on the pancreas (Solvay Pharmaceuticals 1997).

Respiratory symptoms—which have best been described to me by my narrators as trying to breathe through a straw or trying to breathe with a hand over one's mouth while walking up two or three flights of stairs— include decreased pulmonary function, coughing, production of thick sputum, congestion, and shortness of breath. Mucus build-up makes oxygenation of the blood problematic, placing extra strain on the heart and other organs. Those with CF tend to experience cycles of infection and inflammation of increasing frequency and severity, due to the inability to clear mucus, and the scarring of the lungs themselves. Most CF fatalities ultimately result from these opportunistic infections (Solvay Pharmaceuticals 1997).

Pulmonary function usually decreases over time, so that many adults living with CF require full- or part-time supplemental oxygen. Lori, a thirty-six-year-old narrator with joint Canadian-American citizenship who is the author of the second epigraph in this paper, has used portable oxygen tanks with increasing regularity for almost twenty years. She offers an example of the way this encroaches on her life today:

> If I go into a shopping mall and I see someone sixty-five sitting on a park bench there sucking two liters,... I expect that because they're sixty-five, they're seventy. They're old ... When I'm walking in a mall ... I am so self-conscious that I'm half their age and I'm doing the same thing and ... the stares come. Everyone wants to know, "You're young, you're a young girl, what you got that stuff up your nose for?"

Fifty years ago, life expectancy for those with cystic fibrosis was less than two years. With improvements in diagnosis, therapies, nutrition, and medications, life expectancy has risen to slightly more than thirty-two years (Hopkin 1998). In many ways, these dramatic improvements in the treatment of cystic fibrosis *as a disease* mean that the current cohort of adults with CF will experience it *as an illness* in ways that are very different from those of the generations that came before them and those that will come after.[6] Obviously, most of those who came before them did not experience adulthood, but those who are younger today also experience CF differently. In my own interviews with other adults with CF, for example, I have found that even those who are only ten years younger than David and Lori, my oldest narrators, perceive their illness very differently. They have grown up in the era of increased life expectancy and excitement about the discovery of the CF gene, and with an increased hope that a cure will be found.[7] Today it is expected that children with CF will live to adulthood, though that is not always the case. Today's adults with CF grew up in a world where that rarely happened.

THE EMBODIMENT OF TIME

In this essay I focus on the ways in which this disease affects the experience of time for those who have survived into adulthood, and how it does so in ways that are different from those identified by Charmaz. I suggest that time is experienced and has unique meaning in at least two different ways, the combination of which results in the creation of a kind of perpetual present without a non-ill past for those with CF. The first way in which time is experienced—and the one to which I've already referred—is in terms of the absence of a long-term future. Many adults living with CF have lived lives without anticipated futures. Lori, the thirty-six-year-old with dual citizenship, began a number of her descriptions of her future plans with her husband with the unprompted phrase "We're hoping that if I can live to age forty," as in "We're hoping that if I can live to forty" we can do this, or "We're hoping that if I can live to forty" we can do that.[8]

It isn't that Lori and others her age necessarily came into consciousness with the expectation of an early death, but rather that they became conscious in and through the experience of illness. While this may not have meant an early death to them intitially, their parents and family members who understood the disease didn't expect them to live long. In *In the Shadow of Illness* (1996), her account of the experiences of parents and siblings of children with CF, Myra Bluebond-Langner describes the ways in which parents experience the disease. Representative of these accounts is that of a Mrs. Reynolds, who, when asked about what it is like to have a child with the disease, says, "I guess my first thoughts are that it is fatal. It's always uppermost in my mind" (1996, 70). According to Bluebond-Langner, parents sometimes experience guilt at having "given" their child a genetic disease, and anger at the prospect of outliving that same child.

The ways in which this would inform child-rearing are surely complex and diverse. Not only are those with CF "born into time," but their caretakers join them in that temporality. My narrators identify a number of resulting behaviours that range from the decision by parents not to have other children, to the "spoiling" of the child with CF by giving lavish gifts and taking frequent vacations, to avoiding discussions of the future and the making of plans for the future (for either the child or the family). From a number of the narrators, I got the sense that perhaps there were some more subtle effects as well.

Of course, it isn't only parents who communicate the lack of a long-term future. Lori tells of friends' parents who didn't want their children to get "too close" to Lori, and she offers the particularly gruesome account of an experience with an orthodontist that is included as an epigraph in this paper. I suspect that her orthodontist's suggestion to spend her money on her funeral rather than on her braces was offered with the best of intentions.

The second way in which adults with CF live a perpetual present is in their experience of the daily and the short-term. In terms of the daily, many adults with CF live one day at a time (Charmaz 1991, 178).[9] Mike, a twenty-seven-year-old male, does at least four hours of physical therapy per day, every day, even when he is at his healthiest. He must begin each morning with a half hour of chest percussion and end each night with another half-hour session. When especially ill but not hospitalized, he does one- or two-week home IV sequences that last from eight to twelve hours per day. The small, one-bedroom apartment that he shares with his wife is overflowing with the accoutrements of physical and drug therapies.

Lori was interviewed in her room during one of her quarter-annual two-week visits to the hospital, or, as she sarcastically calls it, "the club," which she spends away from her husband and her job. Her days consist of waiting. The rhythm of her time is structured by the forced routines of antibiotic and therapy schedules, and by the "shifts" that regulate nursing and staffing changes (Zerubavel 1979). For Lori, as for Mike, days take forever.

It isn't only days that last forever, however. Short-term projects often do as well, which seems especially cruel for people for whom forever is likely not to last too long. In addition to his daily struggle for survival, Mike also exists from day to day, meaning that he lives with "continued crises that rip life apart" (Charmaz 1991, 185). For example, he was to graduate from a two-year community college the month after we spoke. What is particularly significant about this is that he had matriculated eight years before. Being ill had limited the number of courses he could take per semester, and periods of severe illness and hospitalization had forced him to take frequent incompletes or withdrawals in many of the courses for which he was registered. He simply missed too many days of class to complete a number of those courses. When I asked him if he planned to continue with his education now that he was about to get his associate's degree, there was a long pause before he could tell me no. Though he understood the employment benefits such a credential might provide, he had decided against more schooling. In a passage that shows the convergence of the perpetual short-term and the absence of the long term, he said that:

> Barring a miracle of much-improved CF health ... I won't be able to put the degree to any use. So I'd much rather avoid the stress and just do some computer consulting and make extra money.

Cystic Fibrosis and the Illness Narrative

In conclusion, I return to the notion of the illness narrative. The point of departure for most illness narratives is that illness has somehow disrupted or interrupted or interfered with a perceived future. For adults living with cystic fibrosis, that temporal structure does not work. They have not had a future interrupted by an illness, they have had an illness interrupted—or maybe just extended—by a future. Indeed, the epigraph on the webpage of the Cystic Fibrosis Foundation in the United States is "adding tomorrows everyday." Although these tomorrows are being added faster than ever before, they are for the most part being added one day at a time. If, as Arthur Frank (1995, 55) says, the conventional narrative includes a "past that leads into a present that sets in place a foreseeable future," then adults living with CF certainly do not tell a conventional narrative. Most do not have a foreseeable future today—and they never have. The typical structure of the illness narrative has excluded the experiences of those who have diseases such as cystic fibrosis.

In closing, then, I offer a reflexive use of CF stories to critique narratives in general, and illness narratives in particular. In the spirit of Nancy Mairs (1996), who uses her experiences living "waist-high in the world" to critique the exclusionary aspects of the built spatial environment, I suggest that the stories of adults living with cystic fibrosis can be used to critique the built environments of time, narrative, and, most importantly to us, the illness narrative.

Notes

1. See, for example, Sarah Irwin (2001), as well as the other essays included in Mark Priestley (2001). While it is important to address the specific ways in which the ill and the disabled experience these "stages" of the life course, there has been a tendency in life-course studies to adopt uncritically categories of age that are culturally specific.
2. To illustrate the dilemma that is being old with CF, consider that CF clinics located in hospitals have, until very recently, been housed exclusively in pediatric units. It is only in the last five or ten years that adult clinics have been created. In addition to physical issues related to CF, many of these clinics also address the psychosocial aspects of being an adult with a life-threatening chronic illness. These issues include such things as sexuality, education and employment, and disability and insurance. On these issues, see Bluebond-Langner et al. (2001).
3. For a review that tends to reify the metaphor of intrusion usually found in illness narratives, see Faith McLellan (1994). A slightly different take on the metaphor of immersion is offered by Anatole Broyard (1992), who speaks instead of intoxication.
4. The use of the term narrator, rather than more familiar terms such as subject or interviewee, to identify those who participated in this study is consistent with practice within oral history. Oral historians use the term to acknowledge that the story being told is the participant's rather than the researcher's. This political move is particularly relevant for those doing illness studies precisely because one of the things we have been trying to overcome is the silencing of those who suffer. Additionally, I use the term here to acknowledge and reciprocate the generosity (Frank 2004) of those who told me their stories.
5. Tapes and transcripts of this and all other interviews are deposited in the Community Studies Center at Dickinson College in Carlisle, Pennsylvania. Interviews were completed in compliance with The Oral History Association's *Evaluation Guidelines*.

6 Following Arthur Frank (1995, 187n2), I recognize the problematic nature of this distinction between disease and illness: "The illness experience is in and of a diseased body."
7 Even these younger adults, however, have become less optimistic over time that the discovery of a "cure" for the disease will come in their own lifetimes. Many journalistic accounts of this optimistic generation are now available.
8 For an account of Lori's life that identifies ways in which it is or is not representative of the lives of most people with CF, see Daniel Schubert and Margaret Murphy (2005).
9 While Charmaz (1991) does describe the experience of both the daily and the short term, she does so by contrasting these experiences to the ways in which they were lived prior to chronic illness. Most of those with CF have no such prior experience.

JAMES OVERBOE

ABLEIST LIMITS ON SELF-NARRATION
The Concept of Post-personhood

A few years ago, members of the Intradisciplinary Inquiry into Narratives of Disease, Disability and Trauma project at UBC were asked what narratives of disease, disability, and trauma meant to them. For me, diseased, disabled, and traumatized people are trapped in a glass prison. As we attempt to escape this prison we are recaptured by medical practitioners who shoot us down as we try to go over the wall, and with the greatest of care would patch us up, giving us a prescriptive prognosis that will be the benchmark for our recovery. On the other hand, social scientists lasso us around the neck (effectively silencing us), pull us down to the floor, and, under the auspices of giving us "voice," interpret our stories and, consequently, our lives. Literary theorists cage us, and we become spectacles for them to analyze as they turn our lives into tropes and metaphors of what may go wrong for a fragile humanity. For the most part, the diseased, the disabled, or the traumatized are expected to undergo some form of rehabilitation in order to achieve normality. If normality cannot be achieved, then they must "make sense" of their lives in order to find underlying "meaning" for, or purpose to, their tragic existence.

I have come to the conclusion that the problem is humanism,[1] with its continuum of "pre-person" (allowing for the justification of the eradication of people perceived to be potentially less than human), "less than human" (justifying the public sympathy and support for Robert Latimer, who killed his disabled daughter, Tracy), and the "human" (including disabled people who are seen as "overcoming" their disabilities). The final stage on the continuum is "post-person," which could include myself: the vulnerable who currently are able to be productive but at any time may be deemed as having lives not worth living, so that through some misguided benevolence, others may feel it is charitable to kill us. This paper concerns itself with the concept of post-personhood.

The Compassionate Killing of Post-persons

During the past two years I have attended two academic conferences on narrative where the subject of post-personhood has been discussed. Within the context of narrative, the state of post-personhood comes about when circumstances of disease, disability, or trauma are perceived to rob an individual of his or her personhood. If people are perceived as lacking personhood, then the ethical debate about their "quality of life" begins. The notion of post-personhood frames the debate in a way that presupposes that those people labelled "post-persons" may merely exist and are not fully human. Robert Bogdan and Steven Taylor (1988, 146) conclude that whether disabled people are considered human is dependent upon their interaction with the Other. If the Other accepts the severely disabled person as human, communication is achieved. If the Other assumes that the severely disabled are less than human, then communication is impossible. In either situation, one cannot definitively prove that their perception is flawed because of a faulty belief system.

As a person who experiences dementia, and is often considered a post-person, Gloria Sterin (2002, 8) has identified three reactions. These reactions are "the process of becoming invisible," "the gesture of dismissal," and "the act of smothering"; all are variations on the same theme. Sterin explains,

> Now, nobody wants to be rude; nobody wants to be mean or unkind; but neither do they want to be uncomfortable. I think that's the key word. They are just acutely uncomfortable with you and do not want to deal with that discomfort.
>
> I've seen withdrawal on the part of many people, many old friends who just couldn't handle this disease comfortably, and shied away from contact as much as possible. They are being made very uncomfortable ... For they don't know how to deal with somebody who is not "fully human." So how do you treat such a person? You try not to see them; you avoid them as much you can; or treat them as if they are not there, as if they are invisible.
>
> Let me give you an example, you are sitting in a room and people talk to each other, but they tiptoe around you. When you look at someone, that person looks away from you, and talks to the next person. People simply stop

talking to you in the way that they used to. You are in a different category from the normal population. There's a discomfort and you can almost sense the reason is not that they're angry or upset ... they are just uncomfortable. (8)

At times Sterin has tried to barge in on the conversation; in response, the person answers her very briefly and then turns to another person and engages them. If she addresses a person by name, they will respond to her and listen to what she has to say, but they will not engage her in conversation. She explains,

> Nobody wants to be impolite. But you're not engaged in the process; and that's what makes a person human.... the process. In any other circumstances, for example, if you said, "I broke my leg, it's hard for me to get around," people will be sympathetic and engage you in conversation and say, "How do you manage?" Or "that's too bad, is it going to take long to heal?" And that's within the realm of normal conversation. However, if you say you have Alzheimer's, if you have dementia, it's the kiss of death ... it's that word "dementia." (8)

For Sterin, the second reaction is "the gesture of dismissal" (8–9), which is a series of facial expressions and gestures that devalue her existence. She explains that it is surprising and yet sad to recognize the same gesture and the same tone of voice from different caregivers who otherwise have varied characteristics. Again, Sterin reiterates that there is no malicious intent involved in these interactions. The third reaction is "the act of smothering," where disabled people have no chance to be themselves because their personhood is being suffocated by kindness.

Being "suffocated by kindness," "dismissed by facial expression," or "rendered invisible" are all ways in which those affected see members of society deal with dementia; however, as Sterin points out, these strategies are not working. In Sterin's intersubjective relationship with nondisabled people, the latter are imposing their own subjectivity as the measure of effective communication. As Sterin so eloquently illustrates, it is not the person experiencing post-personhood that has the failure to communicate. It is the "uncomfortableness" of the privileged persons, not the abject other, that causes communication to break down between persons and post-persons. Consequently, what is required is the political will for a paradigm shift that begins to see post-persons as persons who communicate differently.

I make a similar point in my analysis of Jean-Dominique Bauby's autobiography, *The Diving Bell and the Butterfly*, which explores his life with Locked-In Syndrome (LIS):

> The diving-bell for me, does not represent Bauby's imprisonment by LIS but rather the oppressive practices of those who privilege an able-bodied embodiment. They see the problems of the lack of communication, of lesser embodiment and absence of selfhood, as residing with Bauby as a result of LIS. In contrast, I see the problem as lying in such readers' inability to understand his attempts at communication, their failure to appreciate his embodiment, and finally the refusal to recognize his selfhood. (Raoul et al. 2001, 193)

When I have tried to advocate for the personhood of supposedly "inarticulate" post-persons and have invoked my own experience of pre-personhood (having been labelled "retarded" as a baby), I have been criticized as moving beyond my pre-person experience, and by doing so invalidating both my experience and my subsequent opinion. Yet this criticism rests upon the belief that humanity and disability belong on a trajectory, a position that I feel is ableist because it reiterates the belief in both pre-personhood and post-personhood as less-than-human bookends for both the categories of disability and humanism.

Lorraine Code believes that a "rhetorical space" must be developed in order for certain topics to become a matter of public discussion (1995, xvii). Some might argue that this is exactly what discussions about post-personhood attempt to do—open up a rhetorical space for discussion about the lives of people with disabilities. In these discussions I am aware of the privileging of language. For example, literary theorists and social scientists who work in the area of narrative have a great affinity for both the spoken and the written word. I contend that this reification of language, if I dare describe it as such, feeds into their own fears of losing their cherished ability to speak and write, and this skews their ability to make judgements on post-personhood.

Language is political because the forming of grammatically correct sentences is, for the normal individual, the prerequisite for any submission to social laws. If one cannot do so, or is ignorant of grammaticality, one belongs in a special institution. This dominant language or pattern of communication is in itself a strategic site of normality. It paints normality with broad strokes or, under the guise of diversity, it may allow for variations within a range of normality, but it nevertheless rejects any sense of communication that is deemed abnormal. Thus, post-persons who cannot express themselves in either the dominant language or communication style (Deleuze and Guattari 1987, 101; Colebrook 1999, 117) may be eradicated for their own "good."

Discussing conditions under which post-persons exist assumes that the "thing"—that is, post-personhood—exists. Perhaps one might protest that literary theorists and social scientists are only discussing the issue. However, their position as intellectual interpreters (Bauman 1993) gives credence or validity to the concept of post-personhood. At the conferences I attended, the primary focus was on characteristics that signify a state of post-personhood. Given that most people have a greater fear of disability than of death, I argue that the prior assumption that there is some form of "post-personhood" is problematic in itself. Unfortunately, the question of whether the concept of post-personhood reflects an ableist position is rarely considered by scholars who come from a position that privileges an ablebodied perspective.

Often I have found that the seductive sweetness of the potions of compassion, care, and love masks their insidious poison, which robs the disabled, the sick, and the traumatized of their vitality. In his discussion of agape love, Zygmunt Bauman argues that "stooping to" the weak by the self-confident strong is in the end the birth-act of domination and hierarchy: the re-forging of difference into inferiority (1993, 97). From the beginning, Bauman argues, this form of love is contaminated by patronizing and condescending behaviour that is masked by benevolence (97). The re-forging of the cripples, the mad, the diseased, and the traumatized as inferior is based on the belief that they must be recast with care into at least adequate facsimiles of humanity in order to be accepted into the realm of personhood. In extreme cases, as in the case of post-persons, this love, this compassion, manifests itself in their eradication in the name of benefice.

The executioners of the proclamation of post-personhood may have heavy hearts, but they are soothed by the balm that they did all that was humanly possible, and therein lies the problem. Perhaps we have to look beyond our taken-for-granted humanness to see the person within the post-person (as the quotes from Gloria Sterin illuminate). Perhaps we have to step out from behind the empty terms of love and compassion that mask our fear that we too may be closer to post-personhood than we thought. As long as we are able to label others as post-persons, however, we can whisper to each other and to ourselves that, at least for now, we remain human. The encroachment of post-personhood upon our lives is held at bay by the eradication of this loved one (even if this loved one is you, a self-sacrifice for the common good), the constant reminder is gone, and, perhaps over time, even the memories (yours, or those of your loved ones) of post-personhood can be supplanted by the memories of when you or your loved ones were human.

The act of abjecting allows one to make sense of something or someone that is paradoxically meaningless yet disturbing (Kristeva, 1982).

Judith Butler asserts that the strategy of social abjection produces the "*un*symbolizable, the unspeakable, the illegible" (1993, 190). The construction of the human through regulatory and normative practices produces the less than human, the human, and the humanly unthinkable (8). People defined as post-persons are produced as the ultimate "abject other"—the "unsymbolizable, the unspeakable, the illegible," whose lives are "paradoxically meaningless yet disturbing." They may be "humanly unthinkable," but the invocation of "living wills" is the result of the active imagination of people who see the spectre of post-personhood in their future—a life not worth living, a meaningless life, a burden for others—that fuels their belief that they must banish themselves to the realm of death if faced with post-personhood. Or, it is the active memory of a caregiver who can relate to the vibrant person, to the paradoxically distant but ever-present past that haunts the present relationship, in such a way that the caregiver tries to make sense of the inarticulate person's lived experience, but only in terms of what they lack. Whether looking to the future or dealing with a present tinged with a longing for the past, this state of post-personhood is disturbing. In a "compassionate killing," we eradicate the disturbance and restore the person's vitality in memory. We restore order and our faith in humanity, but can we ever be sure that a compassionate killing is better than a "life not worth living?" Unfortunately the dead are silent on this issue.

Death is always interpreted by the living. Zygmunt Bauman writes, "Death means that nothing will happen any more. No miracles, no surprises—no disappointments either" (1993, 100). The death of a loved one is the safety of the lover. They are free without a single "but" to paint the portrait of the dead. With their own palette and their own brushes, they will be able to paint not only the portrait of the dead but also the act of dying, and, perhaps most importantly, they can reinterpret the life of the dead. What comes under their brushes is a death mask that remains forever.

My active imagination has its own fear of the future. I see myself as having LIS and my caregivers believing that I am unable to communicate (none of them have read Bauby's book or the article by Raoul et al.). They believe that my suffering from cerebral palsy has caused me to be shackled with this useless body, and now LIS has robbed me of my mind. After careful consideration, they decide that I have lost the last vestige of my humanity, along with my personhood, and that my life is not worth living. They proclaim, "He has endured enough," and compassionately kill me. These people have no idea that I have returned to a place that I enjoy and knew when I was a pre-person. A place without language, without metaphor, without a need to give my life meaning or purpose. A place where my spasms, my sensations, ran freely without restrictions. As I write this I realize that, perhaps ironically, I am speaking of a place, a state of consciousness, that human beings try to achieve for themselves. Is this state of pre-personhood not similar to a state of meditation? If I am right in my belief that the state of pre-personhood and post-personhood are similar experiences, then might not a state of post-personhood be a meditative experience too? Unfortunately, if we "compassionately kill" post-persons they will be silent on this issue, too.

Having been told many times throughout my life that "my life was not worth living," I am very cautious in making that diagnosis for either myself or others. So pervasive is humanism and ableism that I must be vigilant not to secure my ranking on the scale of humanity by internalizing the belief that some other "gimp" or "crip" is a lesser life form than me. Some other scholars of narrative are becoming aware of the inherent abjection/ableism which they must guard against. The writers of the article "Narrating the Unspeakable" say,

> Literary experts, just like medical specialists, can treat a person/text as a "case" to be dissected and analyzed and, in the process, eliminate the life in the person, denying his or her right to consideration as a unique individual rather than simply as a representative of something "bigger." Similarly, attempts to impose "meaning" on a life and admiration for those who succeed in doing so in difficult circumstances can devalue the lives of those who are not able to express or develop such a coherent "message" about their experiences but nevertheless have lives that are of value. (Raoul et al. 2001, 206)

Yet, within studies of narratives of disease, disability, and trauma, the position of Valerie Raoul and her co-authors is a minority position because of the inherent ableism within the continuum of humanity. Notwithstanding, Gilles Deleuze and Félix Guattari (1994) assert that writers make slits in the canopy of the status quo and allow for fresh air to breathe life into a discipline. On the other hand, commentators maintain the status quo by patching the canopy with clichés and received opinion—a rhetoric that envelops and protects a discipline. Those writers or artists who are willing to think in different ways and with different sensibilities can bring vitality to a stagnant discipline. As Deleuze and Guattari write, "The painter does not paint on a empty canvas, and neither does the writer write on a blank page; but the page or canvas is already covered with pre-existing, pre-established clichés that it is first necessary to erase, to clean, to flatten, or even to shred, so as to let in a breath of fresh air from the chaos that brings us vision" (1994, 204).

From the chaos of being generally diseased, disabled, or traumatized, or relegated specifically to post-personhood, can come a vision that brings fresh air to narratives, but only when the cliché of restrictive humanism with its limited view of personhood and communication is erased. Of course, such an event can only be established when the glass walls are shattered and narrators are willing to question the status quo that continues to frame post-persons as well as other diseased, disabled, and traumatized people as the abject other, to be either restored to, or banished from, humanity. I invite narrators to resist the need to find meaning in "our lives," to reject the need to bring us back into the fold of humanism either by forging us into unreasonable facsimiles of humanity, or giving us "voice." Rather I would ask narrators of disease, disability, and trauma to shift the focus to themselves, and to strip themselves of this restrictive notion of personhood and limited understanding of communication, to facilitate the coming of a "greater health" beyond the normative shadow of humanism.

Note

1 For the purposes of this piece, humanism does not refer to any disciplinary definition. Humanism refers to a taken for granted state of existence or sensibility that requires no proof—normative shadows that are simultaneously nowhere but everywhere. As long as we are judged by others or ourselves as being within the accepted boundaries of humanity, these normative shadows rarely are noticed. However, if we find this sensibility of humanity is or has the potential to be compromised (as in the case of the disabled, the diseased, and the traumatized), normative shadows are constant reminders of the need to restore our humanity in order to stave off becoming the abject other. See Overboe (2004).

NARRATIVE CONCLUSIONS
An Example of Cross-disciplinary Analysis

VALERIE RAOUL, CONNIE CANAM,
GLORIA ONYEOZIRI, CARLA PATERSON

Margaret Edson's Play *Wit*
Death at the End or the End of Death?

At an early stage in our interdisciplinary inquiry into narratives of disease, disability, and trauma, several of us from different disciplines at UBC undertook a collaborative reading of an illness memoir (Jean-Dominique Bauby's *The Diving Bell and the Butterfly*, which recounts the effects of a massive stroke), using Roman Jakobson's model of the functions of communication to guide our analysis. The purpose of this collaboration was to share our respective approaches to narrative analysis, and determine how our disciplinary perspectives diverged and overlapped (Raoul et al., 2001). Subsequently, after seeing Margaret Edson's *Wit*, some of us came together again to see what a similar analysis of a play, rather than a personal memoir, might reveal about how our various disciplinary backgrounds influence our perceptions of a public representation and performance of a narrative of disease.

Wit, a dramatic fiction about a woman dying of ovarian cancer, won the 1999 Pulitzer Prize for drama, and since has played to packed houses across North America. It reached an even wider audience through the film version, directed by Mike Nichols and starring Emma Thompson. Reviewers responded with statements such as "entertainment meets ethics"; "one of the most powerful and moving plays you will ever see"; "powerful and daunting"; "it doesn't have a single boring moment,"[1] and they emphasized Edson's sophisticated use of humor and irony. How can a play about suffering and death manage to make people laugh without trivializing the situation?

In an interview in the *Vancouver Sun* (April 1, 2001), Edson claimed that, for her, "the play isn't really about health care. It just happens to take place in a health-care setting because that was something I knew something about." Could it still have had the same success in a different setting? What difference does it make to the audience's response if it is framed as a thought-provoking entertainment, pedagogical device, or meditation on life and death?

A summary of our discussions on *Wit* can serve to pull together several central issues related to narratives of disease, disability, and trauma that run throughout this book. They relate to the six functions of communication as set out by Jakobson[2] (and Hilde Lindemann Nelson's "things we do with stories," as discussed in our introduction), since they concern the following aspects:

1. the relationship between the story and the narrator who constructs and conveys it (the emotive, expressive, or therapeutic function);
2. the impact on the audience's ideas and behaviour (the conative, didactic, or "reader response" function);
3. the relationship of the content (what is told) to a context recognized by the audience (the referential or documentary function);
4. the role of the form given to the story (the crafted stylistic or poetic function);
5. awareness of the effects of the medium of narration, in this case language and drama (the metalinguistic, self-referential function);
6. elements that ensure that the line of communication is open, in this case interaction between the actor/character and the audience (the phatic function).

In what follows, we will each, in turn, comment in relation to these functions on some aspects of the play that seemed particularly relevant to our discipline.

The Expressive Function: Author-Narrator-Actor in Relation to the Text (Valerie Raoul)

My research focuses on issues raised by autobiographical writing in relation to gender, age, and ethnicity. *Wit* was written by a playwright who does not have cancer, and is generally performed by actors who make no claim to be expressing their own personal experience. It can be contrasted, in this respect, with a play like *My Left Breast*.[3] Edson's "knowledge" of cancer and of hospital life is restricted to having worked as a receptionist in an oncology/AIDS unit (*Vancouver Sun*, April 1, 2001). Nevertheless, she evokes experiences that are recognized by patients and hospital workers as representative of their own. This is the case even though the set is minimalist, and a few symbolic objects serve as metonymies to conjure up a hospital scene. We do not assume that the actor playing the main character, fifty-year-old English professor Vivian Bearing,[4] is actually suffering from the disease, although in the film version she progressively loses her hair as the story proceeds. Her very name, Vivian, indicates that she is a representative of those who want to live and are "bearing" suffering, rather than an actual individual. The audience enters into a willing suspension of disbelief, and accepts that general ideas about illness are being conveyed by means of an imaginary case study.

Since the "autobiographical pact" (Lejeune, 1975/trans. 1989) is not invoked, we do not have to be concerned with the specific "truth" of this case, or consider the need to protect the anonymity of the particular woman concerned. No one is writing her or his own story in search of catharsis or healing; rather, it is the spectators who are required to identify with the character through their imaginations. Their own experiences may be brought to play in their reactions, which may indeed be cathartic or therapeutic for them, but we are dealing with issues of transference rather than "lived experience." The playwright, and the actors, may be considered to be "speaking for others," but this is certainly in a gesture of advocacy (or what is referred to by Ross Chambers as "amplification" of an otherwise unheard message[5]), rather than abrogation of the other's voice or story. Also, paradoxically, the actual presence on stage of a body that appears to change as the illness progresses brings home to us the corporeal, material reality of disease and dying, although we know that the actor will arise from the dead to respond to applause at the end of the play. This dramatic effect recalls the catharsis of classical tragedy, which aimed to evoke both horror and relief. We are not in Vivian's situation—this time—but do we come out of the theatre with a better understanding of it?

The play can be used to illustrate many of the issues raised in Part I of this volume relating to authenticity, authority, and different kinds of "truth" or (dis)simulation in representations of disease, disability, or trauma. It also addresses explicitly the issue of aestheticization, or literary value, in relation to documentary or technical knowledge. It does so by making the principal protagonist a specialist in the poetry of John Donne (with specific reference to his sonnet "Death be not proud ..."), who is forced into confrontation not only with her own death but with a competing, physical (rather than metaphysical), biomedical story about the meaning and value of pain and suffering, and what "conquering death" might mean.

What constitutes the value of life is also called into question by other aspects of Vivian's existence, since she is depicted as a successful but lonely intellectual career woman who has apparently chosen not to have a family or close friends. Interviews inform us that Edson, the author, is a lesbian and a kindergarten teacher.[6] Some autobiographical input might be inferred from her character's unmarried status. Her ovarian cancer (occurring as Bearing arrives at menopause and can no longer "bear" children) could be interpreted as indicative of a failure to perform as a "normal" woman (i.e., mother). In contrast, Vivian's mentor and only visitor, an older female professor, has managed to combine motherhood (and grandmotherhood) with a successful academic career. She is there at the end (along with a homely nurse) as a maternal figure to comfort Vivian when her intellectual knowledge is no longer of any use. While Vivian recalls her close relationship with her father, and that her early fascination for words derived from contact with him, the only mention of her mother is that she died of breast cancer a few years ago. The last book Vivian has read to her is a children's story about a rabbit trying unsuccessfully to evade his mother (or a maternal God?). This straightforward fable promises the comfort of unconditional love, in contrast to Vivian's constant attempts to prove herself worthy and gain paternal/academic approval by tackling the most difficult tasks.

These aspects of the text lend themselves to a psychoanalytic reading, and suggest an interpretation of the play as a defense of maternal emotions and physical contact (Lacan's Imaginary Order or Kristeva's "semiotic") against the paternal, abstract, verbal, and intellectual (Lacan's Symbolic Order and *nom/non du père*), whether the latter be medical or literary. A fierce professor who has never suffered fools gladly, Vivian is infantilized in the clinical environment—attached to umbilical drips, washed and cared for, wheeled about, and finally offered a Popsicle as a soother. This regression can be seen as signifying her (desirable?) re-feminization, as well as serving as a critique of the way patients are treated in hospital. The author may have expressed subjective material related to gender in her text, beyond what is immediately visible, but these elements are part of a broader and more obvious critique of the impersonalized treatment of patients in hospital.

The Conative Function: A Message Addressed to Health Professionals (Connie Canam)

From the perspective of someone working in a university school of nursing, my initial interest in *Wit* was in exploring the play's representation of

Vivian Bearing as a patient and the hospital staff's interactions with her. I noted that this professor's absorption in her work is to the exclusion of all else, including her health. She is depicted as having gone without a medical check-up for several years, and having put off seeing a physician for four months after experiencing symptoms of illness, since her priority was to complete an invited article which was a "great honor" (*Wit*, 1993/1999, 25). She has earned a reputation as a rigorous scholar and teacher, ruthless in her assessments of others' weakness, and just as hard on herself. For her, knowledge is the source of self-esteem ("After twenty years [in Donne studies] I can say with confidence, no one is quite as good as I" [19]), and of personal power ("I could draw so much from the poems. I could be so powerful" [40]). Life is a competition which she believes she has won (16), until she discovers she has cancer.

Vivian's self-esteem is initially boosted by the respectful presence of a clinical fellow, Jason, a former student of hers who failed to achieve top marks in her course. However, her dominant discourse enters into competition with that of the oncology specialist, Dr. Kelekian, who informs Vivian in the opening scene, in a satire of the worst way of breaking bad news, that she has advanced metastatic ovarian cancer. He is abrupt, concise, and factual, paying no attention to her potential emotional response. The initial challenge to her is to master his vocabulary, one that she rises to as another intellectual puzzle to be solved. Similarly, her response to the invitation to take the "full dose" of chemotherapy, however tough, is uncompromising in her readiness to try. The specialist's most persuasive argument is that "as research, it will make a significant contribution to our knowledge," to which she replies, "Knowledge, yes" (12). Later she admits that she knew this treatment would not cure her (53), but she is willing to be a guinea pig in the advance of science.

Vivian assumes that, as a Donne scholar, she knows "all about life and death" (13). However, her attitude as a student was already criticized by the "great" Professor E.M. Ashford, her role model, who accused her of choosing an interpretation of the end of Donne's sonnet on death based on "hysterical punctuation" (14–15): an exclamation mark that implies Death (personified by a capital letter) as the end, rather than death as simply a pause or transition, a comma indicating entry into life everlasting. Vivian refused to follow Ashford's advice to go out and experience life while she was still young, to focus on "simple human truth" rather than "uncompromising scholarly standards" (15). By the end of the play she will admit that she tried to "hide behind the complicated stuff" (49) but that, ultimately, "Now is not the time for verbal swordplay.... Now is a time for simplicity ... for, dare I say it, kindness. I thought being extremely smart would take care of it. But I see that I have been found out" (55–56).

From this perspective, as Edson pointed out in the *Vancouver Sun* interview, it is Vivian's illness or "fall" that redeems her as it forces her to rediscover her own humanity. Jason, the medical fellow, is portrayed as being on the same path as Vivian and Dr. Kelekian, putting research ahead of compassion (47). The nurse, Susie, who is disparagingly referred to as "never very sharp to begin with" (55), has something to teach him and Vivian in this regard. Susie's willingness to be physically close and comforting complements Ashford's attention (through a children's book, *The Runaway Bunny*) to the spiritual, or non-physical, aspects of dying. Affective and experiential knowledge appear to be recognized as more significant than brain power and the mastery of discourse (whether medical or literary), as Vivian "bears/bares" her soul, literally rising silent and naked in the final scene from her abandoned and derelict body.

The play has been used as an instructional tool in thirty leading American medical schools through a program known as the *Wit* Initiative. This drama is of use in educating health care providers from two perspectives. It exposes the effects of poor communication between physicians and patients, appealing to professionals to see those they care for as people rather than as "a specimen jar" (43); and suggests that medical personnel need to consider the non-physical needs of patients, and the fact that pain and suffering have a range of meanings according to varying religious, cultural, or personal values and beliefs. *Wit* reflects the tension in our society between two paradigms of knowledge: the positivist, or scientific, tradition of "objective" facts and progress based on rational cognition, and the humanistic tradition of subjective or affective knowing, which involves a concept of healing and survival that is more than physical. In the play, the former is associated with masculinity (the doctors; Vivian as a defeminized intellectual career woman) and the latter with femininity (the kind nurse; the maternal professor). This distribution may perpetuate stereotypes rather than contest them, although the goal appears to be to emphasize the value of the feminine attributes.

The Referential and Metanarrative Functions: Social and Historical Context (Carla Paterson)

This play, undeniably, is extremely useful for training medical students and nurses in that it can act as a catalyst for discussion of the relationship between disease (in the abstract) and illness (as an individual experience).

It also raises central issues of concern to bioethicists about experimental treatments for the sake of research and when a patient should be allowed to die. Yet, as a historian of medicine, I am troubled by the fact that Vivian Bearing's story does not reflect the realities of what a late-twentieth-century woman suffering from ovarian cancer in North America might actually be expected to have encountered. After-show discussion in Vancouver revealed that many in the audience had or had had cancer, or were accompanying people close to them in that situation. While Vivian's account might resonate with some aspects of their experiences, in other respects it would seem to be very different.

The first area in which this representation is not typical relates to the social context of illness. Vivian is presented as a solitary individual, with only one visitor at the end of her hospital stay. The stage set is always the hospital ward, and we have no knowledge of Vivian's life before or beyond it apart from her own reminiscences. In the film version, an added scene in which she is wearing street clothes is almost shocking for someone who has seen the play and can only imagine her in her hospital bed. In fact, it would be unthinkable for a university professor, still active in her profession and a public figure, to be as isolated as Vivian is. The filmic medium recalls other films about hospitals, in which friends, family, and other people's visitors all form part of the interaction that takes place. The construction of Vivian as an almost abstract "everyman" alone in the face of death is acceptable on stage, where denaturalization is part of a theatrical convention, but the more realistic medium of film exposes the exaggeration of her situation.[7]

The encounter between an individual and the medical system actually entails more intermediaries than it would appear from the play. Not only counselors and social workers are involved, but also patient support groups and organizations advocating on behalf of people with particular diseases. In Vancouver, for example, there are a number of groups (such as The Young and the Breastless, co-founded by one of our research team[8]) that not only provide therapeutic support to patients but lobby for attention to policy issues and often resist dominant medical discourse by experimenting with alternative or complementary medicine. Vivian, although she is a fierce fighter, is portrayed as surprisingly passive and acquiescent in relation to the medical advice she receives; partly because she identifies with fellow "experts," but also because, as a patient with this particular disease, she is depicted as unrealistically alone.

Although she is an intellectual, Vivian does not ask any questions about the origin or cause of her disease, and the references to her family background evoke psychological issues as potential influences, rather than biomedical or environmental ones. In this way, *Wit* might be contrasted with *Refuge* (1991), Terry Tempest Williams' account in which the ovarian and breast cancers suffered by members of the author's family are linked to the testing of atomic weapons in their home state of Utah. Margaret Edson seems, ultimately, more concerned with the metaphysical question raised by Donne (is death the end?) than with physical, material, or social explanations for the experience of disease and its treatment. The end appears to value the "kindness" of Susie (and Professor Ashford as grandmother) over the "knowledge" represented by the doctors. However, a condescending attitude to Susie is implied not only by Vivian's words, but by her racialization in the film (whereas the published text lists her in the cast as having an Irish name, "Susie Monahan"). "Wit" can designate knowledge (wisdom or intelligence) or humorous play with words. Ironically, "wit" in the second sense is used here to critique expert "knowledge," whether it is associated with medicine or literary studies. The power of words paradoxically serves to dissect the illusion of their power over death. The hierarchy established in life by control of a master discourse is not, however, challenged.

The Poetic and Metalinguistic Functions: Language as Power (Gloria Onyeoziri)

As a specialist in rhetoric, and particularly in the use of irony in narrative, I am interested in the way Vivian Bearing applies her intimate relationship with language, cultivated throughout a career devoted to a specific type of poetic discourse, to her present existential predicament. In the play, Vivian uses her knowledge to attempt an analytical and deconstructive treatment of the medical discourse that would otherwise tend to objectify her. Oncological terminology, as used by her research-obsessed doctor and his "brilliant" resident, has the function of escorting her body into an objectified state: diseased, dying, and ultimately a dead thing. Her rereading of that language allows her to turn herself back into a subject of metaphysical speculation. At the same time, that speculation ambiguously parallels the dissecting power of medical language, suggesting a medical tradition itself rooted in the metaphysics of linguistic representation.

The fact that Vivian has to "simplify" her metalinguistic/metaphysical struggle and settle for the "little allegory of the soul" (63) that her former professor reads to her, or enjoys sharing a little laugh with Susie over Susie's ignorance of the etymology of "soporific" (58), leads to several possible, and not necessarily compatible, conclusions. Does Vivian fail in her attempt to deconstruct the medical-research establishment's rhetorical apparatus, since she is forced to accept being the passive object of study? Was her faith in poetic discourse as a source of knowledge misplaced? Is a palliative, soporific end to the process of illness and dying inevitable? In any case, it appears to need to be preceded by a struggle with language, in which the dying subject, the care-giving community, and the audience become engaged.

When Vivian sarcastically gives a professional medical greeting and then opposes her own professional language to it (5), she establishes the principle that she is not negotiating a divide between medicine (the invasive discourse) and her own field of authority (poetic language), but rather a struggle within language itself. Her sense of self can only persist to the extent that she "masters" discourse, which in this context means being able to turn the words of others ironically into her own sense, acting out their significance, and drawing attention to the fact that they are the source of her existence:

> Irony is a literary device that will necessarily be deployed to great effect. I urgently wish this were not so. I would prefer that a play about me be cast in the mythic-heroic-pastoral mode; but the facts, most notably stage-four metastatic ovarian cancer, conspire against that. The *Faerie Queene* this is not. And I was dismayed to discover that the play would contain elements of ... *humor*. (8)

Irony is, for Vivian, the only possible response to a tragicomic situation, since she knows that there will be no Stage/Act Five (13). Her humour is joyless. She provisionally places herself outside her own participation in the code of communication and treats that code as an object of commentary and reflection. The drama and the language are co-conspirators, inseparable in her mind, and the metaphysical, metalinguistic, and poetic are interrelated modes of experience.

"Medical terms are less evocative" (37) than the magical words like "soporific" that have fascinated her since her childhood. Despite this inferiority, they have power as words and therefore have to be reckoned with. Vivian states ironically, "I will grant that in this particular field of endeavour they possess a more potent arsenal of terminology than I. My only defence is the acquisition of vocabulary" (37). The illusory nature of this defence is underscored by the immediate scene change: Vivian has had to return to the hospital suddenly due to an extreme attack of illness (presumably caused by the chemotherapy), and this is the beginning of the end.

The poetic function in the latter part of the play is characterized by a heightened, more overt sarcasm towards the medical profession as language fails as a means of self-defence. As Vivian's attempts to control the metalinguistic and poetic functions of language become more pressing and desperate, we observe an intensified process of syllepsis, whereby medical terms are reinterpreted to add to their conventional figurative sense a more fundamental, life-threatening, literal meaning: For example, "In isolation, I am isolated. For once I can use the term literally" (39). Syllepsis is itself a form of paradox in that it posits both a literal and a figurative meaning, whereas communication centred on non-poetic functions presupposes that context will decide between the two. It seems that Jason is given the final word on poetic language. As he and Susie work together on the inert body of his dying former professor, he explains to her that Donne's paradoxes never lead to a solution, only to "increasing levels of complexity." "Listen, if there's one thing we learned in Seventeenth-Century Poetry, it's that you can forget about that sentimental stuff. Enzyme Kinetics was more poetic than Bearing's classes" (p.77). Jason respects Vivian's discipline (in both senses), elevating it to a scientific status above the "sentimental stuff" represented, in Jason's view, by Susie. Yet the overall message of the play seems to defend the simplicity of kindness and respect for the other as a person, over the verbal pyrotechnics of sophistic poetry or medical jargon. Thanks to Susie, there will be no Code Blue: Vivian will be allowed to die, rather than continue as a painful experiment. The state of *coma* functions as Donne's *comma*, indicating a painless passage from life to death.

The irony and paradox that dominate the play's text leave it open to interpretation: is this an illness narrative destined to be a tool for the enlightenment of medical practitioners, forced to accept the power of literary words and drama? Or is it, on the contrary, a critique of a literary/humanistic view of the world, since the medical practitioners remain in control at the end and Vivian is dead? Her flight into another world/life may convey a spiritual "truth" for those with faith, or represent literally a flight of fancy, an escape from the stage on which her life and death are played out.

The Phatic Function: Narrating and Performing Illness (Valerie Raoul)

The phatic function, according to Jakobson, ensures that lines of communication are open. It works differently for a theatrical production than for reading a dramatic text or watching a film. In this respect, presenting *Wit* as a stage drama has certain advantages, in terms of immediacy, physical engagement, collective response (such as laughter), and after-show discussion. The dramatic devices deployed in *Wit* enable the principal actor to address the audience directly, reminding them that this is a play, and that the pain, suffering, and death depicted are *representations*; copies simulated to provoke reactions. Illness is *performed* in the sense of a masquerade, a metaphorical theatrical show-and-tell, by stand-ins who replace real patients and real hospital staff. The selective action is arranged in order to illustrate certain points. We are told the outcome at the beginning: the heroine will die. At the same time, the playwright's words, spoken by the central actor who is also the commentator, speak for or *represent*, in a metonymical sense (the part for the whole), all those who face death in alienating surroundings. The message is relayed and amplified by the actors' voices, which impart a textual message open to interpretation as we interactively co-construct the story.

Our reactions show that the meaning assigned to the play may vary, according to what we look for in it (or expect to find), and the analytical approaches resulting from our disciplinary training. The story we extract from the performance also reflects the cultural narrative templates (to use Arthur Frank's term) that we choose to apply. The plot can be framed as a defeat for Vivian's world view (pride before a fall); as her salvation through the kindness of others, as an attack on the medical establishment, and as a defence or indictment of Donne's metaphysical ideas on death. Vivian can be seen as a victim or a survivor, a pawn or a warrior in an epic confrontation between science and the humanities, or as a woman who missed out on life in spite of her career success.

If Vivian were a real person, this would not be a *performance* in the theatrical sense. Rather, her designation by medical specialists as a patient with terminal cancer would be *performative*, in the sense developed by speech-act theorist J.L. Austin and popularized by Judith Butler.[9] The diagnosis would turn her into a patient/case rather than an individual person, abolishing her past identity, affecting her present precarious situation, and predicting (or prescribing) her future prospects. Vivian says early in the treatment, "I just hold still and look cancerous. It requires less acting every time" (32), but by the end she cannot hide the effects on her body. The pronouncement of "stage four ovarian cancer" is a death *sentence*, changing utterly her life (as) story. Her only survival (since she has no children) will be through a record of her experience, as told by herself or others. In this sense, *Wit* can also be read as a tribute to all those who have died without leaving a trace, without witnesses or spectators. However one interprets it, this play provides an exceptional example of narrative possibilities in the depiction of illness, illustrating many of the central issues discussed throughout this collection of essays.

Notes

1. Quoted from *The Guardian* (Charlottetown, PEI), May 10, 2001; *Montreal Gazette*, March 21, 2001; *National Post*, March 3, 2001. See Marianne Szegedy-Maszack, "A Lesson before Dying: Med Schools Tackle End-of-Life Issues," *US News and World Report*, June 25, 2001: 48–50.
2. See Jakobson's "Linguistics and Poetics" in S. Chatman and S. Seymour, eds., *Essays in the Language of Literature* (Boston: Houghton Mifflin, 1967).
3. The play and film depict Newfoundlander Gerry Rogers' experience with breast cancer and both have been widely used by the Canadian Cancer Society and others to raise awareness and establish support groups.
4. While Vivian gives her age as fifty (20) in the published text, in the film she is forty-eight (but still two years beyond menopause and not sexually active "at the moment").
5. See Joy James' contribution to this volume.
6. *Vancouver Sun*, April 1, 2001. On Edson's lesbianism, Pamela Renner comments in the *Advocate* (May 25, 1999): "In a watershed moment for gay visibility, four Pulitzer Prizes go to gay and lesbian authors.... the first person she (Edson) called was her partner Linda Merrill" (83). Don Shewey, also in the *Advocate* (August 12, 1998), made a questionable claim: "Although the playwright doesn't specify, we are free to read Dr. Bearing as a lesbian—not just because she's 50 and has never married or been pregnant but because she doesn't identify in relation to a man or any other lover."
7. See Peggy Curran (*Montreal Gazette*, March 21, 2001): "The absence of visitors or get well cards or reading material or discarded trays of inedible food, which worked as a dramatic device in the play, seems contrived in the 'real' world of film." The involvement of laypeople "in shaping the total experience of sickness" is noted by Rosenberg (1992, xviii).
8. Gabi Helms, to whom this book is dedicated. Her experience of cancer and final hospital stay were very different from Vivian's, in terms of support from others. Another story that can be compared with Vivian's is that of Kay, in *Cancer Stories* (Gregory and Russell, 1999). Also suffering from metastasized ovarian cancer (16), and someone who does not want anyone to baby her (112), this patient discovered "the importance of accepting the love and care of others, and to have sympathy for the self" (139).
9. See J.L. Austin (1962), Judith Butler (1990), Andrew Parker and Eve Kosofsky Sedgwick (1995), and Kristin Langellier (2001b, 2004).

VALERIE RAOUL

Postscript
Un-fitting Stories, Un-disciplined Research

The "larger picture" that appears to me on re-reading this volume of essays might be described as a patchwork of studies bound together by a common thread—an interest in a range of narratives that deepen our understanding of disease, disability or trauma. The "patchwork quilt" metaphor is more appropriate than a "mosaic" one would be, as it can be extended to allude to other aspects of the research project represented here. In a quilt, the pieces joined together are traditionally fragments that do not fit in anywhere else. They become part of a design thanks to a connecting frame that imposes coherence on the disparate parts. For many of the writers of these essays, the topic they broach is outside or at the margins of their usual (or former) disciplinary area of research. The importance of their topic to a larger body of knowledge and inquiry only emerged when they met others with similar "unfitting" preoccupations. In the case of this book, the individual essays serve as samplers to illustrate various patterns of analysis and recurring motifs. Each disciplinary or professional approach reveals one aspect of the whole picture, and the product of the combination is multi-layered.

Also, a quilt often is constructed collaboratively by a number of people, usually women, using a supportive frame that subsequently disappears. It is this frame that allows the different layers of the quilt (surface, stuffing, backing) to be held together as a quilting stitch pierces the layers and makes the quilt solid. This stitch (in French the *point de capiton*) is the image Lacan[1] uses to convey the relationship in language between a chain of "signifiers" (such as a narrative) and shifting "signifieds," implying both the "real" experience concerned and the meanings assigned to them. Meanings are elusive, and have to be *pinned down*, provisionally, in specific contexts. One element is joined to another by a tentative thread, a vulnerable stitch (*suture*) that evokes scar tissue. The narrative quilt may also be seen as a protective covering, enabling cicatrization of a "narcissistic wound," a blow to the psyche that may also, in the case of disease, disability, or trauma, be an actual blow to the body. From this psychoanalytic perspective, such narratives convey experiences that are "real" in the Lacanian sense: they intrude into our lives, destroying previous patterns, and we cannot immediately understand them as they do not fit into the symbolic order but disrupt it. Narrative allows their reinstatement into that order by inscribing meaning, and re-asserting control.

The introductions to this volume and to the individual sections draw the parts together by weaving a narrative or script about stories of disease, disability, and trauma. In this postscript, I will discuss the hidden frame that allowed this collaborative endeavour to happen—the process of forming an interdisciplinary team, composed largely of women and drawn together by a desire to understand how narratives function in relation to representations of the body in states of "dis-ease" and "dis-ability" or wounded by trauma. This exercise had a dual impact, as it not only changed what we see, but enabled us to see differently.

As we initially engaged in cross-disciplinary dialogue and debate about the forms and functions of narratives of disease, disability, and trauma, we were all theoretically aware that each discipline adopts a different perspective on what is worth knowing and how to go about pursuing that knowledge; each disciplinary culture tells differing stories about objects and methods of inquiry. In practice, we discovered that it is only by juxtaposing our own familiar narrative with other, competing accounts and interpretations that a multi-faceted, complex structure can be perceived. We undertook explorations of foreign territory, learning each other's language in order to begin to understand, abandoning our previous sense of mastery of a technical discourse and a particular body of knowledge in the process. Some participants did not continue the journey, preferring to return to their home base. Exposing oneself to other people's academic cultures can be alienating. In this sense, research that does not fit into disciplinary parameters can be seen as somewhat analogous to the experience of disease, disability, or trauma, since it may entail a more or less conscious fear of contagion or sense of disempowerment. As Susan Sontag (1977) first suggested, to be ill is to enter an unfamiliar land; to be a stranger or foreigner; to have to redefine not only what we thought we knew, but who we think we are. The same is true of cross-, trans-, or interdisciplinary investigation.

In her essay in this book, Judy Segal discussed the practical obstacles to interdisciplinary research linking the humanities and social sciences with the fields of medicine and health research. Many of the points she raises relate to Julie Thompson Klein's (1990) study of the forms that interdisciplinarity can take.[2] Klein argued that disciplines are provisional mappings of boundaries, initially determined by *what* is studied. Once a group of researchers identify a field of inquiry, they develop a common language and behavioural expectations, building a culture of belonging that excludes those whose fields lie elsewhere and establishing expectations for *how* inquiry will be conducted. Rigorous discipline is applied to ensure that all research deemed suitable for this field will conform to certain rules and standards, restricting *who* will be allowed in. The resulting community develops institutions (associations, journals, conferences, departments) which ultimately bestow respectability and rewards on those who conform to expectations. However, Klein maintains that there is a dialectic of stability and change where disciplinary boundaries are concerned: the units remain provisional, and renewal is possible only when the frontiers are challenged and displaced.

Such challenges can take various forms: researchers may migrate (temporarily or permanently) to another territory (cross-disciplinarity); they may borrow or steal concepts and methods from other areas (mobile transdisciplinarity); they may congregate with foreigners from other disciplines for specific purposes and indulge in various levels of translation or cross-fertilization (problem-oriented multi- or pluri-disciplinarity). This type of collaboration may produce innovations in methods and results, based on hybridity or unconventional partnerships, and such "undisciplined" endeavours may eventually turn into new lineages, as marginalized cultures become disciplines that will in their turn need to be renewed by migration, etc. These shifts, with obvious parallels to theories of nation formation and unstable geopolitical boundaries, involve contact between cultures that interact, with profound effects on the knowledge produced and the people who produce it. Narrative studies, on one hand, and the medical humanities on the other, might both claim to be emerging disciplines since they have their own schools and journals, terminologies, and star performers. Bringing the two together, however, maintains an innovative edge that ensures a self-critical stance.

The dialectic between stability and contestation, leading to an innovative synthesis, applies not only to the establishment, disintegration, and re-establishment of disciplines, but also to the theory and practice of narrative(s). Many theorists have defined "narrative" knowledge and methods in opposition to "scientific" knowledge and method, as exemplified by biomedical disciplines. Laurel Richardson (1990), in reviewing the use of narrative as an object and tool of inquiry in the field of sociology, cites Jerome Bruner's (1986) claim that there are two basic and universal modes of knowledge. One is the impersonal logico-scientific mode, on which the natural sciences are supposed to depend: it favours the abstract, claims to be universal, and assumes that there are facts to be established with certainty and conveyed by transparent terms. The other, typified by narrative, is interpersonal, contextual, embodied, and particular. It recognizes that language is the material of which ideas and images are made, as well as the medium for conveying them. As a specialist in French studies, it strikes me that these two modes are represented in French, unlike English, by two different words for "to know": *savoir*, which means to "know for a fact," based on abstract reasoning (cognition or thinking); and *connaître*, which means to know personally, by familiarity and experience (recognition, implying a relationship between the thinker and the thought). The first mode aims to prove with certainty that something is true, telling an authoritative story of discovery; the second accepts that knowledge is relative and attempts to understand, imparting a tentative tale of recovery. The social sciences, as the name conveys, hover uncomfortably between these two modes of thought, whereas researchers in the humanities may blithely admit to being subjective, sentimental, and "unreliable" as narrators. Yet, as Richardson and many others have demonstrated, scientific discourse is not immune to narrativity, and its assumptions are often the product of empiricist metaphors that camouflage a lack of awareness of the metanarratives they implicitly convey.[3]

These debates about epistemology are central to poststructuralist questioning of certainty in any form, and the deconstruction of metanarratives such as biomedical discourse reveals them as strategic fictions that serve the interests of certain segments of the population (still mostly white middle-class males). It is no coincidence that the majority of health-care professionals other than doctors are female (and often belong to marginalized racial or ethnic groups). Nurses, therapists, dieticians, and medical social workers are the ones dealing with illness as a condition affecting people, while specialized biomedical researchers may perceive themselves to be dealing with abstract diseases to be labelled and contained. This opposition is illustrated strikingly in the play *Wit* discussed in this volume. Femininity is associated with a *healing* that is multifaceted (psychological and spiritual, as well as physical), in contrast with a "masculine" model of *curing* disease, eliminating or correcting disability, and frequently denying the effects of trauma.

It is also no coincidence that women are often assumed to be sick more often or more widely than men. Femininity, as constructed in our society, implies vulnerability and weakness (see Vertinsky, 1990). Yet some illnesses particularly associated with women (such as depression or agoraphobia, discussed in this volume) may be seen as potentially produced by this construction of femininity, rather than as evidence of a prior biological disposition. It is interesting to note how men who tell a story of disease, disability, or trauma (see the Smith and Sparkes essay in this volume) often perceive themselves as demasculinized; as "othered" in a way that women or racialized groups already experience simply by being who they are in relation to white, male "standards" of assessment. Paradoxically, an experience of suffering conveyed through a narrative that elicits a response may enable some women (and others who were "voiceless") to discover a subjectivity and agency previously denied to them.

It is probably also no coincidence that most of the people involved in the Wall project were women. A good deal of work in narrative theory has been undertaken by feminists who aim to destabilize the foundations of hegemonic "knowledge," to redefine identities, and to make changes in the socio-political arena. Some of the collaborators in the project and in this book (women and men) had personal experiences of disease, disability, or trauma (one, psychiatry professor Susan Penfold, already had published her own memoir of abuse). Others had not, and wondered at the outset if for them studying such narratives poses the same risks as, say, men undertaking research on women, or white women on women of colour. We needed not only to acknowledge the privilege of enjoying good health, but the fact that we cannot know how long it will last. This was brought home to us at UBC when one of our colleagues, Gabi Helms, developed breast cancer during the project and subsequently died (see the dedication to this volume). Does it help to have read many narratives of such an experience, when it actually happens to you? Should we regret that she was not able to leave a publishable account of her experience?

The sections of this book reflect the three dimensions that intersect in discussing these issues. The "aesthetic" shaping of an incoherent experience into a public story acknowledged to have meaning serves as a means to establish authority and claim knowledge, on the *epistemological* front. The "therapeutic" effects of storytelling in interactive situations have *ontological* implications in terms of changing identity and re-establishing self-coherence. The pragmatic and political impact of shared stories that reveal and contest the power of metanarratives has *ideological* force, in terms of collective agency and movement towards social change. The shifts in perspective that occur when researchers enter the space between disciplines have far-reaching effects in all three arenas, affecting our ideas about knowledge and how to obtain it, about who we are (in terms of the language we speak and the company we keep as well as our values), and about the aims and effects of what we do. Moving from safe academic ground to the shifting sands of "real life" instances of disease, disability, and trauma, challenges our assumptions in other, even more discomfiting ways. As part of our project, we co-organized a session on traditional Aboriginal healing practices at UBC's First Nations House of Learning, with presentations from an Aboriginal shaman from Siberia and a First Nations healer from BC. This emotionally powerful event provoked spontaneous testimonial story telling and on-the-spot requests for healing. It proved to be a testing experience for some of the academics who attended, as it was very different from our usual conferences. Some felt very uncomfortable, as this type of exchange did not fit into their sense of appropriate intellectual debate. Breaking down divisions between the university and the community and between different types of knowledge, even more than crossing disciplinary boundaries, brings our personal values into question as well as our professional credentials.

For many of us, however, such surprises were an integral part of the excitement and sense of discovery that can be gained from these types of risky exploration, and a reminder of the tension between different types of knowledge. On the one hand, there is still distrust of "narrative knowledge" from proponents of "rigorous, disciplined" inquiry. In response to such critiques, some literary specialists (such as Gerald Prince, 1982) have attempted to turn narrative analysis into a science (narratology) with its own terminology and rules. On the other hand, narrative approaches in the social sciences have been seen by theorists like Patti Lather (1991) to offer an escape from the fiction of scientific rigour into methods that encourage openness and flexibility. From this perspective, narrative is seen as a powerful means to inform a wider audience and to give voice to the marginalized, contesting previous assumptions about which selves can speak and who has knowledge.

Others have, more recently, warned us that the growing belief in the power and ubiquity of narrative[4] may itself constitute a present-day "ideological myth" or master-story (as suggested by Anne Hunsaker Hawkins in the 1999 edition of her 1992 seminal work, *Reconstructing Illness: Studies in Pathography*). It may now seem somewhat conventional, rather than revolutionary, to discuss "damaged identities" and "narrative repair" (the terms used by Hilde Lindemann Nelson, 2001) as essential aspects of recovery from disease, disability, or trauma. Some of the participants in our project (including Richard Ingram and James Overboe, whose work appears in this volume) contest the "order of meaning" that a search for narrative cohesion implies, and question the definition of personhood that being a reliable narrator entails. The postmodern narrator, as what Julia Kristeva[5] calls a *sujet en procès* (a subject in process, in transit, or on trial) tends to produce paradoxical stories with reversible meanings that do not reflect the characteristics previously associated with narrative: that is, coherence, shape, a beginning, middle, and end. Many narrators of stories of disease, disability, or trauma, whether or not they are consciously aware of being postmodern, tend to see their self as not only damaged but often irremediably shattered. Can the fragments that remain constitute a new type of story?

My contention (as a specialist in women's diary writing) is that they can, just as the disparate segments of this volume (or patchwork quilt) together convey a debate that has meaning, even if the ultimate message is that all "meaning" is suspect. Similarly, in contesting previous conceptions of what constitutes a "person" or a "subject," poststructuralist theorists do not imply that embodied selves do not exist. The challenge is, rather, to recognize how the limits of selfhood may be permeable and extended to include previously abject "others": the *unfitting*, whose exclusion may appear to be the condition of survival for those who never doubt their own authority and autonomy. Those who are still (provisionally) "fit" are called on to listen attentively and receptively to the stories told by people who would otherwise be only anonymous specimens in someone else's case study.

Another French linguistic distinction, established by Emile Benveniste (1966), is relevant to the discussion at this point. He pointed to two types of discourse: *récit* (story or narrative) and *discours* (dialogic exchange or commentary), which exist in a dialectical relationship similar to the one invoked above in reference to the renewal of disciplines. The *récit* is written and in the past, it is seen from outside, and the narrator becomes the absent third person to be discussed, while in *discours*, two people, both present, address each other, alternately using the first and second person pronouns. This dialogue may in turn become a *récit* when recounted by someone else (as in this book), provoking further commentary. Stories of disease, disability, and trauma force us to reconsider the relationship of self to other, as the narrators speak to us of their other-ness, and we have to consider that these others could (will?) be us. The fact that a number of writers represented in this volume have themselves experienced disease, disability, or trauma is significant in this regard, as it breaks down the barriers not only between disciplines but between researchers and the objects of research.

This said, we must acknowledge that the authors represented in this volume, even those who have personal experiences of disease, disability or trauma, are mostly white, middle-class academics or professionals, with privileged access to both health care and the discourses of narrativity. While the majority of the writers of these essays are women, and many of the cases discussed are specifically about women's experiences, in some cases gender does not appear to be a significant aspect of the analysis. Economic status is acknowledged as a central issue in several essays (e.g., Jongbloed's), race or ethnicity is a factor in some cases (e.g., Chivers, Procyk and Crowe, and Freiwald), while age is a feature in still other cases (see Schubert). Further work is needed on the intersections of these dimensions, as well as on the particular historical and geographical contexts that affect how illness and suffering are perceived and represented (as illustrated by Diedrich, Reuter, and Muzak). These are aspects that will be addressed more extensively in future projects to be undertaken at the UBC SAGA Centre for Studies in Autobiography, Gender, and Age.

The first stage of our inquiry, which has culminated in this volume, was ambitious, and we are pleased to be able to share our reflections so far on seeking "undisciplined" and "un-fitting" methods in order to listen appropriately to stories of the loss of "fitness": a word that applies to both physical health and social conformity or "fitting in." The narratives analyzed here show that disease, disability, and trauma draw attention to critical perspectives that are usually ignored by discourses evoking "striving for fitness" or "enabling people to fit in." Unfitting stories that cause discomfort as they force us to rethink our assumptions may be the best ones to shake the dominant frames that serve as both supports and straitjackets in research related to health. Some such stories cannot be told in words and an increasingly popular means to represent them is the quilt. Survivors come together to express the value of lives lived with AIDS, breast cancer, or addiction, by creating patchwork memorials.[6] These collective efforts are therapeutic, and they produce aesthetic objects while conveying an ideological message about the need for change. Our project has focused on stories told in words. By juxtaposing a range of approaches to investigating such narratives, we too have aimed to create solidarity from fragments, and a message that we hope can promote change.

NOTES

1 Lacan develops this concept in "Subversion du sujet et dialectique du désir" (*Ecrits*, 793–827). Joël Dor, in his introduction to Lacanian theory (1985), explains how it relates to other aspects of Lacan's reflections on language and the unconscious (49–51).
2 Theories of interdisciplinarity and their effects in Canadian university settings are also illuminated by Brett Fairbairn and Murray Fulton, in *Interdisciplinarity and the Transformation of the University* (2000).
3 Fred Leavitt's *Evaluating Scientific Research. Separating Fact from Fiction* (2001) provides plenty of material for debates over the "objectivity" of scientific knowledge.
4 As exemplified in Robert Fulford's series of Massey lectures (1999) entitled "The Triumph of Narrative."
5 Kelly Oliver (1993) quotes the following comment by Kristeva about the *subject en process*: "it assumes that we recognize, on the one hand, the unity of the subject who submits to a law—the law of communication, among others: yet who, on the other hand, does not entirely submit, cannot entirely submit, does not want to submit entirely." For Oliver, "to recognize the subject-in-process expands our conception of the social. The social becomes both Law and transgression, both meaning and nonmeaning. It becomes a social-in-process/on trial" (184).
6 A Google search for "quilts" provides an impressive range of examples in many places of individual and collective efforts to create testimonies and memorials in this form.

References

Acker, Caroline J. 1993. Stigma or Legitimation? A Historical Examination of the Social Potentials of Addiction Disease Models. *Journal of Psychoactive Drugs* 25 (3): 193–205.

――――. 2002. *Creating the American Junkie: Addiction Research in the Classic Era of Narcotic Control*. Baltimore: Johns Hopkins Univ. Press.

Adams, P.L. 1990. Prejudice and Exclusion as Social Traumata. In *Stressors and the Adjustment Disorders*, ed. Joseph D. Noshpitz and R. Dean Coddington, 362–91. New York: John Wiley.

Adams, Timothy Dow. 1990. *Telling Lies in Modern American Autobiography*. Chapel Hill: Univ. of North Carolina Press.

Aeschylus. 1966. *Agamemnon*. In *The Oresteia*. Trans. Robert Fagles. New York: Penguin.

Alcoff, Linda. 1991. The Problem of Speaking for Others. *Cultural Critique* 20 (Winter 1991–92): 5–32.

――――, and Laura Gray. 1993. Survivor Discourse: Transgression or Recuperation? *Signs: Journal of Women in Culture and Society* 18 (2): 260–90.

American Psychiatric Association. (1980). *The Diagnostic and Statistical Manual for Mental Disorders* (3rd ed.). Washington, DC: American Psychiatric Association Press.

――――. (1987). *The Diagnostic and Statistical Manual for Mental Disorders* (3rd ed., rev.). Washington, DC: American Psychiatric Association Press.

――――. (1994). *The Diagnostic and Statistical Manual for Mental Disorders* (4th ed.). Washington, DC: American Psychiatric Association Press.

――――. (2000). *The Diagnostic and Statistical Manual for Mental Disorders-Text Revision*. Washington, DC: American Psychiatric Association Press.

Anderson, Linda R. 2001. *Autobiography*. New York: Routledge.

Andreason, Nancy C. 1984. *The Broken Brain: The Biological Revolution in Psychiatry*. New York: Harper and Row.

Andrews, William L., ed. 1986. *To Tell a Free Story: The First Century of Afro-American Autobiography, 1760–1865*. Urbana: Univ. of Illinois Press.
Appelfeld, Aharon. 2005. *Story of a Life*. New York: Schocken Books.
Aristotle. *Poetics*. 1961. Trans. S.H. Butcher. New York: Hill and Wang.
Armstrong, Louise. 1993. *And They Call It Help: The Psychiatric Policing of America's Children*. New York: Addison-Wesley.
Arnold, Robert, ed. 1998. *The Definition of Death: Contemporary Controversies*. Baltimore: Johns Hopkins Univ. Press.
Arnott, Peter D. 1989. *Public and Performance in the Greek Theatre*. London: Routledge.
Atkinson, Paul. 1997. Narrative Turn or Blind Alley? *Qualitative Health Research* 7 (3): 325–44.
Atlantic Health Promotion Research Centre. 2005. *Social Sciences and Humanities in Health Research: A Canadian Snapshot of Fields of Study and Innovative Approaches to Understanding and Addressing Health Issues*. Halifax, NS: Dalhousie University.
Atwood, C.E. 1903. Do Our Present Ways of Living Tend to the Increase of Certain Forms of Nervous and Mental Disorder? *New York Medical Journal* 77: 1070–73.
Austin, J.L. 1962. *How to Do Things with Words*. Oxford: Clarendon Press.
Baier, Annette. 1997. Trust and Antitrust. In *Feminist Social Thought: A Reader*, ed. Diana T. Meyers, 604–29. New York: Routledge.
Bal, Mieke. 2002. *Travelling Concepts in the Humanities: A Rough Guide*. Toronto: Univ. of Toronto Press.
Barss, Patchen. 2002. Has the World Gone Mad? *This* 35 (4): 18–22.
Barthes, Roland. 1991. *The Grain of the Voice: Interviews, 1962–1980*. Trans. Linda Coverdale. Berkeley and Los Angeles: Univ. of California Press.
Bauby, Jean-Dominique. 1997. *The Diving Bell and the Butterfly*. Trans. Jeremy Leggatt. New York: Knopf.
Baudrillard, Jean. 1994. *Simulacra and Simulation*. Trans. Sheila Faria Glaser. Ann Arbor: Univ. of Michigan Press.
Bauman, Zygmunt. 1993. *Postmodern Ethics*. Cambridge, MA: Blackwell.
Bayley, John. 1999. *Elegy for Iris*. London: Norton.
———. 2000. *Iris and Her Friends. A Memoir of Memory and Desire*. London: Norton.
Beck, Evelyn T. 1991. Therapy's Double Dilemma: Anti-Semitism and Misogyny. In *Jewish Women in Therapy: Seen But Not Heard*, ed. Rachel Josefowitz Siegel and Ellen Cole, 19–30. New York: Haworth.
Beels, Christian. 2001. *Another Story: The Rise of Narrative in Psychotherapy*. Ithaca, NY: Zeig, Tucker, and Theisen.
Bell, Daniel, and Marilyn Yalom. 1990. *Revealing Lives: Autobiography, Biography, and Gender*. Albany, NY: SUNY Press.
Bell, Rudolph. 1985. *Holy Anorexia*. Chicago: Univ. of Chicago Press.
Bell, Susan E. 1999. Narratives and Lives: Women's Health Politics and the Diagnosis of Cancer for DES Daughters. *Narrative Inquiry* 9 (2): 1–43.

———. 2000. Experiencing Illness in/and Narrative. In *Handbook of Medical Sociology*. 5th ed., ed. Chloe E. Bird, Peter Conrad, and Allen M. Fremont, 184–99. Upper Saddle River, NJ: Prentice Hall.

———. 2001. Photo Images: Jo Spence's Narratives of Living with Illness. *Health* 6 (1): 5–30.

Benner, Patricia E. 1994. Caring as a Way of Knowing and Not Knowing. In *The Crisis of Care: Affirming and Restoring Caring Practices in the Helping Professions*, ed. Susan S. Phillips and Patricia E. Benner, 42–62. Washington, DC: Georgetown Univ. Press.

Benveniste, Emile. 1966. *Problèmes de linguistique générale*. Paris: Gallimard.

Bepko, Claudia. 1991. *Feminism and Addiction*. New York: Haworth.

Berenson, David. 1991. Powerlessness: Liberating or Enslaving? Responding to the Feminist Critique of the Twelve Steps. In *Feminism and Addiction*, ed. Claudia Bepko, 67–84. New York: Haworth.

Berlant, Lauren. 2000. The Subject of True Feeling: Pain, Privacy, and Politics. In *Transformations: Thinking Through Feminism*, ed. Sara Ahmed, Jane Kilby, Celia Lury, Maureen McNeil, and Beverly Skeggs, 33–47. New York: Routledge.

Beutler, Maja. 1980. *Fuss Fassen*. Bern: Zytglogge Verlag.

Beverly, J. 1991. "Through All Things Modern": Second Thoughts on Testimonio. *boundary 2* 18 (2): 1–21.

Bickenbach, Jerome. 1993. *Physical Disability and Social Policy*. Toronto: Univ. of Toronto Press.

Binswager, Ludwig. 1971. *Introduction à l'analyse existentielle*. Paris: Éditions de Minuit.

Blackbridge, Persimmon. 1996. *Sunnybrook: A True Story with Lies*. Vancouver: Press Gang.

Blanchot, Maurice. 1995. *The Writing of the Disaster*. Trans. Ann Smock. Lincoln: Univ. of Nebraska Press.

Blankenburg, Wolfgang. 1991. *La perte de l'évidence naturelle: Une contribution à la psychopathologie des schizophrénies pauci-symptomatiques*. Paris: Presses Univ. de France.

Bloom, Leslie R. 1998. *Under the Sign of Hope: Feminist Methodology and Narrative Interpretation*. Albany, NY: SUNY Press.

Bluebond-Langner, Myra. 1996. *In the Shadow of Illness: Parents and Siblings of the Chronically Ill Child*. Princeton, NJ: Princeton Univ. Press.

———, Bryan Lask, and Denise B. Angst, eds. 2001. *Psychosocial Aspects of Cystic Fibrosis*. London: Oxford Univ. Press.

Bogdan, Robert, and Steven J. Taylor. 1988. Relationships with Severely Disabled People: The Social Construction of Humanness. *Social Problems* 36: 135–48.

Bok, Sissela. 1979. *Lying: Moral Choice in Public and Private Life*. New York: Random House/Vintage Books.

Bordo, Susan. 1993. *Unbearable Weight: Feminism, Western Culture, and the Body*. Berkeley and Los Angeles: Univ. of California Press.

Boskind-White, Marlene. 2000. *Bulimia/anorexia: The Binge/purge Cycle and Self-Starvation*. New York: Norton.

Bourdieu, Pierre, et al. 1993. *The Weight of the World: Social Suffering in Contemporary Society*. Trans. Priscilla Parkhurst Ferguson et al. Stanford, CA: Stanford Univ. Press.

Boyd, J.H., D.S. Rae, J.W. Thompson, B.J. Burns, K. Bourdon, B.Z. Locke, and D.A. Regier. 1990. Phobia: Prevalence and Risk Factors. *Social Psychiatry and Psychiatric Epidemiology* 25 (6): 314–23.

Boyne, Roy. 1990. *Foucault and Derrida: The Other Side of Reason*. London: Routledge.

Braddock, David L., and Dale Mitchell. 1992. *Residential Services and Developmental Disabilities in the United States: A National Survey of Staff Compensation, Turnover, and Related Issues*. Chicago: American Assoc. on Mental Retardation.

Breast Cancer Support Group, Penn State Milton S. Hershey Medical Center. 2001. *Show Me: A Photo Collection of Breast Cancer Survivors' Lumpectomies, Mastectomies, Breast Reconstructions, and Thoughts on Body Image*. 2nd ed. Hershey, PA: Milton S. Hershey Medical Center.

Breckenridge, Carol A., and Candace Vogler. 2001. The Critical Limits of Embodiment: Reflections on Disability Criticism. *Public Culture* 13 (3): 349–57.

Briggs, Laura. 2000. The Race of Hysteria: "Overcivilization" and the "Savage" Woman in Late Nineteenth-Century Obstetrics and Gynecology. *American Quarterly* 52 (2): 246–73.

Brisac, Geneviève. 1994. *Petite*. Paris: Éditions de l'Olivier.

Brodsley, Laurel. 1992. Defoe's *The Journal of the Plague Year*: A Model for Stories of Plagues. In *AIDS: The Literary Response*, ed. Emmanuel Nelson, 11–22. New York: Scribner's Reference.

Brody, Howard. 1987. *Stories of Sickness*. New Haven, CT: Yale University Press.

———. 1991. "My Story Is Broken. Can You Help Me Fix It?": Medical Ethics and the Joint Construction of Narrative. *Literature and Medicine* 13:79–92.

Bronfen, Elisabeth, Birgit Erdle, and Sigrid Weigel. 1999. *Trauma: Zwischen Psychoanalyse und kulturellem Deutungsmuster*. Cologne: Böhlau Verlag.

Brookes, Tim. 1994. *Catching My Breath: An Asthmatic Explores His Illness*. New York: Time/Random House.

Brown, Gillian. 1987. The Empire of Agoraphobia. *Representations* 20: 134–57.

———. 1991. Anorexia, Humanism, and Feminism. *Yale Journal of Criticism* 5 (1): 189–215.

Brown, Laura S. 1995. Not Outside the Range: One Feminist Perspective on Psychic Trauma. In *Trauma: Explorations in Memory*, ed. Cathy Caruth, 100–12. Baltimore: Johns Hopkins University Press.

Broyard, Anatole. 1992. *Intoxicated by My Illness and Other Writings on Life and Death*. New York: Clarkson Potter.

Bruch, Hilde. 1973. *Eating Disorders: Obesity, Anorexia Nervosa, and the Person Within*. New York: Basic Books.

———. 1978. *The Golden Cage: The Enigma of Anorexia Nervosa*. New York: Vintage.

Brumberg, Joan. 1988. *Fasting Girls: The Emergence of Anorexia Nervosa as a Fasting Disease*. Cambridge, MA: Harvard Univ. Press.

Bruner, Jerome. 1996. The Narrative Construal of Reality. In *The Culture of Education*, 130–49. Cambridge, MA: Harvard Univ. Press.
———. 2001. Self-Making and World-Making. In *Narrative and Identity: Studies in Autobiography, Self, and Culture*, ed. Jens Brockmeier and Donal Carbaugh, 25–38. Philadelphia: John Benjamins.
———. 2002. *Making Stories: Law, Literature, Life*. New York: Farrar, Straus and Giroux.
Bury, Michael. 1982. Chronic Illness as Biographical Disruption. *Sociology of Health and Illness* 4 (2): 167–82.
Buss, Helen M. 1993. *Mapping Our Selves: Canadian Women's Autobiography*. Montreal and Kingston: McGill-Queen's Univ. Press.
———. 1999. *Memoirs from Away: A New Found Land Girlhood*. Waterloo, ON: Wilfrid Laurier Univ. Press.
———. 2002. *Repossessing the World: Reading Memoirs by Contemporary Women*. Waterloo, ON: Wilfrid Laurier Univ. Press.
Butler, Judith. 1990. *Gender Trouble: Feminism and the Subversion of Identity*. New York: Routledge.
———. 1993. *Bodies That Matter: On the Discursive Limits of "Sex."* New York: Routledge.
Bynum, Caroline. 1987. *Holy Feast and Holy Fast: The Religious Significance of Food to Medieval Women*. Berkeley and Los Angeles: Univ. of California Press.
Cain, Carole. 1991. Personal Stories: Identity Acquisition and Self-Understanding in Alcoholics Anonymous. *Ethos* 19: 210–53.
Campbell, Nancy. 2000. *Using Women: Gender, Drug Policy, and Social Justice*. New York: Routledge.
Canby, Vincent. 1994. Review of *Rhapsody in August*. In *Perspectives on Akira Kurosawa*, ed. James Goodwin, 222–24. New York: G.K. Hall.
Caplan, Paula J. 1995. *They Say You're Crazy: How the World's Most Powerful Psychiatrists Decide Who's Normal*. New York: Addison-Wesley.
Capps, Lisa, and Elinor Ochs. 1995. *Constructing Panic: The Discourse of Agoraphobia*. Cambridge, MA: Harvard Univ. Press.
Carlson, Marvin. 1996. *Performance: A Critical Introduction*. London: Routledge.
Carricaburu, Danièle, and Janine Pierret. 1995. From Biographical Disruption to Biographical Reinforcement: The Case of HIV-Positive Men. *Sociology of Health and Illness* 17 (1): 65–88.
Caruth, Cathy. 1995a. Trauma and Experience: Introduction. In *Trauma: Explorations in Memory*, ed. Cathy Caruth, 3–12. Baltimore: Johns Hopkins Univ. Press.
———, ed. 1995b. *Trauma: Explorations in Memory*. Baltimore: Johns Hopkins Univ. Press.
———. 1996. *Unclaimed Experience: Trauma, Narrative, and History*. Baltimore: Johns Hopkins Univ. Press.
———, and Thomas Keenan. 1995. The AIDS Crisis Is Not Over: A Conversation with Gregg Bordowitz, Douglas Crimp, and Laura Pinsky. In *Trauma: Explorations in Memory*, ed. Cathy Caruth, 256–71. Baltimore: Johns Hopkins University Press.

Casey, Nell. 2001. *Unholy Ghost: Writers on Depression.* New York: William Morrow.
Cassell, Eric. 2004. *Nature of Suffering and the Goals of Medicine.* New York: Oxford Univ. Press.
Chambers, Ross. 1999. Can the Body Speak? Keynote lecture presented at Facing Life: The Body in Dis/Ease: An Interdisciplinary Symposium, Vancouver, BC.
———. 1991. *Room for Manoeuver: Reading the Oppositional (in) Narrative.* Chicago: Univ. of Chicago Press.
Chambers, Tod, and Martha Stoddard-Holmes, eds. 2005. Narrative, Pain, and Suffering. Special issue, *Literature and Medicine* 24.
Chambliss, Daniel F. 1996. *Beyond Caring: Hospitals, Nurses, and the Social Organization of Ethics.* Chicago: Univ. of Chicago Press.
Chandler, Michael, Chris Lalonde, and Ulrich Teucher. 2003. Culture, Continuity, and the Limits of Narrativity: A Comparison of the Self-narratives of Native and Non-Native Youth. In *Narrative Analysis: Studying the Development of Individuals in Society*, ed. Cynthia Lightfoot & Colette Daiuth, 245–265. Thousand Oaks, CA: Sage.
Charles, R. 2000. An Irish Family Enlivened by a Linguistic Acrobat. *Christian Science Monitor*, March 16.
Charmaz, Kathy. 1987. Struggling for a Self: Identity Levels of the Chronically Ill. In *Research in the Sociology of Health Care: A Research Manual* Vol. 6, ed. J. Roth, and P. Conrad, 283–321. Greenwich, CT: JAI.
———. 1991. *Good Days, Bad Days: The Self in Chronic Illness and Time.* New Brunswick, NJ: Rutgers Univ. Press.
Charon, Rita, and Martha Montello, eds. 2002. *Stories Matter: The Role of Narrative in Medical Ethics.* New York: Routledge.
Chase, S.E. 2005. Narrative Inquiry: Multiple Lenses, Approaches, Voices. In *The Sage Handbook of Qualitative Inquiry* (3rd ed.), ed. N.K. Denzin & Y.S. Lincoln, 651–79. Thousand Oaks, CA: Sage.
Chernin, Kim. 1985. *The Hungry Self: Women, Eating, and Identity.* New York: Times Books.
Childers, Joseph, and Gary Hentzi. 1995. *The Columbia Dictionary of Modern Literary and Cultural Criticism.* New York: Columbia Univ. Press.
Chivers, Sally. 2003. *From Old Woman to Older Women: Contemporary Culture and Women's Narratives.* Columbus: Ohio State Univ. Press.
Clandinin, D. Jean, and F. Michael Connelly. 2000. *Narrative Inquiry: Experience and Story in Qualitative Research.* San Francisco: Jossey-Bass.
Clark, Hilary. Forthcoming. *Depression and Narrative: Telling the Dark.* Albany, NY: SUNY Press.
———. Forthcoming. Teaching Women's Depression Memoirs: Healing, Testimony, and Critique. In *Teaching Life Writing Texts*, ed. Craig Howes and Miriam Fuchs. MLA.
Clark, Janet [Helen MacGill Hughes]. 1961. *The Fantastic Lodge: The Autobiography of a Girl Drug Addict.* Boston: Houghton Mifflin.
Code, Lorraine. 1995. Introduction to *Rhetorical Spaces: Essays on Gendered Locations*, ix–xvii. New York: Routledge.

Colebrook, Claire. 1999. A Grammar of Becoming: Strategy, Subjectivism, and Style. In *Becomings: Explorations in Time, Memory, and Futures*, ed. Elizabeth Grosz, 117–40. Ithaca, NY: Cornell Univ. Press.
Confavreux, C., G. Aimard, and M. Devic. 1980. Course and Prognosis of Multiple Sclerosis Assessed by the Computerized Data Processing of 349 Patients. *Brain* 103: 281–300.
Connerton, Paul. 1989. *How Societies Remember*. Cambridge: Cambridge Univ. Press.
Conrad, Peter, and Heather Jacobson. 2003. Enhancing Biology? Cosmetic Surgery and Breast Augmentation. In *Debating Biology: Sociological Reflections on Health Medicine and Society*, ed. Simon J. Williams, Gillian A. Bendelow, and Linda Berke, 223–34. London: Routledge.
Corin, Ellen. 1990. Facts and Meaning in Psychiatry: An Anthropological Approach to the Lifeworld of Schizophrenics. *Culture, Medicine and Psychiatry* 14: 153–88.
———, ed. 1993. Folies/Espaces de sens. *Anthropologie et sociétés* Special issue, 17 (1–2).
———. 1998. The Thickness of Being: Intentional Worlds, Strategies of Identity, and Experience among Schizophrenics. *Psychiatry* 61.2: 133–46.
———, and Gilles Lauzon. 1992. Positive Withdrawal and the Quest for Meaning: The Reconstruction of Experience among Schizophrenics. *Psychiatry* 55.3: 266–78.
Courtwright, David. 1982. *Dark Paradise: Opiate Addiction in America before 1940*. Cambridge, MA: Harvard Univ. Press.
Couser, G. Thomas. 1997. *Recovering Bodies: Illness, Disability, and Life Writing*. Madison: Univ. of Wisconsin Press.
———. 2001a. Authority. In *Encyclopedia of Life Writing: Autobiographical and Biographical Forms*, ed. Margaretta Jolly, 1: 73–5. Chicago: Fitzroy Dearborn.
———. 2001b. Conflicting Paradigms: The Rhetorics of Disability Memoir. In *Embodied Rhetorics: Disability in Language and Culture*, ed. James C. Wilson and Cynthia Lewiecki-Wilson, 78–91. Carbondale: Southern Illinois Univ. Press.
———. 2003. *Vulnerable Subjects: Ethics and Life Writing*. Ithaca, NY: Cornell Univ. Press.
———. 2005. Disability, Life Narrative, and Representation. *PMLA* 120 (2): 602–606.
Cox, Susan. 2003. Review of *Standing Ovation: Performing Social Science Research about Cancer* by Ross Gray and Christina Sinding. *The Canadian Review of Sociology and Anthropology* (Fall).
Craven, Meaghan. 2002. No Paradise Lost: Academic Honesty in the New Age of Electronic Plagiarism. *Arch: The University of Calgary Alumni Magazine* (Spring): 8–12.
Crimp, Douglas. 1990. Mourning and Militancy. In *Out There: Marginalization and Contemporary Culture*, ed. Russell Ferguson, Martha Gever, Trinh T. Minh-ha, and Cornel West, 233–45. New York: New Museum of Contemporary Art.

———, and Adam Rolston. 1990. *AIDS DemoGraphics*. Seattle: Bay.
Crossley, Michele L. 2000. *Introducing Narrative Psychology*. Buckingham, UK: Open University Press.
Cushing, Pamela. 2003a. Shaping the Moral Imagination of Caregivers: Disability, Difference and Inequality in L'Arche. PhD diss., McMaster University.
———. 2003b. Policy Approaches to Framing Social Inclusion and Social Exclusion: An Overview (international), ed. C. Crawford. North York, ON: Roeher Institute.
Daiute, Colette, & Cynthia G. Lightfoot. (2004). *Narrative Analysis: Studying the Development of Individuals in Society*. Thousand Oaks, CA: Sage.
Danica, Elly. 1988. *Don't: A Woman's Word*. Charlottetown, PEI: Gynergy.
———. 1996. *Beyond Don't: Dreaming Past the Dark*. Charlottetown, PEI: Gynergy.
Davies, Carole Boyce. 1992. Collaboration and the Ordering Imperative in Life Story Production. In *De/Colonizing the Subject: The Politics of Gender in Women's Autobiography*, ed. Sidonie Smith and Julia Watson, 3–19. Minneapolis: University of Minnesota Press.
Davis, Lennard J. 2002. *Bending Over Backwards: Disability, Dismodernism, and Other Difficult Positions*. New York: New York Univ. Press.
Deleuze, Gilles, and Félix Guattari. 1987. *A Thousand Plateaus: Capitalism and Schizophrenia*. Trans. Brian Massumi. Minneapolis: Univ. of Minnesota Press.
———. 1994. *What Is Philosophy?* Trans. Hugh Tomlinson and Graham Burchill. New York: Columbia Univ. Press.
DePaul, Michael. 1993. *Balance and Refinement: Beyond Coherence Methods of Moral Inquiry*. London: Routledge.
Derrida, Jacques. 1970. Structure, Sign, and Play in the Discourse of the Human Sciences. In *The Languages of Criticism and the Sciences of Man: The Structuralist Controversy*, ed. Richard Macksey and Eugenio Donato, 247–72. Baltimore: Johns Hopkins Univ. Press.
———. 1976. *Of Grammatology*. Trans. Gayatri Chakravorty Spivak. Baltimore: Johns Hopkins Univ. Press.
———. 1978. Cogito and the History of Madness. In *Writing and Difference*, 31–63. Trans. Alan Bass. London: Routledge.
DeSalvo, Louise. 1997. *Breathless: An Asthma Journal*. Boston: Beacon.
Diedrich, Lisa. 2004. "Without Us All Told": Paul Monette's Vigilant Witnessing to the AIDS Crisis. *Literature and Medicine* 23 (1): 112–27.
———. Forthcoming. *Treatments: Negotiating Bodies, Language, and Politics in Illness Narratives*. Minneapolis: Univ. of Minnesota Press.
Dillingham, W.P. 1911. *Reports of the Immigration Commission: Dictionary of Races or Peoples*. Washington, DC: United States Immigration Commission.
Doane, Janice, and Devon Hodges. 2001. *Telling Incest: Narratives of Dangerous Remembering from Stein to Sapphire*. Ann Arbor: Univ. of Michigan Press.
Donley, Carol, and Sheryl Buckley, eds. 2000. *What's Normal?: Narratives of Mental & Emotional Disorders*. Kent, OH: Kent State Univ. Press.
Dor, Joël. 1985. *Introduction à la lecture de Lacan*. Paris: Denoël.

Dorazio-Milgliore, Margaret, and Marsha Henry. 2002. *Making Women Visible*. Vancouver: BC Centre of Excellence for Women's Health.
Doubrovsky, Serge. 1970. *Fils*. Paris: Galilée.
———, Jacques Lecarme, and Philippe Lejeune, eds. 1993. *Autofictions et cie*. Paris: Université de Paris X, Centre de Recherches sur les Textes Modernes.
Doubt, Keith. 1996. *Towards a Sociology of Schizophrenia: Humanistic Reflections*. Toronto: Univ. of Toronto Press.
Don, Timothy. 1990. *Telling Lies in Modern American Autobiography*. Chapel Hill: Univ. of Carolina Press.
Dreyfus, Hubert L. 1987. Foucault's Critique of Psychiatric Medicine. *Journal of Medicine and Philosophy* 12: 311–33.
Driscoll, Ellen. 1993. The Politics of Recovery. In *Consuming Passions: Feminist Approaches to Weight Preoccupation and Eating Disorders*, ed. Catrina Brown and Karin Jasper, 251–73. Toronto: Second Story.
Durkheim, Emile. 1933 [1893]. *The Division of Labor in Society*. New York: Free Press.
Eakin, Paul John. 1999. *How Our Lives Become Stories: Making Selves*. Ithaca, NY: Cornell Univ. Press.
———, ed. 2004. *The Ethics of Life Writing*. Ithaca, NY: Cornell University Press.
Eco, Umberto. 1996. *Six promenades dans les bois du roman et d'ailleurs*. Paris: Éditions Grasset and Fasquelle.
Edlund, M.J. 1990. The Economics of Anxiety. *Psychiatric Medicine* 8 (2): 15–26.
Edson, Margaret. 1993/1999. *Wit*. New York: Dramatists Play Service.
Ellmann, Maud. 1993. *The Hunger Artists: Starving, Writing, Imprisonment*. Cambridge, MA: Harvard Univ. Press.
Euripides. 1963. *Electra*. In *Medea and Other Plays*. Trans. Philip Vellacott. London: Penguin.
Everett, Barbara. 2000. *A Fragile Revolution: Consumers and Psychiatric Survivors Confront the Power of the Mental Health System*. Waterloo, ON: Wilfrid Laurier Univ. Press.
Fairbairn, Brett, and Murray Fulton. 2000. *Interdisciplinarity and the Transformation of the University*. Saskatoon: Univ. of Saskatchewan, Centre for the Study of Cooperatives.
Famighetti, Robert, ed. 1994. *World Almanac and Book of Facts, 1995*. New York: St. Martin's.
Farrell, Kirby. 1998. *Post-traumatic Culture: Injury and Interpretation in the Nineties*. Baltimore: Johns Hopkins Univ. Press.
Fawcett, Gail. 1996. *Living with Disability in Canada: An Economic Portrait*. Hull, QC: Human Resources Development Canada.
Fee, Dwight, ed. 2000. *Pathology and the Postmodern: Mental Illness as Discourse and Experience*. London: Sage.
Felman, Shoshana, and Dori Laub. 1992. *Testimony: Crises of Witnessing in Literature, Psychoanalysis, and History*. New York: Routledge.
Finney, Gail. 1989. *Women in Modern Drama: Freud, Feminism, and European Theatre at the Turn of the Century*. Ithaca, NY: Cornell Univ. Press.

———. 2006. *Visual Culture in Twentieth-Century Germany: Text as Spectacle.* Bloomington: Indiana Univ. Press.

Fiore, Robin N., and Hilde Lindemann Nelson, eds. 2003. *Recognition, Responsibility, and Rights: Feminist Ethics and Social Theory.* New York: Rowman and Littlefield.

Folkenflik, Robert, ed. 1993. *The Culture of Autobiography: Constructions of Self-Representation.* Stanford, CA: Stanford Univ. Press.

Foucault, Michel. 1961. *Folie et déraison: Histoire de la folie à l'âge classique.* Paris: Plon.

———. 1973. *The Birth of the Clinic: An Archaeology of Medical Perception.* Trans. A.M. Sheridan Smith. New York: Pantheon.

———. 1978. *History of Sexuality.* Vol. 1. Trans. Robert Hurley. New York: Vintage.

———. 1994. *Dits et écrits.* Vol. 4. Paris: Gallimard.

Frähm, Anne E., with David J. Frähm. 1992. *A Cancer Battle Plan: Six Strategies for Beating Cancer from a Recovered "Hopeless Case."* Colorado Springs: Pinon.

Frank, Arthur W. 1991. *At the Will of the Body: Reflection on Illness.* Boston: Houghton Mifflin.

———. 1995. *The Wounded Storyteller: Body, Illness, and Ethics.* Chicago: Univ. of Chicago Press.

———. 2000. Illness and the Interactionist Vocation. *Symbolic Interaction* 23: 321–33.

———. 2002. Approaches to Narrative Inquiry. Panel discussion at *Narratives of Disease, Disability, and Trauma,* Vancouver, BC.

———. 2004. *Renewal of Generosity: Illness, Medicine and How to Live.* Chicago: Univ. of Chicago Press.

Frans, Douglas. 1994. Social Work, Social Science, and the Disease Concept: New Directions for Addiction Treatment. *Journal of Sociology and Social Welfare* 21 (2): 71–89.

Freedman, Jill, and Gene Combs. 1996. *Narrative Therapy: The Social Construction of Preferred Realities.* New York: Norton.

Freud, Sigmund. 1939. *Moses and Monotheism.* Trans. Katherine Jones. New York: Vintage.

———. 1948. *An Autobiographical Study.* Trans. James Strachey. London: Hogarth and the Institute of Psycho-Analysis.

———. *Totem and Taboo.* 1950. Trans. and ed. James Strachey. New York: Norton.

———. 1960. *Letters of Sigmund Freud, 1873–1939.* Ed. Ernst L. Freud. Trans. Tania and James Stern. New York: Basic Books.

———. 1961. *Beyond the Pleasure Principle.* Ed. and trans. James Strachey. New York: Norton.

———. 1963. 'Civilized' Sexual Morality and Modern Nervousness. In *Sexuality and the Psychology of Love,* ed. Philip Rieff, 10–30. New York: Collier Books.

Friedling, Melissa Pearl. 2000. *Recovering Women: Feminisms and the Representation of Addiction.* Boulder, CO: Westview.

Fulford, Robert. 1999. *The Triumph of Narrative. Storytelling in the Age of Mass Culture.* Toronto: House of Anansi.

Gale, Augusta Hicks. 1996. *Older Than My Mother: A Nurse's Life and Triumph over Breast Cancer.* Seattle: Ananse.

Gamble, Vanessa N. 1993. A Legacy of Distrust: African Americans and Medical Research. *American Journal of Preventive Medicine* 9: 35–38.

———. 1997. Under the Shadow of Tuskegee: African Americans and Health Care. *American Journal of Public Health* 87 (11): 1773–78.

Gammel, Irene, ed. 1999. *Confessional Politics: Women's Self-Representations in Life Writing and Popular Media.* Carbondale: Southern Illinois Univ. Press.

Garfinkel, Paul. 2001. Interview with Michael Enright. *Sunday Morning.* CBC Radio. 10 June.

Geertz, Clifford. 1994. The Uses of Diversity. In *Assessing Cultural Anthropology*, ed. Robert Borofsky, 454–66. Columbus, OH: McGraw-Hill.

Geracimos, A. 2000. Christopher Nolan: Against All Odds. *Publishers Weekly*, March 13: 57–58.

Gerschick, Thomas J., and Adam Stephen Miller. 1995. Coming to Terms: Masculinity and Physical Disability. In *Men's Health and Illness: Gender, Power, and the Body*, ed. Donald E. Sabo, and David F. Gordon, 183–204. London: Sage.

Giddens, Anthony. 1991. *Modernity and Self-Identity: Self and Society in the Late Modern Age.* Cambridge: Polity.

Gilman, Sander L. 1988. *Disease and Representation: Images of Illness from Madness to AIDS.* Ithaca, NY: Cornell Univ. Press.

———. 2000. *The Fortunes of the Humanities.* Stanford, CA: Stanford Univ. Press.

Gilmore, Leigh. 1994. *Autobiographics: A Feminist Theory of Women's Self-Representation.* Ithaca, NY: Cornell Univ. Press.

———. 2001. *The Limits of Autobiography: Trauma and Testimony.* Ithaca, NY: Cornell Univ. Press.

———. 2003. Jurisdictions: *I, Rigoberta Menchù*, *The Kiss*, and Scandalous Self-Representation in the Age of Memoir and Trauma. *Signs: Journal of Women in Culture and Society* 28 (21): 695–718.

Glaser, Barney, and Anselm Strauss. 1967. *The Discovery of Grounded Theory.* Chicago: Aldine.

Goffman, Erving. 1963. *Stigma: Notes on the Management of Spoiled Identity.* Englewood Cliffs, NJ: Prentice Hall.

Gonzalez, David. 2003. It Was a Brilliant Cure—But We've Lost the Patient! The Stigma of Cinemania. 26 February. <http://www.cinemaniastigma.com>.

———. 2005. *The Stigma of Cinemania*, December 4. <http://www.cinemaniastigma.com>.

Good, Byron J., and Mary-Jo DelVecchio Good. 1993. "Learning Medicine": The Constructing of Medical Knowledge at Harvard Medical School. In *Knowledge, Power, and Practice: The Anthropology of Medicine and Everyday Life*, ed. Shirley Lindenbaum and Margaret Lock, 81–107. Berkeley and Los Angeles: Univ. of California Press.

Goodwin, James. 1994. Akira Kurosawa and the Atomic Age. In *Perspectives on Akira Kurosawa*, ed. James Goodwin, 81–107. New York: G.K. Hall.

Goshen-Gottstein, Esther. 1990. *Recalled to Life: The Story of a Coma*. New Haven, CT: Yale Univ. Press.

Government of Canada. 1996. *Equal Citizenship for Canadians with Disabilities: The Will to Act. Federal Task Force of Disability Issues*. Hull, QC: Human Resources Development Canada.

Graham, Jory. 1982. *In the Company of Others*. New York: Harcourt Brace Jovanovich.

Gregory, David M., and Cynthia K. Russell. 1999. *Cancer Stories: On Life and Suffering*. Montreal: McGill-Queen's Univ. Press.

Grob, Gerald N. 1985. *The Inner World of American Psychiatry, 1890–1940: Selected Correspondence*. New Brunswick, NJ: Rutgers Univ. Press.

Guattari, Félix. 1995. *Chaosophy*. Ed. Sylvère Lotringer. New York: Semiotext(e).

Gubrium, Jaber F., and James A. Holstein. 1998. Narrative Practice and the Coherence of Personal Stories. *Sociological Quarterly* 39: 163–87.

———. 1999. At the Border of Narrative and Ethnography. *Journal of Contemporary Ethnography* 28 (5): 561–73.

Gullette, Margaret Morganroth. 2004. *Aged by Culture*. Chicago: Univ. of Chicago Press.

Habermas, Jürgen. 1995. *Sociologie et théorie du langage*. Paris: Armand Colin.

Hacking, Ian. 1995. *Rewriting the Soul: Multiple Personality and the Sciences of Memory*. Princeton, NJ: Princeton Univ. Press.

Haiken, Elizabeth. 1997. *Venus Envy: A History of Cosmetic Surgery*. Baltimore: Johns Hopkins Univ. Press.

Hammersley, Martyn S., and Paul Atkinson. 1983. *Ethnography: Principles in Practice*. New York: Tavistock.

Hartman, Geoffrey. 2004. Response: Narrative and Beyond: Psychoanalysis and Narrative Medicine. *Literature and Medicine* 23 (2): 334–45.

Hawkins, Anne Hunsaker. 1997. Medical Ethics and the Epiphanic Dimension of Narrative. In *Stories and Their Limits: Narrative Approaches to Bioethics*, ed. Hilde Lindemann Nelson, 150–70. New York: Routledge.

———. 1999. *Reconstructing Illness: Studies in Pathography*. 2nd ed. West Lafayette, IN: Purdue Univ. Press.

Hawkins, Anne Hunsaker, and Marilyn Chandler McEntyre, eds. 2000. *Teaching Literature and Medicine*. New York: MLA Publications.

Henderson, Mae Gwendolyn. 1998. Speaking in Tongues: Dialogics, Dialectics, and the Black Woman Writer's Literary Tradition. In *Women, Autobiography, Theory: A Reader*, ed. Sidonie Smith and Julia Watson, 343–51. Madison: University of Wisconsin Press.

Henke, Suzette. 1998. *Shattered Subjects: Trauma and Testimony in Women's Life-Writing*. New York: St. Martin's.

———. 2001. Literary Life-Writing in the Twentieth Century. *Poets and Writers* (May/June): 40–46.

Herman, Judith Lewis. 1992. *Trauma and Recovery*. New York: Basic Books.

———, and Lisa Hirschman. 1981. *Father–Daughter Incest*. Cambridge, MA: Harvard Univ. Press.

Heschel, Susannah. 1991. Jewish Feminism and Women's Identity. In *Jewish Women in Therapy: Seen but Not Heard*, ed. Rachel Josefowitz Siegel and Ellen Cole, 31–39. New York: Haworth.

Heywood, Leslie. 1996. *Dedication to Hunger: The Anorexic Aesthetic in Modern Culture*. Berkeley and Los Angeles: Univ. of California Press.

Hinchman, Lewis P., and Sandra K. Hinchman, eds. 1997. *Memory, Identity, Community: The Idea of Narrative in the Human Sciences*. Albany: SUNY Press.

Hollway, W. 2000. *Doing Qualitative Research Differently: Free Association, Narrative and the Interview Method*. London: Sage.

Holstein, James A., and Jaber F. Gubrium. 2000. *The Self We Live By: Narrative Identity in a Postmodern World*. New York: Oxford Univ. Press.

Hopkin, Karen. 1998. *Understanding Cystic Fibrosis*. Jackson: Univ. Press of Mississippi.

Horsman, J. 1999. *Too Scared to Learn: Women, Violence and Education*. Toronto: McGilligan Books.

Hunter, Kathryn Montgomery. 1991. *Doctors' Stories: The Narrative Structure of Medical Knowledge*. Princeton, NJ: Princeton Univ. Press.

Hyden, L.C. 1997. Illness and Narrative. *Sociology of Health and Illness* 19 (1): 48–69.

Ignatieff, Michael. 2000. *The Rights Revolution*. Toronto: Anansi.

———. (1984). *The Needs of Strangers: An Essay on Privacy, Solidarity, and the Politics of Being Human*. New York: Penguin.

Ingram, Richard A. 2005. Troubled Being and Being Troubled: Subjectivity in the Light of Problems of the Mind. PhD dissertation, University of British Columbia.

Irwin, Sarah. 2001. Repositioning Disability and the Life Course: A Social Claiming Perspective. In *Disability and the Life Course: Global Perspectives*, ed. Mark Priestley, 15–25. Cambridge, UK: Cambridge University Press.

Iser, Wolfgang. 1989. *Prospecting: From Reader Response to Literary Anthropology*. Baltimore: Johns Hopkins Univ. Press.

Jakobson, Roman. 1967. Linguistics and Poetics. In *Essays on the Language of Literature*, ed. Seymour Benjamin Chatman and Samuel R. Levin. Boston: Houghton Mifflin.

James, Adam. 2001. *Raising Our Voices: An Account of the Hearing Voices Movement*. Gloucester, UK: Handsell.

Janoff-Bulman, Ronnie. 1992. *Shattered Assumptions: Towards a New Psychology of Trauma*. New York: Free Press.

Jezer, Marty. 1997. *Stuttering: A Life Bound Up in Words*. New York: Basic Books.

Jones, Ann Hudson. 1997. "Literature and Medicine: Narratives of Mental Illness." *Lancet* 350: 359–61.

Jongbloed, Lyn. 1996. Factors Influencing Employment Status of Women with Multiple Sclerosis. *Canadian Journal of Rehabilitation* 9: 213–22.

Jonnes, Jill. 1996. *Hep-Cats, Narcs, and Pipe Dreams: A History of America's Romance with Illegal Drugs*. Baltimore: Johns Hopkins Univ. Press.

Johnson, Julia, ed. 2004. *Writing Old Age*. London: Centre for Policy on Ageing.

Joseph, Norma Baumel. 1995. Jewish Education for Women: Rabbi Moshe Feinstein's Map of America. *American Jewish History* 83 (2): 205–22.

Jurga, Antoine, and Jean-Christophe Planche. 1997. *Écritures autobiographiques: "Petite" de Geneviève Brisac*. Calais: CRDP du Nord.

Kaemmerling, Richard. 2002. Das Ich und seine Gesamtausgabe: Zum Problem der Autobiographie. *Kursbuch* 148: 99–109.

Kaganoff, P. 1990. Review of *I Raise My Eyes to Say Yes*. *Publisher's Weekly* 23 November.

Kandall, Stephen R. 1996. *Substance and Shadow: Women and Addiction in the United States*. Cambridge, MA: Harvard Univ. Press.

Kaplan, Caren. 1998. Resisting Autobiography: Out-Law Genres and Transnational Feminist Subjects. In *Women, Autobiography, Theory: A Reader*, ed. Sidonie Smith and Julia Watson, 208–16. Madison: Univ. of Wisconsin Press.

Kaplan, E. Ann. 1999. Trauma and Aging: Marlene Dietrich, Melanie Klein, and Marguerite Duras. In *Figuring Age: Women, Bodies, Generations*, ed. Kathleen M. Woodward, 171–94. Bloomington: Indiana University Press.

———. and Ban Wang, eds. 2004. *Trauma and Cinema: Cross-Cultural Explorations*. Hong Kong: Hong Kong Univ. Press.

Karp, David Allen. 1996. *Speaking of Sadness: Depression, Disconnection, and the Meanings of Illness*. New York: Oxford Univ. Press.

Kauffman, Jeffrey. 2002. Safety and the Assumptive World: A Theory of Traumatic Loss. In *Loss of the Assumptive World: A Theory of Traumatic Loss*, ed. J. Kauffman, 205–12. New York: Brunner-Routledge.

Kavinoky, Bernice. 1966. *Voyage and Return: An Experience with Cancer*. New York: Norton.

Kayal, Philip M. 1993. *Bearing Witness: Gay Men's Health Crisis and the Politics of AIDS*. Boulder, CO: Westview.

Kaye, Dennis. 1993. *Laugh, I Thought I'd Die: My Life with ALS*. Toronto: Viking Penguin.

Kaysen, Susanna. 1993. *Girl, Interrupted*. New York: Vintage.

Kertész, Imre. 1992. *Fateless*. Trans. Christopher C. Wilson and Katharina M. Wilson. Evanston, IL: Northwestern Univ. Press.

King, Nicholas. 2002. Immigration, Race, and Geographies of Difference in the Tuberculosis Pandemic. In *Return of the White Plague: Global Poverty and the New Tuberculosis*, ed. Matthew Gandy and Alimuddin Zumla, 39–55. London: Verso.

Kingfisher, Catherine Pélissier. 1996. *Women in the American Welfare Trap*. Philadelphia: Univ. of Pennsylvania Press.

Kirsch, Anke. 2001. *Trauma und Wirklichkeit: Wiederauftauchende Erinnerungen aus Psychotherapeutischer Sicht*. Stuttgart: Kohlhammer.

Kittay, Eva F. (1999). *Love's Labor: Essays on Women, Equality, and Dependency*: New York, Routledge.

Kleiber, Douglas A., and Susan M. Hutchinson. 1999. Heroic Masculinity in the Recovery from Spinal Cord Injury. In *Talking Bodies: Men's Narratives of the Body and Sport*, ed. Andrew C. Sparkes and Martti Silvennoinen, 135–55. University of Jyvaskyla: SoPhi.

Kleinman, Arthur. 1988. *The Illness Narratives: Suffering, Healing, and the Human Condition.* New York: Basic Books.

———. 1995a. The Social Course of Chronic Illness: Delegitimation, Resistance, and Transformation in North American and Chinese Societies. In *Chronic Illness: From Experience to Policy*, ed. S. Kay Toombs, David Barnard, and Ronald A. Carson, 176–88. Bloomington: Indiana Univ. Press.

———. 1995b. *Writing at the Margin: Discourse between Anthropology and Medicine.* Berkeley and Los Angeles: Univ. of California Press.

———, and Joan Kleinman. 1994. How Bodies Remember: Social Memory and Bodily Experience of Criticism, Resistance, and Delegitimation Following China's Cultural Revolution. *New Literary History* 25:710–21.

Koehn, Daryl. 1999. *Rethinking Feminist Ethics: Care, Trust and Empathy.* New York: Routledge.

Kondracke, Morton. 2001. *Saving Milly: Love, Politics, and Parkinson's Disease.* NY: Perseus Books Group.

Kosaka, B. 2002. Cognitive Issues and Lupus. *Lupus Lighthouse: Official Newsletter of the BC Lupus Society* 24: 24–27.

Kriegel, Leonard. 1987. The Cripple in Literature. In *Images of The Disabled: Disabling Images*, ed. Alan Gartner and Tom Joe, 31–46. New York: Praeger.

Kristeva, Julia. 1984. *Powers of Horror: An Essay on Abjection.* New York: Columbia Univ. Press.

Krystal, Henry. 1995. Trauma and Aging: A Thirty-Year Follow-Up. In *Trauma: Explorations in Memory*, ed. Cathy Caruth, 76–99. Baltimore: Johns Hopkins University Press.

L'Arche. 2006. L'Arche Canada Vision. http://www.larche.ca/en/home/vision/

Labov, William. 1982. Speech Actions and Reactions in Personal Narrative. In *Analyzing Discourse: Text and Talk*, ed. Deborah Tannen, 219–47. Washington DC: Georgetown University Press.

Lacan, Jacques. 1966. *Ecrits.* Paris: Seuil.

LaCapra, Dominick. 2001. *Writing History, Writing Trauma.* Baltimore: Johns Hopkins Univ. Press.

Laing, Ronald David. 1969. *The Divided Self: An Existential Study in Sanity and Madness.* New York: Pantheon.

Langellier, Kristin M. 1989. Personal Narratives: Perspectives on Theory and Research. *Text and Performance Quarterly* 9: 4, 243–76.

———. 2001a. Personal Narrative. In *Encyclopedia of Life Writing: Autobiographical and Biographical Forms.* Vol. 2, ed. Margaretta Jolly, 699–701. London: Fitzroy Dearborn.

———. 2001b. 'You're Marked': Breast Cancer, Tattoo and the Narrative Performance of Identity. In *Narrative and Identity: Studies in Autobiography, Self, and Culture*, ed. Jens Brockmeier and Donal Carbaugh, 145–84. Philadelphia: John Benjamins.

———, and Eric E. Peterson. 2004. *Storytelling in Daily Life: Performing Narrative.* Philadelphia: Temple Univ. Press.

Langer, Lawrence. 1991. *Holocaust Testimonies: The Ruins of Memory.* New Haven, CT: Yale Univ. Press.

Lanham, Richard A. 1968. *A Handlist of Rhetorical Terms: A Guide for Students of English Literature*. Berkeley and Los Angeles: Univ. of California Press.

Laub, Dori. 1995. "Truth and Testimony: The Process and the Struggle." In *Trauma: Explorations of Memory*, ed. Cathy Caruth, 61–75. Baltimore: Johns Hopkins Univ. Press.

Lawrence, Marilyn. 1984. *The Anorexic Experience*. London: Women's Press.

Lazarre, Jane. 1998. *Wet Earth and Dreams: A Narrative of Grief and Recovery*. Durham, NC: Duke Univ. Press.

Leavitt, Fred. 2001. *Evaluating Scientific Research. Separating Fact from Fiction*. Upper Saddle River, NJ: Prentice Hall.

Leder, Drew. 1990. *The Absent Body*. Chicago: Univ. of Chicago Press.

Lejeune, Philippe. 1975. *Le pacte autobiographique*. Paris: Seuil.

———. 1989. *On Autobiography*. Trans. Katherine Leary. Minneapolis: Univ. of Minnesota Press.

———. 2005. *Signes de vie. Le Pacte autobiographique 2*. Paris: Seuil.

Lévinas, Emmanuel. 1981. *Otherwise Than Being: Or Beyond Essence*. Trans. Alphonso Lingis. The Hague: Martinus Nijhoff.

———. 1993. Philosophy and the Idea of the Infinite. In *To the Other: An Introduction to the Philosophy of Emmanuel Levinas*, trans. Adriaan Peperzak, 88–119. West Lafayette, IN: Purdue Univ. Press.

Leys, Ruth. 2000. *Trauma: A Genealogy*. Chicago: Univ. of Chicago Press.

Lieblich, Amia, Rivka Tuval-Maschiach, and Tamar Zilber. 1998. *Narrative Research: Reading, Analysis, and Interpretation*. London: Sage.

Lifton, Robert Jay. 1967. *Death in Life: Survivors of Hiroshima*. Charlottesville: Univ. of North Carolina Press.

———. 1973. *Home from the War*. New York: Simon and Schuster.

———. 1979. *The Broken Connection: On Death and the Continuity of Life*. New York: Simon and Schuster.

Lim, D. 1985. Nursing Care Study. Imprisoned by Fear. *Nursing Mirror* 161: 18–19.

Longmore, Paul K. 2003. *Why I Burned My Book and Other Essays on Disability*. Philadelphia: Temple Univ. Press.

Lonsdale, Susan. 1990. *Women and Disability: The Experience of Physical Disability among Women*. London: Macmillan.

Lorde, Audre. 1980. *The Cancer Journals*. San Francisco: Aunt Lute Books.

———. 1988. A Burst of Light. In *A Burst of Light*, 49–134. Ithaca, NY: Firebrand Books.

Lunsky, Yona (2002). *Psychosocial Risk Factors for Mental Health Problems in Adults with Developmental Disabilities*. Ontario Association for Developmental Disabilities Research conference, Richmond Hill, Ontario. p. 10.

Lupus Canada. http://www.lupuscanada.org.

Lyotard, Jean François. 1984. *The Postmodern Condition: A Report on Knowledge*. Minneapolis: Univ. of Minnesota Press.

Macsween, Morag. 1993. *Anorexic Bodies: A Feminist and Sociological Perspective on Anorexia Nervosa*. New York: Routledge.

Maerz, Ursula. 2001. Revolte und Requiem. *Die Zeit* 34 (16 August): 35.

Mairs, Nancy. 1986. On Living behind Bars. In *Plaintext*, 125–54. Tucson: Univ. of Arizona Press.

———. 1996. *Waist-High in the World: A Life among the Nondisabled*. Boston: Beacon.

Marx, Karl. 1964 [1884]. *The Economic and Philosophic Manuscripts of 1844*. New York: International Publishers.

Massumi, Brian. 1992. *A User's Guide to Capitalism and Schizophrenia: Deviations from Deleuze and Guattari*. Cambridge, MA: MIT Press.

Mattingly, Cheryl. 1991. The Narrative Nature of Clinical Reasoning. *American Journal of Occupational Therapy* 45 (11): 998–1005.

———. 1998. *Healing Dramas and Clinical Plots: The Narrative Structure of Experience*. New York: Cambridge Univ. Press.

———, and Linda C., eds. 2000. *Narrative and the Cultural Construction of Illness and Healing*. Berkeley and Los Angeles: Univ. of California Press.

———, and Mary Lawlor. 2001. The Fragility of Healing. *Ethos* 21 (1): 30–57.

Maynard, Fredelle Bruser. 1985. *Raisins and Almonds*. 2nd ed. Markham, ON: Penguin.

———. 1989. *The Tree of Life*. Markham, ON: Penguin.

McLellan, Faith. 1994. From Book to Byte: Narratives of Physical Illness. *Medical Humanities Review*. 8 (2): 9–21.

Menand, Louis. 1997. The Demise of Disciplinary Authority. In *What's Happened to the Humanities?*, ed. Alvin Kernan, 201–19. Princeton, NJ: Princeton Univ. Press.

Metzger, Deena. 1992. *Writing for Your Life: A Guide and Companion to the Inner Worlds*. San Francisco: HarperSanFrancisco.

Metzl, Jonathan. 2003. *Prozac on the Couch: Prescribing Gender in the Age of Wonder Drugs*. Durham, NC: Duke Univ. Press.

Michel, Doris. 1984. *"Fuss Fassen: Worin?" Krisen und Krisen Bestehen in Schreiben Über Sich Selbst*. Ed. Peter von Matt. Zürich: Univ. of Zurich Press.

Miedema, Baukje, and Janet Stoppard, eds. 2000. Asylum or Cure? Women's Experiences of Psychiatric Hospitalization. *Women's Bodies, Women's Lives*, ed. Baukje Miedema, Janet Stoppard, & Vivienne Anderson, 103–20. Toronto: Sumach Press.

Mishler, Elliot G. 1984. *The Discourse of Medicine: Dialectics of Medical Interviews*. Norwood, NJ: Ablex.

———. 1995. Models of Narrative Analysis: A Typology. *Journal of Narrative and Life History* 5 (2): 87–123.

———. 1999. *Storylines: Craft Artists' Narratives of Identity*. Cambridge, MA: Harvard Univ. Press.

Mitchell, David T. 2000. Body Solitaire: The Singular Subject of Disability Autobiography. *American Quarterly* 52 (2): 311–15.

Mitchell, S. Weir. 1904. The Evolution of the Rest Treatment. *Journal of Nervous and Mental Disease* (June): 368–73.

Monette, Paul. 1988a. *Borrowed Time: An AIDS Memoir*. San Diego: Harcourt Brace Jovanovich.

———. 1988b. *Love Alone: Eighteen Elegies for Rog.* New York: St. Martin's.
———. 1992. *Becoming a Man: Half a Life Story.* San Diego: Harcourt Brace Jovanovich.
———. 1994. *Last Watch of the Night: Essays Too Personal and Otherwise.* New York: Harcourt Brace.
Monks, John. 1989. Experiencing Symptoms in Chronic Illness: Fatigue in Multiple Sclerosis. *International Disability Studies* 11: 78–83.
Moorhouse, Jocelyn. 1997. *A Thousand Acres.* United States: Buena Vista Studios.
Morris, David B. 1998. *Illness and Culture in the Postmodern Age.* Berkeley and Los Angeles: Univ. of California Press.
Morrison, Martha. 1989. *White Rabbit: A Doctor's Own Story of Addiction, Survival, and Recovery.* New York: Crown.
Moss, Pamela, and Isabel Dyck. 2002. *Women, Body, Illness: Space and Identity in the Everyday Lives of Women with Chronic Illness.* New York: Rowman and Littlefield.
Murray, Timothy. 1997. *Drama Trauma: Spectres of Race and Sexuality in Performance, Video, and Art.* London: Routledge.
Musto, David. 1999. *The American Disease: Origins of Narcotics Control.* 3rd ed. New York: Oxford Univ. Press.
Muszynski, Leon. 1988. Improving on Welfare. *Policy Options* (March): 26–31.
Myers, Kimberly, ed. Forthcoming. *Illness in the Academy.* Purdue Univ. Press.
Nader, Kathleen, Nancy Dubrow, and B. Hudnall Stamm, eds. 1999. *Honoring Differences: Cultural Issues in the Treatment of Trauma and Loss.* Philadelphia: Taylor and Francis.
Narcotics Anonymous World Services. World Service Board of Trustees Bulletin #17, "What Is Addiction?" http://www.na.org/bull17-r.htm.
Nash, Christopher, ed. 1994. *On Narrative.* Chicago: Univ. of Chicago Press.
Neimeyer, Robert A. 1998. *Lessons of Loss: A Guide to Coping.* New York: McGraw-Hill.
———. ed. 2001. *Meaning Reconstruction and the Experience of Loss.* Washington, DC: American Psychological Association.
Nelson, Hilde Lindemann, ed. 1997. *Stories and Their Limits: Narrative Approaches to Bioethics.* New York: Routledge.
———. 2001. *Damaged Identities, Narrative Repair.* Ithaca, NY: Cornell Univ. Press.
———. 2002. 7 Things to Do with Stories. Paper presented at the Peter Wall Institute of Advanced Studies/University of British Columbia conference, "Narratives of Disease, Disability and Trauma." Vancouver, BC.
———. 2002. Context: Backward, Sideways, and Forward. In *Stories Matter: The Role of Narrative in Medical Ethics*, ed. Rita Charon and Martha Montello, 39–47. New York: Routledge.
Nietzsche, Friedrich. 1992. *Ecce Homo: How One Becomes What One Is.* Trans. R.J. Hollingdale. London: Penguin.
———. 1999. On Truth and Lying in a Non-Moral Sense. In *The Birth of Tragedy and Other Writings.* Ed. Raymond Geuss and Ronald Speirs. Trans. Ronald Speirs, 139–53. Cambridge: Cambridge Univ. Press.

———. 1974. *The Gay Science*. Trans. Walter Kaufmann. New York: Vintage.
Noe, Denise. 1996. The Mute Speak. *The Humanist* 56: 13–17.
Nolan, Christopher. 1987. *Under the Eye of the Clock: The Life Story of Christopher Nolan*. London: Weidenfeld and Nicolson.
Nuland, Sherwin B. 1993. *How We Die: Reflections on Life's Final Chapter*. New York: Vintage.
Oliver, Kelly. 1993. *Reading Kristeva. Unravelling the Double-bind*. Bloomington: Univ. of Indiana Press.
Oliver, Michael. 1996. *Understanding Disability: From Theory to Practice*. London: Macmillan.
Oral History Association. 1992. *Oral History Association Evaluation Guidelines*. Los Angeles: Oral History Association.
Orbach, Susie. 1986. *Hunger Strike: The Anorectic's Struggle as a Metaphor for Our Age*. New York: Norton.
Ortner, Sherry B. 1995. Resistance and the Problem of Ethnographic Refusal. *Comparative Studies in Society and History* 37 (1): 173–93.
Overboe, James. 2004. Articulating a Sociology of Desire: Exceeding the Normative Shadow. PhD diss., Univ. of British Columbia.
Pahor, Boris. 1995. *Pilgrim among the Shadows*. Orlando: Harcourt Brace.
Parker, Andrew, and Eve Kosofsky Sedgwick, eds. 1995. *Performativity and Performance*. New York: Routledge.
Parry, Alan, and Robert Doan. 1994. *Story Re-visions: Narrative Therapy in the Postmodern World*. New York: Guilford.
Parsons, Talcott. 1954. *Essays in Sociological Theory*. Glencoe, IL: Free Press.
Pascal, Roy. 1960. *Design and Truth in Autobiography*. Cambridge, MA: Harvard Univ. Press.
Patterson, Wendy, ed. 2002. *Strategic Narrative: New Perspectives on the Power of Personal and Cultural Storytelling*. Lanham, MD: Lexington Books.
Patton, Cindy. 2002. *Globalizing AIDS*. Minneapolis: Univ. of Minnesota Press.
Pearl, N. 2000. Beyond the McCourts: Irish Memoirs. *Library Journal* 125(20): 224.
Peavey, Fran. 1990. *A Shallow Pool of Time: An HIV-Positive Woman Grapples with the AIDS Epidemic*. Philadelphia: New Society.
Penfold, Susan. 1998. *Sexual Abuse by Health Professionals: A Personal Search for Healing and Meaning*. Toronto: Univ. of Toronto Press.
Pennebaker, James W. 1990. *Opening Up: The Healing Power of Expressing Emotions*. New York: Guilford Press.
———. 2000. Telling Stories: The Health Benefits of Narrative. *Literature and Medicine* 19 (1): 3–18.
Peterson, Eric E. 2000. Narrative Identity in a Solo Performance: Craig Gingrich-Philbrook's "The First Time." *Narrative Inquiry* 10 (1): 229–51.
Phillips, Susan S., and Patricia E. Benner, eds. 1994. *The Crisis of Care: Affirming and Restoring Caring Practices in the Helping Professions*. Washington, DC: Georgetown Univ. Press.
Plath, Sylvia. 1963. *The Bell Jar*. London: Faber and Faber.

Plummer, Ken. 1995. *Telling Sexual Stories: Power, Change, and Social Worlds.* New York: Routledge.
Poirier, Suzanne. 2002. Voice in the Medical Narrative. In *Stories Matter: The Role of Narrative in Medical Ethics*, ed. Rita Charon and Martha Montello, 48–58. New York: Routledge.
Polkinghorne, Donald E. 1989. *Narrative Knowing and the Human Sciences.* Albany, NY: SUNY Press.
Porter, Roy. 1997. *The Greatest Benefit to Mankind: A Medical History of Humanity from Antiquity to the Present.* New York: Norton.
Poser, C.M., D.W. Paty, W.I. McDonald, L. Scheinberg, and G.G. Ebres. 1984. *The Diagnosis of Multiple Sclerosis.* New York: Thieme-Stratton.
Potter, L.T. 1882. Agoraphobia: A Contribution to Clinical Medicine. *Chicago Medical Journal and Examiner* 45: 472–75.
Priestley, Mark, ed. 2001. *Disability and the Life Course: Global Perspectives.* Cambridge: Cambridge Univ. Press.
Prince, Gerald. 1982. *Narratology: The Form and Functioning of Narrative.* Berlin: Mouton.
Prince, Michael J. 1991. *The Disability Income System in Canada: A Literature Review and Policy Analysis.* Community Services Task Team of the Premier's Advisory Council for Persons with Disability, Victoria, British Columbia.
Prince, Stephen. 1999. *The Warrior's Camera: The Cinema of Akira Kurosawa.* Rev. ed. Princeton, NJ: Princeton Univ. Press.
Profitt, Norma Jean. 2000. *Women Survivors, Psychological Trauma, and the Politics of Resistance.* New York: Haworth.
Radley, Alan. 1989. Style, Discourse and Constraint in Adjustment to Chronic Illness. *Sociology of Health and Illness* 11 (3): 230–52.
———, and Diane Taylor. 2003. Images of Recovery: A Photo-Elicitation Study on the Hospital Ward. *Qualitative Health Research* 13 (1): 77–99.
Radner, Gilda. 1989. *It's Always Something.* New York: Avon Books.
Raoul, Valerie, Connie Canam, Gloria Onyeoziri, James Overboe, and Carla Paterson. 2001. Narrating the Unspeakable: Interdisciplinary Readings of Jean-Dominique Bauby's *The Diving Bell and the Butterfly. Literature and Medicine* 20 (2): 128–208.
Reiff, Philip. 1966. *The Triumph of the Therapeutic: Uses of Faith after Freud.* New York: Harper and Row.
Rhodes, Lorna A. 1993. The Shape of Action: Practice in Public Psychiatry. In *Knowledge, Power, and Practice: The Anthropology of Medicine and Everyday Life*, ed. Shirley Lindenbaum and Margaret Lock, 129–46. Berkeley and Los Angeles: Univ. of California Press.
Richardson, Laurel. 1990. Narrative and Sociology. *Journal of Contemporary Ethnography.* 19 (1): 116–135.
———. 1997. Narrative Knowing and Sociological Telling. In *Fields of Play: Constructing an Academic Life*, 26–35. New Brunswick, NJ: Rutgers University Press.
Ricoeur, Paul. 1985. *Temps et récit 3. Le temps raconté.* Paris: Éditions du Seuil.

———. 1990. *Soi-même comme un autre*. Paris: Éditions du Seuil.
Riessman, Catherine Kohler. 1990a. *Divorce Talk: Women and Men Make Sense of Personal Relationships*. New Brunswick, NJ: Rutgers Univ. Press.
———. 1990b. Strategic Uses of Narrative in the Presentation of Self and Illness. *Social Science and Medicine* 30 (11): 1195–1200.
———. 1992. Making Sense of Marital Violence: One Woman's Narrative. In *Storied Lives: The Cultural Politics of Self-Understanding*, ed. George C. Rosenwald and Richard L. Ochberg, 231–49. New Haven, CT: Yale Univ. Press.
———. 1993. *Narrative Analysis*. Qualitative Research Methods Series Vol. 30. Newbury Park, CA: Sage.
———. 1997. A Short Story about Long Stories. *Journal of Narrative and Life History* 7 (1–4): 155–59.
———. 2002a. Accidental Cases: Extending the Concept of Positioning in Narrative Studies. *Narrative Inquiry* 12 (1): 37–42.
———. 2002b. Analysis of Personal Narratives. In *Handbook of Interview Research: Context and Method*, ed. Jaber F. Gubrium and James A. Holstein, 695–710. Newbury Park, CA: Sage.
———. 2002c. *Illness Narratives: Positional Identities*. Invited Annual Lecture, Cardiff University, Health Communication Research Centre, Cardiff, Wales, May.
———. 2003. Performing Identities in Illness Narrative: Masculinity and Multiple Sclerosis. *Qualitative Research* 3 (1): 5–33.
Rimstead, Roxanne. 2001. *Remnants of Nation: On Poverty Narratives by Women*. Toronto: Univ. of Toronto Press.
Rioux, Marcia, Leon Muszynski, and Cameron Crawford. 1992. *Comprehensive Disability Income Security Reform*. Downsview, ON: Roeher Institute.
Robbins, Jill. 1991. *Prodigal Son/Elder Brother: Interpretation and Alterity in Augustine, Petrarch, Kafka, Lévinas*. Chicago: Univ. of Chicago Press.
Roberts, Brian. 1999. Some Thoughts on Time Perspectives and Auto/biography. *Auto/Biography* 7: 21–25.
Rodriguez, Lourdes. 2000. Les fils tenus du sens. Narration et soutiens socioculturels dans la constitution d'une position subjective face à l'expérience psychotique. PhD diss., UQAM.
Roe, Emery. 1994. *Narrative Policy Analysis*. Durham, NC: Duke Univ. Press.
Rose, Nikolas. 1994. Medicine, History, and the Present. In *Reassessing Foucault: Power, Medicine and the Body: Studies in the Social History of Medicine*, ed. Colin Jones and Roy Porter, 48–72. New York: Routledge.
Rosenbaum, J.F., R.A. Pollock, M.W. Otto, and M.H. Pollack. 1995. Integrated Treatment of Panic Disorder. *Bulletin of the Menninger Clinic* 59, 2 Suppl A: A4–26.
Rosenberg, Charles E. 1992. "Introduction" in *Framing Diseases: Studies in Cultural History*, ed. Charles E. Rosenberg and Janet Golden, xiii–xxvi. New Brunswick, NJ: Rutgers Univ. Press.
Rosenwald, George C., and Richard L. Ochberg, eds. 1992. *Storied Lives: The Cultural Politics of Self-Understanding*. New Haven, CT: Yale Univ. Press.

Roth, Tim. 1999. *The War Zone*. United States: New Yorker Films.
Rutland, Barry, ed. 1997. *Gender and Narrativity*. Ottawa: Centre for Textual Analysis, Discourse, and Culture.
Sacks, Oliver. 1984. *A Leg to Stand On*. New York: Summit.
———. 1985. *The Man Who Mistook His Wife for a Hat*. New York: Summit.
Sanchez-Hucles, Janis V. 1998. Racism: Emotional Abusiveness and Psychological Trauma for Ethnic Minorities. *Journal of Emotional Abuse* 1 (2): 69–87.
Sakalys, Jurate A. 2000. The Political Role of Illness Narratives. *Journal of Advanced Nursing*. 31 (6): 1469–475.
Schaub, Danielle. 1997. 'Released Sorrows Long Held in Check': Quest for Self-Knowledge in Fredelle Bruser Maynard's *Raisins and Almonds* and *The Tree of Life*. In *Union in Partition: Essays in Honor of Jeanne Delbaere*, ed. Gilbert Debusscher and Marc Maufort, 141–52. Liège, Belgium: Université de Liège.
Schechtman, Marya. 1996. *The Constitution of Selves*. Ithaca, NY: Cornell Univ. Press.
Scheff, Thomas J., ed. 1975. *Labelling Madness*. Englewood Cliffs, NJ: Prentice Hall.
Schiwy, Marlene. 1996. Healing Dimensions of the Journal. In *Voice of Her Own: Women and the Journal-Writing Journey*, 113–42. New York: Simon and Schuster.
Schmidt, Maja Saj. 1998. Literary Testimonies of Illness and the Reshaping of Social Memory. *A/b: Auto/Biography Studies* 13 (1): 71–91.
Schneider, Barbara. 2003. Narratives of Schizophrenia: Constructing a Positive Image. *Canadian Journal of Communication* 28 (2): 185–201.
———. 2005. Mothers Talk about Their Children with Schizophrenia: A Performance Autoethnography. *Journal of Psychiatric and Mental Health Nursing* 12: 333–40.
Schneider, B., H. Scissons, L. Arney, G. Benson, J. Derry, K. Lucas, M. Misurelli, D. Nickerson, and M. Sunderland. 2004. Communication between People with Schizophrenia and Their Medical Professionals: A Participatory Research Project. *Qualitative Health Research* 14 (4), 562–77.
Schor, Naomi. 1995. Depression in the Nineties. In *Bad Objects: Essays Popular and Unpopular*, 159–63. Durham, NC: Duke Univ. Press.
Schubert, J. Daniel, and Margaret Murphy. 2005. The Struggle to Breathe: Living at Life Expectancy with Cystic Fibrosis. *Oral History Review* 32 (1): 35–56.
Scott, Joan W. 1992. Experience. In *Feminists Theorize the Political*, ed. Judith Butler and Joan W. Scott, 22–40. New York: Routledge.
Sedgwick, Eve Kosofsky. 1993. Epidemics of the Will. In *Tendencies*, 130–42. Durham, NC: Duke Univ. Press.
Segal, Judy Z. *Health and the Rhetoric of Medicine*. Carbondale: Southern Illinois Univ. Press, 2005.
Semprún, Jorge. 1982. *What a Beautiful Sunday!* Trans. Alan Sheridan. San Diego: Harcourt Brace Jovanovich.
———. 1997. *Literature or Life*. Trans. Linda Coverdale. New York: Viking-Penguin.

———. 2001a. *Der Tote mit meinem Namen*. Trans. Eva Moldenhauer. Frankfurt/Main: Suhrkamp.

———. 2001b. *Die Ohnmacht*. Trans. Eva Moldenhauer. Frankfurt/Main: Suhrkamp.

———, and Elie Wiesel. 1997. *Schweigen ist Unmöglich*. Trans. Wolfram Bayer. Frankfurt/Main: Suhrkamp.

Seymour, Wendy. 2002. Time and the Body: Re-embodying Time in Disability. *Journal of Occupational Science* 9 (3): 135–42.

Shapiro, Kenneth A. 1985. *Dying and Living: One Man's Life with Cancer*. Austin: Univ. of Texas Press.

Shay, Jonathan. 1994. *Achilles in Vietnam: Combat Trauma and the Undoing of Character*. New York: Atheneum.

Sheldon, Barbara H. 1997. *Daughters and Fathers in Feminist Novels*. Frankfurt/Main: Peter Lang.

Shephard, Ben. 2000. *A War of Nerves*. London: Jonathan Cape.

Sherrid, Pamela. 1988. The Prison of Paralysis, the Freedom of Words: Cerebral Palsy Victim Christopher Nolan Writes of His Experiences. *US News and World Report*, March 14: 60.

Sherwin, Susan. 1998. *The Politics of Women's Health: Exploring Agency and Autonomy*. Philadelphia: Temple Univ. Press.

———. 1992. *No Longer Patient: Feminist Ethics and Health Care*. Philadelphia: Temple Univ. Press.

Shimrat, Irit. 1997. *Call Me Crazy: Stories from the Mad Movement*. Vancouver, BC: Press Gang.

Shorter, Edward. 1997. *A History of Psychiatry: From the Era of the Asylum to the Age of Prozac*. New York: John Wiley.

Sienkiewicz-Mercer, Ruth, and Steven B. Kaplan. 1989. *I Raise My Eyes to Say Yes*. West Hartford, CT: Whole Health Books.

Simmel, Georg. 1950. *The Sociology of Georg Simmel*. Ed. and trans. Kurt H. Wolff. Glencoe, IL: Free Press. (Orig. pub. 1903.)

———. 1978. *The Philosophy of Money*. Boston: Routledge and Kegan Paul. (Orig. pub. 1907.)

Simmons, Harvey G. 1982. *From Asylum to Welfare*. Toronto: National Institute on Mental Retardation [now the Roeher Institute—Eds.].

Simon, Bennett. 1988. *Tragic Drama and the Family: Psychoanalytic Studies from Aeschylus to Beckett*. New Haven, CT: Yale Univ. Press.

Singer, Linda. 1993. *Erotic Welfare: Sexual Theory and Politics in the Age of Epidemic*. New York: Routledge.

Sitte, Camillo. 1965. *City Planning According to Artistic Principles*. Trans. George R. Collins and Christiane Crasemann Collins. New York: Random House.

Skultans, Vieda. 2000. Narrative, Illness, and the Body. Special issue, *Anthropology and Medicine* 7 (1): 5–13.

Slater, Lauren. 1996. *Welcome to My Country: Journeys into the World of a Therapist and Her Patients*. New York: Anchor-Doubleday.

———. 1998. *Prozac Diary*. New York: Penguin.

———. 2001. *Lying: A Metaphorical Memoir*. New York: Random House.
———. 2003. *Love Works Like This: Travels through a Pregnant Year*. New York: Bloomsbury.
Smith, Brett, and Andrew C. Sparkes. 2002. Men, Sport, Spinal Cord Injury, and the Construction of Coherence: Narrative Practice in Action. *Qualitative Research* 2 (2): 143–71.
———. 2004. Men, Sport, and Spinal Cord Injury: An Analysis of Metaphors and Narrative Types. *Disability and Society*, 19 (6): 509–612.
———. 2005a. Men, Sport, Spinal Cord Injury and Narratives of Hope. *Social Science & Medicine* 61 (5): 1095–105.
———. 2005b. Analyzing Talk in Qualitative Inquiry: Exploring Possibilities, Problems, and Tensions. *Quest*, 57 (2): 213–42.
Smith, Dorothy. 1996. Telling the Truth after Postmodernism. *Symbolic Interaction* 19 (3): 171–202.
———. 1999. The Ruling Relations. In *Writing the Social: Critique, Theory, and Investigations*. Toronto: Univ. of Toronto Press. 73–95.
Smith, Sidonie. 1993. *Subjectivity, Identity, and the Body: Women's Autobiographical Practices in the Twentieth Century*. Bloomington: Indiana Univ. Press.
Solvay Pharmaceuticals. 1997. *Growing Older with CF: A Handbook for Adults*. Vol. 1. N.p.: Solvay Pharmaceuticals.
Somers, Margaret R. 1994. The Narrative Constitution of Identity: A Relational and Network Approach. *Theory and Society* 23: 605–49.
Sontag, Deborah, and Lynda Richardson. 1997. Doctors withhold HIV Pill Regimen from Some. *New York Times*, 2 March.
Sontag, Susan. 1977. *Illness as Metaphor*. New York: Vintage-Random House.
———. 1989. *AIDS and Its Metaphors*. London: Penguin.
———. 1990. *Illness as Metaphor* and *AIDS and Its Metaphors*. New York: Doubleday.
Sophocles. 1977. *Oedipus the King*. In *The Three Theban Plays*. Trans. Robert Fagles. New York: Penguin.
Sparkes, Andrew C. 1998. Athletic Identity: An Achilles' Heel to the Survival of Self. *Qualitative Health Research* 8 (5): 644–64.
———. 1999. Exploring Body Narratives. *Sport, Education, and Society* 4 (1): 17–30.
———. 2005. Narrative Analysis: Exploring the Whats and the Hows of Personal Stories. In *Qualitative Research in Health Care*, ed. M.Holloway, 91–109. Milton Keynes: Open Univ. Press.
———, and Brett Smith. 2002. Sport, Spinal Cord Injury, Embodied Masculinities, and the Dilemmas of Narrative Identity. *Men and Masculinities* 4 (3): 258–85.
———, and Brett Smith. 2003. Men, Sport, Spinal Cord Injury and Narrative Time. *Qualitative Research* 3 (3): 295–320.
Spivak, Gayatri Chakravorty. 1988. "Can the Subaltern Speak?" In *Marxism and the Interpretation of Culture*, ed. Cary Nelson and Larry Grossberg, 271–318. Urbana: Univ. of Illinois Press.

———. 1999. *A Critique of Postcolonial Reason: Toward a History of the Vanishing Present.* Cambridge, MA: Harvard Univ. Press.

Stacey, Jackie. 1997. *Teratologies: A Cultural Study of Cancer.* London: Routledge.

Steinhoff-Smith, Roy H. 1999. *The Mutuality of Care.* St. Louis, MO: Chalice.

Sterin, Gloria. 2002. Essay on a Word. *Dementia: The International Journal of Social Research and Practice* 1 (1): 7–10.

Stone, Deborah. 1984. *The Disabled State.* Philadelphia: Temple Univ. Press.

Stoppard, Janet M., and Linda M. McMullen, eds. *Situating Sadness: Women and Depression in Social Context.* New York: New York Univ. Press, 2003.

Strawson, Galen. 2004. A Fallacy of Our Age: Not Every Life Is a Narrative. *Times Literary Supplement,* 15 October: 13–15.

Styron, William. 1990. *Darkness Visible: A Memoir of Madness.* New York: Random House.

Suckling, C.W. 1890. Agoraphobia and Allied Morbid Fears. *American Journal of the Medical Sciences* 99: 476–83.

Sullivan, Andrew. 1996. When Plagues End: Notes on the Twilight of an Epidemic. *The New York Times Magazine,* 10 November, 52–62, 76–77, 84.

Sutherland, H. 1877. On 'Agoraphobia' (so called). *Journal of Psychological Medicine and Mental Pathology* 3: 265–69.

Szasz, Thomas. 1972. *The Myth of Mental Illness: Foundations of a Theory of Personal Conduct.* London: Paladin.

———. 1974. *Ceremonial Chemistry: The Ritual Persecution of Drugs, Addicts, and Pushers.* New York: Anchor/Doubleday.

Tal, Kalí. 1996. *Worlds of Hurt: Reading the Literatures of Trauma.* New York: Cambridge Univ. Press.

Taylor, Charles. 1994. Philosophical Reflections on Caring Practices. In *The Crisis of Care: Affirming and Restoring Caring Practices in the Helping Professions,* ed. Susan S. Phillips and Patricia E. Benner, 174–88. Washington, DC: Georgetown Univ. Press.

Teucher, Ulrich. 2001.Writing in the Face of Death: Norbert Elias and Autobiographies of Cancer. In *Norbert Elias and Human Interdependencies,* ed. T. Salumets, 159–74. Montreal and Kingston: McGill-Queen's Univ. Press.

———. 2003. The Therapeutic Psychopoetics of Cancer Metaphors: Challenges in Interdisciplinarity. Free Space: Reconsidering Interdisciplinary Theory and Practice, ed. Tamara Seiler & Bruce Janz. Special issue. *History of Intellectual Culture,* 3 (1): 1–15.

———. 2006. Renegade Cells: Patricia Blondal's Last Poem. In *The Winnipeg Connection: Writing Lives at Mid-Century,* ed. Birk Sproxton, 305–10. Univ. of Winnipeg: Prairie Fire Press.

Theriot, Nancy. 1997. Women's Voices in Nineteenth-Century Medical Discourse: A Step toward Deconstructing Science. In *History and Theory: Feminist Research, Debates, Contestations,* ed. B. Laslett, R.B. Joeres, M. Mayres, E.B. Higginbotham, and J. Barker-Nunn, 156–86. Chicago: Univ. of Chicago Press.

Thomas, John, and Wilfrid Waluchow. 1998. *Well and Good: A Case Study Approach to Biomedical Ethics.* Peterborough, ON: Broadview.

Thorpe, Geoffrey. 1998. Agoraphobia. In *The Encyclopaedia of Mental Health*, ed. Howard S. Friedman, 39–51. San Diego: Academic Press.
Titchkosky, Tanya. 2003. *Disability, Self, and Society*. Toronto: Univ. of Toronto Press.
Tönnies, Ferdinand. 1957. *Community and Society*. New York: Harper Torchbooks. (Orig. pub. 1887.)
Toombs, S. Kay. 1992. *The Meaning of Illness: A Phenomenological Account of the Different Perspectives of Physician and Patient*. Boston: Kluwer Academic.
———. 1995. Sufficient Unto the Day: A Life with Multiple Sclerosis. In *Chronic Illness: From Experience to Policy*, ed. S. Kay Toombs, David Barnard, and Ronald A. Carson, 3–23. Bloomington: Indiana Univ. Press.
Torjman, Sherri. 1988. *Income Insecurity: The Disability Income System in Canada*. Downsview, ON: Roeher Institute.
Torrey, E. Fuller. 1974. *The Death of Psychiatry*. Radnor, PA: Chilton.
———. 1996. *Out of the Shadows: Confronting America's Mental Illness Crisis*. New York: John Wiley.
———. 2001. *Surviving Schizophrenia: A Manual for Families, Consumers, and Providers*. New York: HarperCollins.
Trent, James W. 1994. *Inventing the Feeble Mind: A History of Mental Retardation in the United States*. Berkeley and Los Angeles: Univ. of California Press.
Turner, Victor W. 1986. Dewey, Dilthey, and Drama: An Essay in the Anthropology of Experience. In *The Anthropology of Experience*, ed. Victor W. Turner and Edward M. Bruner, 33–44. Urbana: Univ. of Illinois Press.
Ungerson, Clare. 1999. Personal Assistants and Disabled People. *Work, Employment and Society* 13: 583–600.
US Census Bureau. 2000. Statistical Abstract of the United States: 2000 (Table No. 191). 120th edition. Washington, DC.
US Department of Health and Human Services. (1986). *Health Status of the Disadvantaged Chartbook 1986* (DHHS Publication No. [HRSA] HRS-P-DV86-2). Washington, DC: Bureau of Health Professions/Division of Disadvantaged Assistance.
———. (1987). *Health Care Coverage by Sociodemographic and Health Characteristics, United States, 1984, Data from the National Health Survey Series 10, No. 162*. Hyattsville, MD: National Center for Health Statistics.
Van der Kolk, Bessel A. 1996. Trauma and Memory. In *Traumatic Stress: The Effects of Overwhelming Experience on Mind, Body, and Society*, ed. Bessel A. van der Kolk, Alexander C. McFarlane, and Lars Weisaeth, 279–302. New York: Guilford.
———, Alexander C. McFarlane, and Onno van der Hart. 1996. A General Approach to Treatment of Posttraumatic Stress Disorder. In *Traumatic Stress: The Effects of Overwhelming Experience on Mind, Body, and Society*, ed. Bessel A. van der Kolk, Alexander C. McFarlane, and Lars Weisaeth, 417–40. New York: Guilford.
———, Lars Weisaeth, and Onno van der Hart. 1996. History of Trauma in Society. In *Traumatic Stress: The Effects of Overwhelming Experience on Mind,*

Body, and Society, ed. Bessel A. van der Kolk, Alexander C. McFarlane, and Lars Weisaeth, 47–76. New York: Guilford.

———, Onno van der Hart, and Charles R. Marmar. 1996. Dissociation and Information Processing in Posttraumatic Stress Disorder. In *Traumatic Stress: The Effects of Overwhelming Experience on Mind, Body, and Society*, ed. Bessel A. van der Kolk, Alexander C. McFarlane, and Lars Weisaeth, 303–27. New York: Guilford.

Van Horn, A.K. 1886. A Case of Agoraphobia. *Chicago Medical Journal and Examiner* 52: 600–604.

Vanier, Jean. 1995. *An Ark for the Poor: The Story of L'Arche*. Toronto: Novalis.

———. 1998. *Becoming Human*. Toronto: House of Anansi.

Vertinsky, Patricia A. 1990 *The Eternally Wounded Women: Women, Doctors, and Exercise in Late Nineteenth Century.* Manchester, U.K.: Manchester Univ. Press.

Vidler, Anthony. 1991. Agoraphobia: Spatial Estrangement in Georg Simmel and Siegfried Kracauer. *New German Critique* 54: 31–45.

———. 1993. Bodies in Space/Subjects in the City: Psychopathologies of Modern Urbanism. *differences* 5 (3): 31–51.

Visker, Rudi. 2000. The Price of Being Dispossessed: Lévinas's God and Freud's Trauma. In *The Face of the Other and the Trace of God: Essays on the Philosophy of Emmanuel Levinas*, ed. Jeffrey Bloechl, 243–75. New York: Fordham Univ. Press.

Vos, E.A.D. 2003. *Cross-Cultural Dimensions in Conscious Thought: Narrative Themes in Comparative Context*. Lanham, MD: Rowman and Littlefield.

Waddington, Miriam. 1989. *Apartment Seven: Essays Selected and New*. Toronto: Oxford Univ. Press.

Walker, Janet. 1999. Textual Trauma in *Kings Row* and Freud. In *Endless Night: Cinema and Psychoanalysis, Parallel Histori*es, ed. Janet Bergstromm, 171–87. Berkeley and Los Angeles: Univ. of California Press.

———. 2005. *Trauma Cinema: Documenting Incest and the Holocaust*. Berkeley and Los Angeles: Univ. of California Press.

Walker, Margaret U. 1998. *Moral Understandings: A Feminist Study in Ethics*. New York: Routledge.

Walton, J. Michael. 1987. *Living Greek Theatre: A Handbook of Classical Performance and Modern Production*. New York: Greenwood Press.

Warhol, Robyn R., and Helena Michie. 1996. Twelve-Step Teleology: Narratives of Recovery/ Recovery as Narrative. In *Getting a Life: Everyday Uses of Autobiography*, ed. Sidonie Smith and Julia Watson, 327–50. Minneapolis: Univ. of Minnesota Press.

Warley, Linda. 1992. Inhabiting Contradiction: The Female Subject in *Don't: A Woman's Word*. *Open Letter* 8 (2): 70–80.

Webber, S.G. 1872. Agoraphobia Again. *Boston Medical and Surgical Journal* 10 (18): 445–47.

Weber, Max. 1958. *The Protestant Ethic and the Spirit of Capitalism*. Trans. Talcott Parsons. New York: Charles Scribner and Sons. (Orig. pub. 1904–1905.)

Weinfeld, Morton. 2001. *Like Everyone Else ... But Different: The Paradoxical Success of Canadian Jews*. Toronto: McClelland and Stewart.

Weissman, Myrna M. 1990. Epidemiology of Panic Disorder and Agoraphobia. *Psychiatric Medicine* 8 (2): 3–13.

Welter, Barbara. 1966. The Cult of True Womanhood: 1820–1860. *American Quarterly* 18 (2) (pt.1): 151–74.

Wendell, Susan. 1996. *The Rejected Body. Feminist Reflections on Disability*. New York: Routledge.

White, Michael, and David Epston. 1989. *Literate Means to Therapeutic Ends*. Adelaide: Dulwich Centre Publications.

———. 1990. *Narrative Means to Therapeutic Ends*. New York: Norton.

Widdicombe, Susan. 1998. Identity as an Analysts' and a Participants' Resource. In *Identities in Talk*, ed. Charles Antaki and Susan Widdicombe, 191–206. London: Sage.

Widerman, Eileen, Lois Millner, William Sexauer, and Stanley Fiel. 2000. Health Status and Sociodemographic Characteristics of Adults Receiving a Cystic Fibrosis Diagnosis after Age 18 Years. *Chest* 118: 427–33.

Wiesel, Elie. 1960. *Night*. New York: Bantam.

Wikan, Uni. 1992. Beyond the Words: The Power of Resonance. *American Ethnologist* 19: 460–79.

———. 1995. The Self in a World of Urgency and Necessity. *Ethos* 23 (3): 259–85.

Williams, Gareth. 1984. The Genesis of Chronic Illness: Narrative Re-construction. *Sociology of Health and Illness* 6 (2): 175–200.

———. 1993. Chronic Illness and the Pursuit of Virtue in Everyday Life. In *Worlds of Illness: Biographical and Cultural Perspectives on Health and Disease*, ed. Alan Radley, 92–108. London: Routledge.

Williams, Terry Tempest. 1991. *Refuge*. New York: Pantheon.

Williamson, Janice. 1993. Elly Danica: "An Enormous Risk, but It's Got to Be Done." In *Sounding Differences: Conversations with Seventeen Canadian Women Writers*, ed. Janice Williamson, 77–86. Toronto: Univ. of Toronto Press.

Winter, Angela R. 1996. "Faith in the Process": Reading Elly Danica's *Don't: A Woman's Word*. *Essays on Canadian Writing* 60: 187–98.

Wolff, J. 1989. The Invisible *Flâneuse*. Women and the Literature of Modernity. In *The Problems of Modernity: Adorno and Benjamin*, ed. by A. Benjamin, 141–156. New York: Routledge.

Wortham, Stanton E.F. 2001. *Narrative in Action: A Strategy for Research and Analysis*. New York: Teachers College Press.

Wurmser, Leon. 1978. *The Hidden Dimension: The Psychodynamics of Compulsive Drug Use*. Lanham, MD: Rowman and Littlefield.

Yoshimoto, Mitsuhiro. 2000. *Kurosawa: Film Studies and Japanese Cinema*. Chapel Hill, NC: Duke Univ. Press.

Young, Allan. 1993. A Description of How Ideology Shapes Knowledge of a Mental Disorder. In *Knowledge, Power, and Practice: The Anthropology of Medicine and Everyday Life*, ed. Shirley Lindenbaum and Margaret Lock, 108–28. Berkeley and Los Angeles: Univ. of California Press.

Young, Katherine. 2000. Gesture and the Phenomenology of Emotion in Narrative. *Semiotica* 131 (1–2): 79–112.
Zerubavel, Eviatar. 1979. *Patterns of Time in Hospital Life: A Sociological Perspective*. Chicago: Univ. of Chicago Press.
Zimmermann, Jeffrey, and Victoria Dickerson. 1996. *If Problems Talked: Narrative Therapy in Action*. New York: Guilford.
Zizek, Slavoj. 1989. *The Sublime Object of Ideology*. New York: Verso.
Zola, Irving Kenneth. 1982. *Missing Pieces: A Chronicle of Living with a Disability*. Philadelphia: Temple Univ. Press.
Zussman, Robert. 2000. Introduction. Autobiographical Occasions. Special issue, *Qualitative Sociology* 23 (1): 5–8.

Notes on Contributors

HELEN M. BUSS is a Professor Emeritus of English, University of Calgary, and has published novels, literary criticism, and books on women's autobiographical practices, as well as her own story, *Memoirs from Away: A New Found Land Girlhood*. Buss continues to read memoirs, but currently is occupied in writing a fiction based on her recent experience of the effects on self definition occasioned by the medical diagnosis of a chronic blood disorder. The study of Lauren Slater's approaches to narrating her challenges with mental illness are instructive in this regard, as contemporary experiments in memoir are teaching fiction writers new strategies. Transferring insights from one genre to another has always been a form of cross-disciplinary discovery, yet the art of fiction has so dominated literary study that little attention has been given to the way in which autobiographical tradition has contributed to how fictions are made. Slater brings together various narrative strategies chosen from medicine, science, and psychotherapy, as well as from fiction, poetry, and creative non-fiction, to make her memoir texts. In doing so she allows us to appreciate how a personal story authorizes itself, and gains its readers' trust and belief in the writer's sincerity.

SALLY CHIVERS, who was at UBC during the Wall project, is now a member of the English department at Trent University, where she also teaches Canadian studies. Her essay is part of her ongoing research into the cultural and social connections between aging and disability, which are more complicated than one initially might expect. Representation continues to be central in her research, which combines literary and film analysis, critical theory, focus group interviews, and work on social movements. In putting these elements together, narrative and narratology are useful in demonstrating the cultural and social stories that make disability and old age meaningful, in positive and negative ways. She is particularly interested in how artistic forms contribute to critical thought and social movements, especially in the growing field of disability studies and the Canadian disability movement.

HILARY CLARK (Department of English, University of Saskatchewan) has long been preoccupied with depression both as an ongoing condition in her life and a subject central to her research and teaching. She teaches a course for the Women's and Gender Studies Department entitled "Women, Depression, and Writing," focusing particularly on how personal narratives interpret and construct the experience of depression and the encounters depression entails with medication and therapies, an account of which is in *Teaching Life Writing Texts*, edited by Craig Howes and Miriam Fuchs (forthcoming). Her teaching includes the two narratives discussed in this volume, which analyze the experience of psychiatric hospitalization for depression. Her personal account of living with depression as an academic will appear in *Illness in the Academy*, edited by Kimberly Myers (forthcoming). Currently, she is assembling a volume of essays by contributors from a wide range of disciplines on depression and narrative. She also works on modernist writing from the perspective of trauma theory.

PAMELA CUSHING currently teaches courses in sociology, social justice, and peace, as well as disability studies, at King's University College, University of Western Ontario. While rooted in critical anthropological theory and ethnographic methods, her research in the area of impairment has been cross-disciplinary by necessity, given her interest in caregiving and developmental impairment(s). In this area, experimental narrative approaches are emerging to address issues of voice and representation, especially for people who do not use words to communicate. In her contribution, Cushing examines the ways in which informal narratives about everyday life can help those who work and share life with people with impairments, by facilitating continuity and contributing to an understanding of the histories of those who need care. Her research was extended in 2005 by fieldwork done with youth with complex developmental impairments and their co-workers in Scottish Camphill residential schools, using participant observation and co-created narratives about the youths' experiences of inclusion/exclusion there and elsewhere.

LISA DIEDRICH (Department of Women's Studies, SUNY–Stony Brook) is currently completing a book, *Treatments: Negotiating Bodies, Language, and Politics in Illness Narratives* (forthcoming, 2007, University of Minnesota Press). In it, she analyzes contemporary memoirs as both effective and affective histories, while being attentive to both the rhetoric and practices of politics as well as the poetics and practices of suffering. She calls her method for reading illness narratives "treatments," a term with multiple meanings, including "the process or manner of behaving towards or dealing with a person or thing"; "the application of medical care or attention to a patient, ailment, etc."; "a manner or instance of dealing with a subject or work of literature, art, etc."; and "a discussion or arrangement of terms, negotiation." Utilizing this method, she asks the following questions: What sort of subject is formed in the practice of writing memoirs in general, and illness narratives in particular? What sorts of knowledges are articulated in such writing? How does language both capture and fail to capture the "scenes of loss" portrayed in illness narratives? And, finally, what sort of ethics emerges out of such writing?

GAIL FINNEY. The essay by Gail Finney (Department of German, University of California-Davis) is part of a book project, tentatively titled *Children of Oedipus: Staging Family Trauma in Contemporary Cinema*, in which she currently is engaged. Her work was inspired by the marked increase in American cinematic depictions of extreme family trauma—radical alienation between family members, addictions of all kinds, child and spousal abuse, child molestation and parent–child incest, sibling incest, loss of one's child, suicide, and murder—since the early 1990s. This study of film grew out of her earlier work on narrative, as reflected in her books *The Counterfeit Idyll: The Garden Ideal and Social Reality in Nineteenth-Century Fiction* (1984) and *Christa Wolf* (1999), as well as in her study of Freudian theory (*Women in Modern Drama: Freud, Feminism, and European Theater at the Turn of the Century*, 1989); it also benefits from a collection she has edited entitled *Visual Culture in Twentieth-Century Germany: Text as Spectacle* (2006).

BINA TOLEDO FREIWALD teaches courses on women's writing, critical theory, and contemporary practices of self-representation in the English department at Concordia University. Her research approaches life-narratives in a variety of genres as privileged sites for the construction and interrogation of collective identities, where innovative writing practices convey agency and resistance. A central activity of her research has been to examine how oppressed, excluded, and often traumatized liminal subjects critique the dominant social order and negotiate *be/longing*: the subject's longing to belong so that s/he may "be." Her essay connects her earlier work on contemporary Canadian women's autobiography to her present project on the construction of national and diasporic identities in Jewish women's life narratives in pre-state Israel and Canada. Relevant publications include "Nation and Self-Narration: A View from Québec/Quebec" in *Canadian Literature* 172 (Spring 2002): 17–38; "Minnie Aodla Freeman's *Life Among the Qallunaat* and the Ethics of Subjectivity," in the edited volume *Postmodernism and the Ethical Subject*, ed. B. Gabriel and S. Ilcan (Montreal: McGill-Queen's University Press, 2004), 273–301; and "Gender, Nation, and Self-Narration: Three Generations of Dayan Women in Palestine/Israel," in the edited volume *Tracing the Autobiographical*, ed. M. Kadar, J. Perrault, S. Egan, and L. Warley (Waterloo: Wilfrid Laurier University Press, 2005), 165–88.

BARBARA HAVERCROFT. A member of the Department of French and the Centre for Comparative Literature at the University of Toronto, Barbara Havercroft has published extensively (mainly in French) on contemporary French, Québécois, and German autobiographical writings, especially those by women authors, and on the encounter between feminism and postmodernism in relation to literary theory. She is currently completing a book entitled *Voix intimes: sujet, sexe et genre dans les écrits autobiographiques contemporains*. As well as editing a number of special journal issues on related topics, she recently completed a SSHRC-funded research project on forms of discursive agency in recent women's autobiographical texts. Her latest project is entitled *"Unspeakable" Wounds: Social Trauma in Contemporary Women's Autobiographical Writings*," and deals with various forms of gender-related trauma (incest, family violence, anorexia, etc.), as represented in recent texts by francophone women writers from France, Québec, and Belgium.

ANNE HUNSAKER HAWKINS has long been fascinated with what she calls pathographies—narratives (most of them book-length) in which people describe their illness experience. In 1993, she published a story of these narratives as *Reconstructing Illness: Studies in Pathography*. At that time she took on a full-time appointment in the humanities department at the Penn State College of Medicine, where she now teaches courses in humanities to medical students and, sometimes, to clinicians. An important aspect of her work is trying to help medical students understand the patient's perspective on illness and treatment at the same time that students are being immersed (indoctrinated) into the culture of medicine. One dramatic way to help students come to an understanding of the patient's perspective on illness and treatment is to invite patients into the classroom. This essay stems from such an encounter, which raised concerns about the benefits and perils, to the teller, of narrating the story of a painful and disorienting experience. This discussion returns to the subject of her earlier book—autobiographies about illness—through the lens of trauma theory.

RICHARD INGRAM, who was a research assistant for the Wall project while working on his doctoral dissertation in interdisciplinary studies at UBC, has since been a post-doctoral research fellow in disability studies in the Department of Educational Studies, also at UBC. This essay is based on the second of four papers, presented at conferences in the United States, Canada, and England, and all concerned with societal demands to demonstrate an ability to conform to narrative. He has continued to reflect on the "order of making sense" (a concept introduced to describe the technique of power operating in and through narrative reason) as being at once a regime and a code of conduct, a mode of governance and an ethical injunction. Beyond his commitment to interdisciplinarity, he considers indiscipline to be necessary for the disruption of narrative reason, whether the latter is institutionalized in procedures of psychiatrization or academic learning. He believes in creating the conditions needed for more people to come out as psychiatric survivors, and this essay is dedicated to the memory of non-survivors, and to survivors isolated by fear.

JOY JAMES teaches in the Women's Studies Program at the University of British Columbia, and in the School of Critical, Cultural, and Historical Studies at the Emily Carr Institute of Art+Design+Media in Vancouver. Her essay is part of a larger transdisciplinary project on the politics of aesthetics in the formation of individual and collective subjectivities. James's research began with a study of the battles between art and psychiatry at the end of the nineteenth century, and continues on in her current investigation into how recent collaborative projects linking art, science, and new media technologies are impacting public policy decisions in Canada. Articulating how paradoxically productive limitations of narrative theory relate to the constitution of the "human" represents one of the ongoing concerns of her work.

HEIDI JANZ is a post-doctoral fellow with the interdisciplinary Vulnerable Persons and End of Life Care New Emerging Team (VP-Net) project in the Disability Studies Programme at the University of Manitoba. For her post-doctoral work, she is collecting journalistic narratives about some recent high profile cases involving people with disabilities and end-of-life issues. This essay is part of her ongoing project, which examines the dual roles that people with disabilities are often compelled to perform when they pursue careers in the TAB-dominated fields of academia or writing.

LYN JONGBLOED's work focuses on the interrelationships between disability and the social, economic, and political environment, and her essay examines the ways in which social policies shape individual narratives of disability. She and Mary Ann McColl are co-editors of a book entitled *Disability and Social Policy in Canada* (forthcoming, Captus Press). Her current work focuses on disability policies and she is planning a project which examines policy options related to the provision of assistive equipment and devices to people with disabilities in BC. As a faculty member in the School of Rehabilitation Sciences at UBC, she is concerned with helping occupational therapy students to learn to listen to the narratives of people with whom they work. She considers herself to be a cross-disciplinary researcher.

JANET MACARTHUR is a member of the English department at the University of British Columbia (Okanagan), where she teaches auto/biography and Renaissance literature. Most recently, she has presented and published papers on narratives of illness and disability. She is currently working on a collection of settlement-era life-writing and fiction by indigenous and non-indigenous women who lived in the Okanagan in the late nineteenth century.

JOANNE MUZAK is in the process of completing a doctoral dissertation entitled *High Lives/Low Lives: Women's Memoirs of Drug Addiction*, for the Department of English and Film Studies at the University of Alberta. This interdisciplinary project examines published memoirs of upper- and middle-class white women whose recountings of their lives as self-proclaimed "junkies" reflect medical discourses of addiction. In the late twentieth and early twenty-first century, this means that addicted women come to understand themselves as "sick" with the "disease" of addiction, as illustrated by the memoir discussed in her essay. Research in the cross-disciplinary terrain of addiction has recently led Muzak to explore the discursive resemblances between women's depression and drug addiction, and her article on Elizabeth Wurtzel's memoirs is included in Hilary Clark's forthcoming collection of essays on depression and narrative from SUNY Press.

GLORIA ONYEOZIRI, who was a member of the Wall project, teaches francophone, African, and Caribbean literature in the Department of French, Italian, and Hispanic Studies at UBC. Her current research is on the uses of irony, particularly as it developed in postcolonial texts that challenge the status quo. She has also written recently on her own experience of becoming blind.

JAMES OVERBOE teaches at Wilfrid Laurier University, in the Department of Sociology. In his work, he has adopted an interdisciplinary approach to sociology and to his research into marginalized bodies and subjectivity. His current research joins nuanced readings of poststructuralist theory with radical theories of subjectivity to discuss rupture as a productive force. His work in progress considers the complex relationship between disability and narrative, while some of his articles address the ways in which narrative can endorse ableism, while nevertheless having the potential to affirm "exposed" disabilities. He is also taking a critical look at bioethics, considering how metanarrative and case studies are often based on humanistic values that devalue disabled sensibilities as expressions of life.

ROBERT PROCYK AND CHRISTINE CROWE. Since their chapter was written, the Saskatchewan Indian Federated College was renamed the First Nations University of Canada and thus became the only First Nations-controlled university in North America. While retaining their commitment to the mission and mandate of the First Nations University of Canada, both Robert Procyk and Christine Crowe (née Watson) have since left FNUC. Procyk now coordinates the off-campus program for the University of Saskatchewan in Prince Albert, SK, while Crowe works for the Centre for Continuing Education at the University of Regina. In their new professional roles, both authors continue to work directly with Aboriginal students who are struggling to overcome personal, historical, and socio-cultural trauma in order to achieve academic success at the post-secondary level. As universities across Canada attempt to recruit and retain a growing number of Aboriginal students on their campuses, it is imperative that these post-secondary institutions devote resources to assisting students who are often found at the margins of academia and left behind by traditional university approaches to education. The challenge for universities today is to acknowledge the narratives of trauma that these students arrive with and, through careful attention to support programs and cultural environments, nourish a sense of community and safety that will allow these students to write new narratives of personal and academic post-secondary success.

JULIE RAK (Department of English and Film Studies, University of Alberta), focuses on non-fictional narratives (autobiography, biography and memoir) in print media, as well as in online environments and on television.

Her areas of scholarship include feminist and queer studies, minority writing, and popular culture in North America. Currently, she is working on an interdisciplinary project about the ways in which autobiography and biography produced for mass markets circulate as identity's form of capital. Her essay in this book forms part of her commitment to the study of life narratives by people who have experienced discrimination. As part of her desire to make the academy more accessible and equitable for everyone, she has co-taught with Heidi Janz at the University of Alberta. She also teaches Aboriginal students in the University of Alberta's Transitional Year Program (TYP).

SHELLEY Z. REUTER (Concordia University) teaches courses on the sociology of health and medicine, "race," knowledge, and feminist theories. The psychiatric narrative that she describes in her contribution to this volume is explored further in her book, *Narrating Social Order: A Reinterpretation of Agoraphobia* (forthcoming in 2007 from University of Toronto Press). She is continuing her interest in medical discourse as a narrative of social order in her current research on racialism in the discourse of genetics, which focuses in particular on the construction and reification of Tay-Sachs as a "Jewish genetic disease." Though a sociologist by training, her work tends to be interdisciplinary, drawing from and contributing to scholarship in the history of medicine, anthropology, geography, cultural studies, science studies, and women's studies.

LOURDES RODRIGUEZ DEL BARRIO (Department of Sociology, Université de Montréal) is director of the Mental Health and Culture Research and Action team there (Équipe de recherche et action en santé mentale et culture–ERASME). Her research deals with the points of view, speech, and practices of people living with mental health problems, a group that, largely, has been ignored by researchers, stakeholders, and policy and program makers. She has developed a research program designed to listen to, understand, and make heard these forgotten voices. Her work involves collecting and analyzing the subjective experiences of personal and social suffering and exclusion by people with mental health issues, and uses critical and hermeneutic theory to study both the alteration of personal identity and the impact of social support practices. From these perspectives, she currently is leading a number of assessment studies aimed at understanding the role played by a range of mental health practices and services in the life trajectories and everyday experiences of service users.

BARBARA SCHNEIDER (Faculty of Communication and Culture, University of Calgary) began her work on the discourses of mental illness after her son was diagnosed with schizophrenia in 2000. Her interdisciplinary work has gone in two directions: one path focuses on narrative and identity in the talk of people with schizophrenia and of the parents of schizophrenics (Schneider 2003, 2005), while the other involves participatory action research with a group of people who have schizophrenia. This collaboration has resulted in a project on communication between people with schizophrenia and their medical professionals (Schneider et al. 2004) and a new SSHRC-funded project on housing for people with severe mental illnesses. Both research projects have used performance as a way to present schizophrenia narratives to audiences. The members of the participatory group constructed a theatre presentation based on their experiences that they since have performed numerous times for groups of medical professionals. Schneider also developed a solo performance, based partly on her experience, to present the narratives of mothers of people with schizophrenia (Schneider 2005), which will play a strong role in the analysis and presentation of a current housing project.

J. DANIEL SCHUBERT is a faculty member in the Department of Sociology at Dickinson College in Carlisle, Pennsylvania. His work on cystic fibrosis represents a convergence of his professional work (a Bourdieuian approach to the sociologies of knowledge and deviance) and his personal life—Dan is a CF sibling. Metaphorically, he understands society as text and therefore works to integrate narrative research into the still largely positivistic discipline of American sociology. Currently, he is continuing his work on chronic illness and is also involved in research on the sociology of disaster. Along with a geologist at Dickinson, he recently took students to Montserrat to do an interdisciplinary study of the sociological and geological effects of the Soufriere Hills Volcano on that island. He believes that those who do work in illness studies and disaster studies could have much to say to and learn from each other about suffering, and the ways in which those who suffer tell their stories.

JUDY Z. SEGAL is a member of the Department of English at UBC, and participated in the Wall project. Her recently published monograph, *Health and the Rhetoric of Medicine*, takes up persuasion both as a neglected element in studies of health and medicine and as a transdisciplinary topic. Her current work is on pharmaceutical advertising as a rhetoric of values, with a special interest in representations and regulations of pleasure, especially social pleasure, in pharmaceutical ads. Judy teaches graduate and undergraduate courses in the history and theory of rhetoric and in the rhetoric of science and medicine at UBC, where she collaborates with philosophers, historians, scientists, and social scientists on projects in science and technology studies and sits on the President's International Advisory Committee of the Canadian Institutes of Health Research. All her work promotes wide-ranging studies of health, including questions, methodologies, and perspectives from the humanities.

BRETT SMITH AND ANDREW C. SPARKES. Brett Smith is a member and Andrew C. Sparkes is director of the Qualitative Research Unit in the School of Sport and Health Sciences at the University of Exeter, UK. The general research interests of this research group revolve around issues of embodiment, identity, and culture in sport and physical activity, which are focused upon via a range of approaches that include ethnography, auto/biography, life history, and narrative analysis. Current research projects, which are cross-disciplinary and interdisciplinary, include the lived experiences of becoming disabled through sport and the narrative reconstruction of selves; ageing bodies and sporting selves; body–self relationships in sporting auto/biographies; and the transformation of body–self relationships through the practice of Eastern movement forms. The group aspires to (re)present its findings to diverse audiences by utilizing a variety of genres that include realist tales, autoethnography, confessional tales, poetic representations, ethnodrama, and fictional representations.

SHARON DALE STONE (Lakehead University) is a sociologist also affiliated with the women's studies and gerontology programs. Her research focuses on experiences of living with chronic impairments, and issues that arise as a result of those impairments. She draws on work in the humanities, social sciences, social work, nursing, and medicine. Recently, she has begun to conceptualize her research in terms of occupational science—an interdisciplinary field that problematizes what people do, how they do it, why they do it, and to what effect. Narrative research is important in this context, because it examines the meaning of telling stories of traumatic illness and survival. This essay was written at an early stage of data collection for a project examining the narratives of women who survived a hemorrhagic stroke at a young age. Since then, Stone has interviewed many more women and has begun to publish analyses about different aspects of their experiences. Why women are motivated to tell their stories, and why they tell them as they do, remain important questions for investigation.

ULRICH TEUCHER (Department of Psychology, University of Saskatchewan) is a core member of the Program for Culture and Human Development there. His interdisciplinary and cross-cultural research builds on his work as a pediatric oncology nurse and his academic training in psychology and comparative literature. Using qualitative and quantitative analyses, he explores how narrative accounts of health and identity construct meaning with the help of narrative tropes such as metaphor. The discussion in her essay concerns the difficulties authors face in writing about "limit experiences" such as cancer, "factual" representation, and the limits of language. Fictionalization and other artful strategies may enable them to approximate more closely what seems incomprehensible and unrepresentable. Currently, Teucher is interviewing young Cree and non-Aboriginal cancer patients, collecting metaphors, drawings, and oral accounts in order to better understand children's cross-cultural experiences of illness. He is also collecting life-narratives from Aboriginal elders, and participating in a tri-cultural study of self-knowledge in British, Japanese, and Canadian Aboriginal children.

INDEX

able-bodied. *See* TAB (temporarily ablebodied)
ableism, and concept of post-personhood, 278–79, 281
Aboriginal peoples, colonization of, 204–205; and creation of First Nations college, 217–18; and importance of education, 220–21, 222; as problematic for students, 217–18, 222, 223–24. *See also* Saskatchewan Indian Federated College
Aboriginal post-secondary students: and curriculum, 220–21, 222; family problems of, 220, 221, 222–23; financial/housing support for, 221, 223; financial problems of, 220, 221, 223; as graduates/employees, 219; narratives of, 219–24; and need for community, 222, 223; withdrawal of, 218, 220, 225. *See also* Saskatchewan Indian Federated College
academic workplace: anti-Semitism in, 228; and difficulty of asking for help, 177, 178; exhausting pace of, 176–77; and fear of cognitive impairment, 177; as not accepting of illness/disability, 175–79; and obsession with knowledge/intellect, 288, 289–90, 291–92. *See also* Saskatchewan Indian Federated College

Aeschylus, 89, 90
aesthetic function of narrative, 6, 7, 25–31, 74–75, 301
age and aging. *See* elders
agencing, concept of (Chambers), 149, 151–52, 153, 157
agoraphobia, 49, 205–206, 247–54; and class, 251–52; as discussed in *DSM*, 252–54; as distinguished from shell shock, 251; first clinical account of, 247–48; and gender, 249–51; and race, 251–52; and urban life/social change, 248–49
AIDS, 53–60, 206; drug treatments for, 54, 57–59, 60nn8–9; early crisis years of, 26–27, 53–54, 57–58; and environment, 125; and Freudian theory of latency/trauma, 54; and narrative of shared experience, 53–57; and political activism, 57–58; possible end of, 59–60; as state of being "between two deaths," 55, 58; and testimonial/act of bearing witness, 53–54
Alzheimer's disease, 177, 277
American Psychiatric Association, 99, 118, 229, 240, 252. *See also DSM*
amplification, concept of (Chambers/Couser), 110, 149, 151, 153, 287
anorexia, 27; and mind/body opposition, 61–62, 66–67; and paradox of

349

self-control/self-destruction, 63–64; as protest against patriarchy, 63; and testimonial/act of bearing witness, 62, 64, 68; as woman's disease, 62–63, 64–65. See also *Petite*
"anti-psychiatry" movement, 238, 240, 242–43. See also mental illness; psychiatry
anti-Semitism: in academic workplace, 228; as experienced by Freud, 230–31; and Jewish identity, 227, 228, 231–33; prairie landscape, as symbol of, 232–33; in rural Canada, 227, 231–32; serial autobiography, as narrative of, 205, 227, 228–29, 230, 231–33; and sexism, 228, 230, 231–32, 233; as social trauma, 229–30
anti-Semitism narrative: confessional/testimonial functions of, 205; and Jewish identity, 227, 228, 231–33; and post-traumatic stress disorder, 229–30; prairie imagery in, 232–33; serial autobiography as, 205, 227, 228–29, 230, 231–33; unresolved ending of, 233
Aristotle, 89–90
assemblage, concept of (Deleuze/Guattari), 153, 155, 156, 157
atomic bombing of Japan, trauma caused by: as delayed reaction, 99, 116; and memory/suppression of memory, 29, 98–99, 100, 102, 104; and mental confusion, 97, 99, 102, 104; and reliving of catastrophic events, 97, 102–103; as shared by entire generation, 29, 99. See also Nagasaki; *Rhapsody in August*
Autobiographical Study, An (Freud), 230–31
autobiography, 80–81; confessional/testimonial functions of, 205, 234–35; and trauma recovery process, 117. See also disabled, autobiographies by
autobiography, serial, 205, 227–35; and anti-Semitism/Jewish identity, 205, 227, 228–29, 230, 231–33; and incest, 205, 227, 228–29, 233–35
autopathography, 25, 123, 171, 173. See also illness narrative; pathography

Bauby, Jean-Dominique, 6, 277–78, 280, 285
Baudrillard, Jean, 239–40, 241
Bearing, Vivian. See *Wit* (Edson), protagonist of
Belchertown State School (Massachusetts), 83, 86
Bell Jar, The (Plath), 46
Beutler, Maja, 27, 71, 73, 74–78
Beyond Don't: Dreaming Past the Dark (Danica), 227, 229, 234–35
Beyond the Pleasure Principle (Freud), 95
biomedical discourse. See medical discourse
Blackbridge, Persimmon, 110, 149–57. See also *Sunnybrook: A True Story with Lies*
Bluebond-Langner, Myra, 267, 270
"borderline personality disorder," 26, 46, 48
Borrowed Time (Monette), 27, 53, 54, 56; as quest narrative, 57–58
breast cancer, 113–14, 127
Brisac, Geneviève, 27, 62–63, 67–68, 110. See also anorexia; *Petite*

Canada/Quebec Pension Plan, disability benefits from, 210, 211, 212, 214, 215
Canadian Institutes of Health Research (CIHR), 9, 11–12
cancer, 18, 27, 71, 72–73
cancer, breast, 113–14, 127
cancer, ovarian. See *Wit*
cancer narrative, 71–78; and aestheticization of disease, 74; and difficulty of writing, 71–73; fictionalization of, 75–76; lack of closure in, 74; medical chronology of, 73. See also *Fuss Fassen*; *Wit*
Chambers, Ross, 110, 149, 151–53, 157, 287
Charmaz, Kathy, 266–67, 269
childhood immunization, 18–19
chronic illness: abjection of, 173; cultural/pathographic interest in, 42, 124; and definition of trauma, 118; and end-of-life issues, 266; as invisible, 174–75, 178; "journey" narrative of, 178–79; and "mind over matter"

myth, 175; as ongoing "interruption" of life, 266–67; as "Other," 171, 172; and testimonial narrative, 171. *See also* cystic fibrosis; lupus; multiple sclerosis
city life/social change, and agoraphobia, 248–49
communication, functions of (Jakobson), 6, 286. See also *Wit*
confessional narrative, 36–37, 38–39; autobiography as, 205, 234–35; psychoanalysis as, 254n3
Confessions (Rousseau), 80
cosmetic surgery, 19
"crips" (disabled), 80; personhood of, 281; and "supercrip" stereotype, 82–84, 87
cross-disciplinarity, 13, 298, 299; in narrative analysis, 207–208, 285–304. See also *Wit*
cystic fibrosis, 206, 265–72; description of, 268–69; and diminished future expectations, 269–71; and discovery of gene, 268, 269; illness narrative of, 266, 267, 268–69, 271–72; and life expectancy, 266, 269; as "normal" experience, 267, 271; oxygen supplements for, 268–69; parents' experience of, 270; people's reactions to, 265, 269; and routines of therapy/health care, 270–71; and sense of time, 267–68, 269–71

Danica, Elly, 205, 227, 228–29, 230, 233–35. *See also* incest narrative
Dantean journey, as image/theme, 46–47, 118
Darkness Visible: A Memoir of Madness (Styron), 46, 46–47
Death of Psychiatry, The (Torrey), 238
Deleuze, Gilles, 153, 240, 278, 281. *See also* Guattari, Félix
dementia, 276–77
depression, 45–46, 49
Derrida, Jacques, 242
Diagnostic and Statistical Manual for Mental Disorders. See *DSM*
diary, as narrative form, 38
disability income, for women with multiple sclerosis, 204, 209–16

disability narrative, 3–6, 25, 27–28, 124; coherence of, 111–12, 197–99. *See also* disabled, autobiographies by; L'Arche; multiple sclerosis; post-personhood; post-persons; spinal cord injuries
disabled: and able-bodied world, 79–80, 81–82, 84–86; "celebration"/romanticization of, 79–80, 82, 85, 87; as "crips"/"supercrips," 80, 82–84, 87; gender differences, in reactions of, 111; government assistance for, 209–16; institutions for, 86–87; "invisible" symptoms of, 211–12, 214; "normal" lives of, 85–86; society's obligation to, 215–16; stigma/negative perceptions of, 160–61. *See also* multiple sclerosis; post-personhood; post-persons; spinal cord injuries
disabled, autobiographies by, 27–28, 79–87; as facilitated by able-bodied world, 81, 83, 84–85; and normalcy of subjects' lives, 85–86; political intentions of, 81–82, 83, 86–87; and stereotype of "supercrip," 82–84, 87
disease narrative. *See* illness narrative
Diving Bell and the Butterfly, The (Bauby), 6, 277–78, 280, 285
doctors, characterization of, 47–48, 289, 290, 292, 294
Donne, John, 287, 289, 292, 294, 295
Don't: A Woman's Word (Danica), 227, 228, 233–34
drug addiction: early demographics of, 256–57; early views of, 256; and federal drug legislation, 256–57; imprisonment and institutionalization for, 257; as postwar white middle-class phenomenon, 257–58, 259; "reinvention" of, as disease, 258
drug addiction as disease, concept of, 206, 255–63; as biological/physiological, 258; early history of, 256–57; feminist criticism of, 260; as legitimizing white middle-class drug use, 255–56, 258, 262, 263; as postwar phenomenon, 257–58, 259; as promoted by therapy groups, 260, 264n8; "symptoms" of, 259. *See also* Morrison, Martha

drugs/drug treatments: for cancer, 72; for HIV/AIDS, 54, 57–59, 60nn8–9; for mental illness, 36–37, 48, 49, 50; for multiple sclerosis, 213; for schizophrenia, 135, 145, 146, 147

DSM (*Diagnostic and Statistical Manual for Mental Disorders*), 237; as "apparatus of capture," 240, 244n5; diagnostic categories of, 239–41; racial context of, 252; and shift away from psychoanalysis, 252–54; 3rd ed. (*DSM-III*), 99, 118–19, 252; 3rd rev. ed. (*DSM-III-R*), 99, 119, 239; 4th ed. (*DSM-IV*), 119, 124; 4th rev. ed. (*DSM-IV-TR*), 229, 239

Durkheim, Emile, 248

Early Psychosis Intervention Program (Vancouver/Richmond), 240–41, 243

Ecce Homo (Nietzsche), 154

Edson, Margaret, 207–208, 285–86, 292; background of, 286–87, 288. See also *Wit*

elders: and intergenerational relationships, 97–98, 100, 101, 102–103; as narrators of past history, 98, 100, 101, 104; and shared experience of catastrophe, 99. See also atomic bombing of Japan; Nagasaki; *Rhapsody in August*

elders, as war survivors: delayed reaction of, 99; and memory/suppression of memory, 98–99, 100, 102, 104; mental confusion of, 97, 99, 102, 104; as reliving catastrophic events, 97, 102–103. See also atomic bombing of Japan; Nagasaki; *Rhapsody in August*

Euripides, 89, 90

family trauma: in film, 90–91; in Greek drama, 89–91. See also incest

film treatments of narratives, 26, 28–29. See also *Rhapsody in August*; *War Zone*; *Wit*

First Nations. See Aboriginal peoples

First Nations University of Canada (Saskatchewan), 204. See also Saskatchewan Indian Federated College

Foucault, Michel, 242

Frank, Arthur, 107, 176, 191; on illness, 174, 177, 178, 267; and illness narrative, 108, 265, 272; and narrative templates, 20, 108, 111, 295; and quest narrative, 57, 111, 199; and restitution narrative, 111, 192

Freud, Sigmund, 54, 80, 91, 165: anti-Semitism towards, 230–31; and study of hysteria, 230–31; on stress of urban life, 248; trauma theory of, 54, 91, 92, 95, 115–16, 230–31

functions of communication (Jakobson), 6, 286. See also *Wit*

Fuss Fassen [*Gaining a Foothold*] (Beutler), 71, 74–78; and aestheticization of cancer, 27, 74, 76–78; change as continuity in, 77–78; as compared to Holocaust narratives, 74–75; fragmented narration of, 76–77; and writing as survival strategy, 77–78

Geneviève, Saint, 67–68

Girl, Interrupted (Kaysen), 26, 45–46, 47–49

Gonzalez, David, 238–39

Greek drama, and subject of family trauma, 89–91

Guattari, Félix, 153, 240, 241–42, 278, 281

Harrison Anti-Narcotic Act (U.S.), 257

hemorrhagic stroke, women as survivors of, 111, 181–88; and exclusion from popular discourse, 181, 188; and experiences of child/young victims, 183–84, 185–87; impacts on, as generally positive, 184–88; and journey metaphor, 186–87, 188; and misdiagnosis, 183; overview of, 182

Herman, Judith, 93, 120–21, 122, 125, 126, 229

Hiroshima, bombing/survivors of, 116, 117

Holocaust: Freud's comments on, 230–31; and importance of testimony, 121–22; narrative of, as artistic construct, 74–75; survivors of, 56; trauma caused by, 116, 121, 122

Horwitz, Roger, 53

hospitalization narrative, 45–52; characterization of doctors in, 47–48, 50; in context of sexist society, 46, 49, 50–51; as descent into hell, 46–47; humour/satire in, 46, 48–49; lack of closure in, 46, 51–52; and lost/missing time, 46, 47, 49–50, 52; and medical report as narrative form, 47, 48; survival in, 48–49; as testimonial/act of bearing witness, 46, 51; as therapeutic, 46, 51. *See also* psychiatric hospitals; psychosis; *Sunnybrook: A True Story with Lies*

hospitals and institutions: conditions/abuse in, 83, 86, 125, 160; for disabled, 83, 86–87; doctors in, 47–48, 50; and narratives by caregivers, 163–64; and postwar deinstitutionalization, 238; survival in, 48–49. *See also* disabled; disabled, autobiographies by; hospitalization narrative; L'Arche; psychiatric hospitals; *Sunnybrook: A True Story with Lies*

human connection, need for, 124–25, 143, 145. See also *Wit*

humour/satire: in confessional narrative, 39; in hospitalization narrative, 46, 48–49, 157

hysteria, 230–31, 251

illness: as associated with women, 301; battle myth of, 172; as "call for stories," 71; as identity, 45, 87, 129–37; as "other" place, 171; as puzzle rather than mystery, 179; as unfamiliar land, 298. *See also specific illnesses*

illness, chronic: abjection of, 173; cultural/pathographic interest in, 42, 124; and definition of trauma, 118; and end-of-life issues, 266; as invisible, 174–75, 178; "journey" narrative of, 178–79; and "mind over matter" myth, 175; as ongoing "interruption" of life, 266–67; as "Other," 171, 172; and testimonial narrative, 171. *See also* cystic fibrosis; lupus; multiple sclerosis

illness narrative, 3–6, 25, 26–27, 42–43. *See also* pathography; *see also specific illnesses*

incest, film depictions of, 28, 91–92; and Freudian theory of trauma, 91, 92, 95; and experience of witness, 95–96; as graphic, 94–96; and patriarchal power, 93; and recollection by victims, 92–93; as symbolic, 93–94; through settings, 93–94, 95–96

incest narrative: confessional/testimonial functions of, 205, 234–35; as moving from healing process to political action, 234; and post-traumatic stress disorder, 229–30; and racism, 227, 228, 233–34; serial autobiography as, 205, 227, 228–29, 233–35; and social trauma, 229–30

"indelible image" of trauma, 102, 117, 118, 120, 127

institutions and hospitals: conditions/abuse in, 83, 86, 125, 160; for disabled, 83, 86–87; doctors in, 47–48, 50; and narratives by caregivers, 163–64; and postwar deinstitutionalization, 238; survival in, 48–49. *See also* disabled; disabled, autobiographies by; hospitalization narrative; L'Arche; psychiatric hospitals; *Sunnybrook: A True Story with Lies*

interdisciplinarity, 12–13, 299; challenges of, 299; examples of, 13; problems of, for researchers, 14–16

interdisciplinarity, in health research, 11–22, 299; dissemination of, 15; examples of need for, 17–19; expertise required for, 15; funding for, 14; and peer review, 14; and postdisciplinarity, 16–22; and university appointments/tenure, 14–15

I Raise My Eyes to Say Yes (Sienkiewicz-Mercer), 79, 81, 82–83, 85–86

It's Always Something (Radner), 73–74

Jakobson, Roman, 6, 285, 286

journey, image/myth of: in chronic illness narrative, 178–79; and hemorrhagic stroke, 186–87, 188; and psychiatric hospitalization, 46–47; and trauma recovery process, 117–18

Kaysen, Susanna, 26, 45–46, 47–49, 50, 51, 52; "borderline personality

disorder" of, 26, 46, 48; characterization of doctors by, 47–48; drugs given to, 48, 49; humour/satire of, 46, 48–49; and lost/missing time, 46, 47, 49–50, 52; survival tactics of, 48–49
Kleinman, Arthur, 172, 175, 227, 229, 267
Kurosawa, Akira, 29, 97, 98–100. *See also Rhapsody in August*

Lacan, Jacques, 54, 55, 56, 173, 288, 297–98
language: and Aboriginal identity, 218; Joycean, as used by Christopher Nolan, 86, 87; regenerative potential of, 77–78; spoken/written, as prerequisite for personhood, 278; as therapy for schizophrenia, 35; as used to counter/resist medical discourse, 292–94
L'Arche, and use of narrative/storytelling by caregivers, 159–60; to counter negative attitudes towards disabled, 160–61, 166–67; to demonstrate inclusion/value of disabled, 159–60, 163, 164–65; to develop residents' histories, 164, 166; examples of, 161–63, 164–65, 166–69; and "narrative gap" of institutional care, 163–64; social function of, 163; as sometimes problematic, 168–69; teaching function of, 165–66; to understand/acknowledge differences, 163
latency and trauma, Freudian theory of, 54, 92
Lazarre, Jane, 42–43
letter, as narrative form, 38
Lifton, Robert J., 117–18, 120, 124–25
Locked-In Syndrome (LIS), 6, 277–78, 280
Love Alone (Monette), 53
Lowell, Robert, 46
lupus, 110–11, 171–79; and academic workplace, 175–79; active phase of, as "Other," 172–73, 176; cognitive dissonance of, 173, 175; as difficult to diagnose, 174; and disruption of daily life/identity, 173–74; flares of, 172, 173; as invisible illness, 174–75; living with, in able-bodied world, 173, 174–75, 176; nature of, 171, 172, 173; self-blame for, 174; and "self-in-life"/"self-in-illness," 171–73
lying, 39–40, 150
Lying: A Metaphorical Memoir (Slater), 26, 33, 34, 39–42, 43, 110

"mad movement," 238, 240, 242–43. *See also* mental illness; psychiatry
Mairs, Nancy, 26, 45–47, 49–52, 272; characterization of doctors by, 50; drugs given to, 50; and lost/missing time, 49–50, 52; and permanent societal "prison" of, 51–52; as subjected to shock therapy, 49–50, 51; survival tactics of, 50
Marx, Karl, 248
Maynard, Fredelle Bruser, 205, 227, 228–29, 230, 231–33. *See also* anti-Semitism; serial autobiography
McLean Hospital (Massachusetts), 46, 47
medical discourse: as antithesis of narrative, 6, 20, 46, 47, 299–300; and chronology of cancer narratives, 73; and schizophrenic identity narrative, 129–37; of trauma, as problematic, 229; as white middle-class male construct, 300. *See also DSM*
medical reports/documents, as narrative form, 38–39, 47, 48, 76
memoir. *See* Slater, Lauren
mental illness: "borderline personality disorder," 26, 46, 48; concept of, as rejected by "mad movement," 238, 240; in context of sexist society, 46, 49; and diagnostic categories of *DSM*, 239–41; hospitalization for, 45–52; "making sense of," 241–43; and postwar expansion of psychiatry, 237–41. *See also* psychiatric narrative; psychiatry; psychosis; schizophrenia
metanarrative, 111, 203–208; as white middle-class male discourse, 300; in *Wit*, 290–92. *See also* Aboriginal peoples; anti-Semitism; drug addiction as disease; *DSM*; incest narrative; medical discourse; multiple sclerosis; postpersonhood; psychiatric narrative; racism

Metropolitan State Hospital (Massachusetts), 46
Monette, Paul, 26–27, 53–60; as being "between two deaths," 55, 58; and quest for "magic bullet," 57–58, 59; and shared experience of AIDS/death, 53–57; as survivor, 54, 56
Morrison, Martha, 206, 255–56, 258–63; background and family life of, 261–62; drug addiction of, as legitimized by white middle-class privilege, 261–62, 262–63; early drug use "symptoms" of, 259; as embracing concept of addiction as disease, 260–61, 262; and gender/class stereotypes of addiction, 262–63; life story/social identity constructed by, 256, 259–60, 260–61, 263; marriage of, as signalling recovery, 262, 263; "street junkie" persona of, 262–63; tough/tomboy persona of, 262. *See also* drug addiction
multidisciplinarity, 12–13
multiple sclerosis, women with, 204, 209–16; and access to disability benefits, 211–12; and adequacy of disability benefits, 212–13, 215; as denied part-time work, 214–15; drug costs/coverage for, 213; employment/unemployment situations of, 211–12, 213, 214–15; fatigue of, 211–12, 214; insurance coverage of, 213, 215; physicians' assessment of, 211–12, 214; and problem of "invisible" disability, 211–12, 214; provincial social assistance for, as inadequate, 215; reduced social activities of, 212–13; and society's obligation to disabled, 215–16
Munchausen syndrome, 41
Murdoch, Iris, 29
My Left Breast (play/film), 286

Nagasaki, bombing of, 29, 97–98; as experience of entire generation, 29, 99; flash of, 102; as juxtaposed with present events, 97, 101, 102, 103–104; memorials to, 97, 98, 100; physical/mental effects of, 97, 98, 101–102; as recalled by survivor, 29, 97, 100; as relived by survivor, 97, 102–103. *See also* atomic bombing of Japan; elders; *Rhapsody in August*
Narcotics Anonymous, 260, 262, 264n8
narrative, 3; aesthetic function of, 6, 7, 25–31, 74–75, 301; coherence of, 303; of disability, 3–6, 25, 27–28, 124; feminist work in, 301; as giving voice to "unfitting"/marginalized, 303; of illness, 3–6, 25, 26–27, 42–43; medical discourse, as antithesis of, 6, 20, 46, 47, 299–300; and "order of meaning," as contested, 303; polemical function of, 6, 7, 8, 203–208; political/social context of, 203–208, 301; templates of, 20, 108, 111, 295; of trauma, 3–6, 25, 28–29, 119–23. *See also* therapeutic function of narrative. *See also specific illnesses and types of narrative*
narrative, as literary/artistic construct, 25–31, 74–75; coherence of, 28; documentary value of, 29–31, 109; film treatments of, 26, 28–29, 285, 291; functions of, 6–7, 286; medical discourse, as antithesis of, 6, 20, 46, 47, 300; and postdisciplinary research, 19–22; as testimonial/act of bearing witness, 45, 49, 53–54, 62, 64, 68; as therapeutic, 46, 51, 62–63, 64, 71. *See also* metanarrative; qualitative research and therapeutics; *Wit*
"narrative gap," of institutional care, 163–64
narrative templates (Frank), 20, 108, 111, 295; quest narrative, 57–58, 111, 199; restitution narrative, 111, 192, 193, 194, 196, 197–99
narrative therapy, as moral imperative, 243. *See also* mental illness; psychiatric narrative; psychiatry
Nietzsche, Friedrich, 149, 150, 153–55, 156
Nolan, Christopher, 28, 79–80, 81, 82–87; and able-bodied "saviours," 84–85; "celebration"/romanticization of, 79–80, 85, 87; as "charity cripple," 84; as defined by disability, 87; normalcy of, 86; and stereotype of

"supercrip," 82–84, 87; use of Joycean language by, 86, 87. See also disabled, autobiographies by

"On Living Behind Bars" (Mairs), 45, 49–52
"On Truth and Lying in a Non-Moral Sense" (Nietzsche), 150
Oprah Winfrey Show, The, 36
"Other": as able-bodied, 276; as face of chronic illness, 171–72, 176
ovarian cancer. See Wit

Pahor, Boris, 74, 75
pain, 12, 30, 115, 172, 175, 247, 267, 290, 294
pathography, 5, 20, 25, 42, 113, 117; and need for human connection, 124–25; and social/political activism, 125–26; topics of, 124; and trauma theory, 120, 123–26. See also illness narrative. See also specific illnesses
personhood: degrees of, 275–76; life stories of, 206–207; spoken/written language, as prerequisite for, 278. See also post-personhood; post-persons; pre-personhood
Petite (Brisac), 27, 61–68; as exemplum, 68; heroic figures in, 67–68; and mind/body opposition, 66–67; mouth, as symbol in, 65–66; narration of, 62, 64, 67–68; and paradox of self-control/self-destruction, 63–64; and reading as nourishment, 66–67; and symbolism of lean syntax, 62, 65; as testimonial/act of bearing witness, 62, 64, 68; as therapeutic, 62–63, 64; title of, 64–65
pharmaceutical industry, 238; and narrative, 243, 244
Pilgrim among the Shadows (Pahor), 74, 75
plague narrative, 58. See also AIDS; Monette, Paul
polemical function of narrative, 6, 7, 8, 203–208
political/social activism: by AIDS patients, 57–58; by disabled, 81–82, 83, 86–87; by incest survivors, 234; and pathography, 125–26

political/social context of narrative, 203–208, 301
postdisciplinarity, in health research, 16–22; examples of need for, 17–19; and narrative, 19–22
post-personhood, concept of, 206–207, 275–82; as ableist, 278–79, 281; and "living wills," 280; narratives of, as problematic, 278, 281–82; and privileging of language, 278; as reinforced by compassion, 277, 279–81; as rooted in fear of disability, 278, 279, 280; reactions to, 276–77. See also personhood; pre-personhood
post-persons: abjection of, 279–80; "compassionate killing" of, 279–81; dismissal of, 277; and interaction with able-bodied "Other," 276; as invisible, 276–77; reduced language skills of, 278; as "suffocated by kindness," 277. See also personhood; pre-personhood
post-traumatic stress disorder (PTSD), 118–19, 124, 229
pre-personhood, 275, 278, 280–81. See also personhood; post-personhood; post-persons
prosopopoeia, 151–52, 153, 154. See also Sunnybrook: A True Story with Lies
protease inhibitors, 54, 58–59
Prozac, 241, 243
Prozac Diary (Slater), 33, 34, 36–39, 43
psychiatric hospitals, 46, 47; admission to, as death threat, 144–45; alternatives to, 145–46, 147; doctors in, 47–48, 50; drugs given in, 48, 49, 50, 135, 145, 146, 147, 240; involuntary commitment/treatment in, 240; lost/missing time in, 46, 47, 49–50, 52; shock therapy administered in, 49–50, 51, 240; solitary confinement in, 49; stopped time in, 144, 145; survival in, 48–49. See also hospitalization narrative; mental illness; psychosis
psychiatric narrative: of agoraphobia, 247–54; as based on concept of mental illness, 237–41; and narrative therapy, as moral imperative, 243; and need for critique of, 244; and "order of making sense," 241–43; and phar-

maceutical industry, 243, 244; rejection of, by "mad movement," 238, 240, 242–43; and shift from psychoanalysis to biopsychiatry, 252–54
psychiatry: and *DSM*, 239–40; and "making sense" of mental illness, 241–43; and opposition of "mad movement," 238, 240, 242–43; postwar expansion of, 205, 238–39; and ties with pharmaceutical industry, 238, 243, 244; and "war" on mental illness, 237–41
psychoanalysis, decline of, 252–54
psychosis, 109–10, 139; concept of, as rejected by "mad movement," 238, 240; intervention program for, 240–41, 243; "making sense of," 241–43; negative public view of, 237. *See also* mental illness; psychiatric narrative; psychiatry; schizophrenia
psychosis, life history narrative of, 141–42, 205; garden image in, 143–44, 146; hospitalization in, as death threat, 144–45; and isolation from "real"/"normal" life," 141, 143, 144, 145, 147; and need for human connection, 143, 145; personal space in, 146; and prayer, as therapeutic, 146; street image in, 142–43, 144, 145, 146, 147; time and space in, 140, 146–47; timeline of, 140–42; violence in, 141, 142–43, 144, 145. *See also* schizophrenia
"psych wars," 205, 237–44. *See also* mental illness; psychiatric narrative; psychiatry
PTSD (post-traumatic stress disorder), 118–19, 124, 229

qualitative research and therapeutics, narrative in, 107–12; "broken stories" of, 112; as compared to artistic narrative, 108, 109; and "narrative templates," 108–109
quest narrative, 111, 199; AIDS narrative as, 57–58

racism: and Aboriginal peoples, 204–205, 217–18, 222; as experienced with sexism, 204, 205, 228, 230, 231–32, 233; and health research on women, 204; serial autobiography, as narrative of, 205, 227, 228–29, 230, 231–33; and study of agoraphobia, 251–52. *See also* anti-Semitism; Danica, Elly; Maynard, Fredelle Bruser
Radner, Gilda, 73–74
Raisins and Almonds (Maynard), 227, 228, 231–32
Refuge (Williams), 292
restitution narrative, 111; of spinal cord injury victims, 192, 193, 194, 196, 197–99
Rhapsody in August (film), 29, 97–104; closing scene of, 99, 102–103; indirect storytelling of, 99, 101–102; and theme of recollection, 98. *See also* atomic bombing of Japan; elders; Nagasaki
Roland (medieval hero), 67
rugby, injuries suffered in. *See* spinal cord injuries

Sacks, Oliver, 117–18
SAGA (Centre for Studies in Autobiography, Gender, and Age), 9–10
SARS outbreak (Toronto), 17–18; and stigma attached to patients, 20, 21
Saskatchewan Indian Federated College (SIFC): and colonization trauma, 217–18, 222, 223–24; as community, 222, 223, 224–25; creation of, 217–18; curriculum of, as culturally relevant, 220–21, 222; graduates/employees of, 219–24; withdrawal rate at, 218, 225
Saving Milly (Kondracke), 29
schizophrenia, 109, 129; drugs for, 135, 145, 146, 147; language as therapy for, 35. *See also* psychosis
schizophrenia, as identity: denial of, 135; and medical discourse, 130–35; and rejection of illness model, 135–36; as source of fear and isolation, 141. *See also* psychosis
schizophrenic identity narrative, as medical discourse, 130–32; as contested/resisted, 135–36; examples of, 132–35. *See also* psychosis
Semprún, Jorge, 73, 74–75

serial autobiography, 205, 227–35; and anti-Semitism/Jewish identity, 205, 227, 228–29, 230, 231–33; and incest, 205, 227, 228–29, 233–35
sexism: and psychiatric patients, 46, 49, 50–51; and racism, 204, 205, 228, 230, 231–32, 233. *See also* women
sexual abuse/assault. *See* incest, film depictions of; incest narrative
shell shock, 116, 251
Shilts, Randy, 58
Show Me (breast cancer book), 127
Sienkiewicz-Mercer, Ruth, 28, 79–80, 81, 82–83, 85–87; and able-bodied collaborator, 81, 83, 85; "celebration"/romanticization of, 82, 87; as defined by disability, 87; institutional abuse of, 83, 86; normalcy of, 85–86; political intentions of, 83, 86–87; and stereotype of "supercrip," 82–83. *See also* disabled, autobiographies by
Simmel, Georg, 249
Slater, Lauren: and authorization of self, 33–34, 36, 37–39, 41–42; and confessional narrative, 36–37, 38–39; and de-authorization, 36, 39, 41; drug given to, 36–37; and medical report as narrative form, 38–39; and memoir as both fact and fiction, 39–42; and self-knowledge through others, 34–36; as survivor, 42
Slater, Lauren, books by: *Love Works Like This*, 43; *Lying*, 26, 33, 34, 39–42, 43, 110; *Prozac Diary*, 33, 34, 36–39; *Welcome to My Country*, 33, 35–36
social change, and agoraphobia, 248–49
social/political activism: by AIDS patients, 57–58; by disabled, 81–82, 83, 86–87; by incest survivors, 234; and pathography, 125–26
social/political context of narrative, 203–208
social trauma, 227–35; alienation/estrangement and, 230; as experienced by Freud, 230–31; and need for community-based recovery, 230; and problems of medical discourse, 229; and stressors "of human design," 229–30. *See also* anti-Semitism; incest narrative

Sontag, Susan, 21–22, 54, 74, 110, 171, 298
Sophocles, 89, 90
spinal cord injuries, as suffered by rugby players, 111, 191–99; and coherence, in narratives of, 111, 197–99; and concept of heroic masculinity, 193–94; and continuing presence/awareness of body, 192, 195; and disruption of pre-injury time, 195–97; identity dilemmas of, 192–94; and rejection of alternative body–self narratives, 194, 197–99; and restitution narrative, 193, 194, 196, 197–99; and self-devaluation, 192–93
Statistical Manual for the Use of Institutions for the Insane, 251
stigma: of AIDS patients, 54; of psychiatric patients, 45, 46; of SARS patients, 20, 21
stroke, hemorrhagic. *See* hemorrhagic stroke
stroke, ischemic, 181, 189n1
Styron, William, 46, 46–47
Sullivan, Andrew, 59–60
Sunnybrook: A True Story with Lies (Blackbridge), 110, 149–57; art installation associated with, 150; and character of Diane/Persimmon, 156–57; and concept of agencing, 149, 151–52, 153, 157; and concept of assemblage, 153, 157; and fragmentation of text, 150, 152; as giving voice to institutionalized/outcasts, 150–51, 152; humour in, 157; images and text in, 155–56; multiplicity of voices in, 150, 152–53, 155–56; narrative coherence of, 150, 152; Nietzschean reading of, 149, 150, 153–55, 156; shadow forms in, 156–57; use of typography in, 155–56
survival: of AIDS patients, 54, 56, 59; of atomic bomb victim, 97–104; as diminished existence, 56; in hospitalization narrative, 48–49; in memoir, 42–43

TAB (temporarily able-bodied): and disabled, 79–80, 81–82, 84–86; and lupus sufferers, 173, 174–75, 176

Tal, Kalí, 121–22, 125, 126
testimonials/acts of bearing witness: in AIDS narrative, 53–54; in anorexia narrative, 62, 64, 68; autobiography as, 205, 234–35; as balanced against therapeutic function, 113–15, 119–23, 124; in hospitalization narrative, 46, 51; as important to trauma recovery, 121–22; as rooted in legal world, 115, 122; and social/political activism, 125–26
therapeutic function of narrative, 6–7, 7–8, 71, 108, 122–23, 301; as balanced against testimony, 113–15, 119–23, 124; in literary/artistic narrative, 46, 51, 62–63, 64, 71; as rooted in medical world, 115
A Thousand Acres (film), 28, 91, 92–94
Tönnies, Ferdinand, 248
Totem and Taboo (Freud), 91
transdisciplinarity, 13, 298, 299
trauma, 89; and catastrophic events, 99; contemporary theory/treatment of, 119–23; in family, 90–91; Freudian theory of, 54, 91, 92, 95, 115–16, 230–31; "indelible image" of, 102, 117, 118, 120, 127; and journey image/myth, 117–18; as metaphor, 121–22; and need for human connection, 124–25; as part of "human experience," 118–19, 124; recovery from, 116, 117–18, 121–22; of soldiers, 116, 118, 251; of war/genocide victims, 73, 116, 121, 122. *See also* atomic bombing of Japan; elders; incest; Nagasaki; post-traumatic stress disorder
trauma, social, 227–35; alienation/estrangement and, 230; as experienced by Freud, 230–31; and need for community-based recovery, 230; and problems of medical discourse, 229; and stressors "of human design," 229–30. *See also* anti-Semitism; incest narrative
trauma narrative, 3–6, 25, 28–29; as discussed by trauma theorists, 119–23
trauma theory: contemporary, 119–23; Freudian, 54, 91, 92, 95, 115–16,

230–31; historical, 115–19; and pathography, 120, 123–26; and publication of illness narratives, 114–15
Tree of Life, The (Maynard), 227, 232–33
typography, innovative use of, 155–56

Under the Eye of the Clock (Nolan), 79, 81, 83–85
urban life/social change, and agoraphobia, 248–49

Vietnam War, 116, 118, 121, 255

war: and effect on returning soldiers, 116, 118, 251, 255; "indelible images" of, 102, 118; and trauma of victims, 73, 116, 121, 122. *See also* atomic bombing of Japan; Holocaust; Nagasaki
War Zone, The (film), 28, 91, 94–96
Weber, Max, 248
Welcome to My Country: A Therapist's Memoir of Madness (Slater), 33, 35–36, 43
Westphal, Carl Otto, 247–48
"When Plagues End" (Sullivan), 59–60
White Rabbit: A Doctor's Own Story of Addiction, Survival, and Recovery (Morrison), 206, 255–56, 258–63. *See also* drug addiction; Morrison, Martha
Wiesel, Elie, 73, 122
Wit (Edson), 207–208, 285–304; and aestheticization of cancer, 287; as fictional case study, 286–87; film version of, 285, 287, 291; as instructional tool, 290; kindness/humanity in, as feminine, 288, 289–90, 292, 294, 300; meanings of, 295; medical discourse in, 292–94; and poetry of Donne, 287, 289, 292, 294, 295; as representation of cancer experience, 291–92; scientific knowledge in, as masculine, 289, 290, 292, 294, 300; and significance of title, 292; as stage drama, 285–86; 294–95; use of language in, 292–94. *See also* Edson, Margaret
Wit (Edson), and functions of communication (Jakobson), 286; conative/didactic, 288–90; expressive/emotive,

286–88; phatic, 294–96; poetic/metalinguistic, 292–94; referential/metanarrative, 290–92

Wit (Edson), protagonist of: death of, 294; doctor of, 289, 290, 292; as Donne scholar, 287, 289; independence/toughness of, 288, 289, 291; irony/sarcasm of, 293–94; isolation of, 291; knowledge/intellect of, 288, 289–90, 291–92; medical resident of, 289, 290, 292, 294; mentor of, as maternal figure, 288, 289, 290, 292; name of, 287; nurse of, as comfort to, 288, 290, 292, 294; objectification of, 292; parents of, 288, 291–92; as survived only by narrative, 295–96; treatment of, in hospital, 288, 291; and use of language, to counter/resist medical discourse, 292–94

women: Aboriginal, 221–24; as agoraphobics, 247, 249–51, 252, 253–54; as anorectics, 62–63, 64–65; and borderline disorder diagnosis, 46; as frontline health care workers, 300; as hemorrhagic stroke survivors, 111, 181–88; hospitalization of, in context of sexist society, 46, 49, 50–51; as incest victims, 89–96, 205, 227, 228–29, 233–35; with lupus, 110–11, 171–79; with multiple sclerosis, 204, 209–16; racism and sexism towards, 204, 205, 228, 230, 231–32, 233; role of, as discussed in *DSM*, 253–54; societal view of, as weak/vulnerable, 301